Cruises

Cruising the Caribbean, Mexico, Hawaii, New England, and Alaska

ECONOGUIDE.COM | 2000–01

Corey Sandler

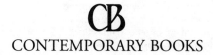

CONTEMPORARY BOOKS

Econoguide is a registered trademark of Word Association, Inc.

Cover photograph copyright © Arnulf Husmo/Tony Stone Images

Published by Contemporary Books
A division of NTC/Contemporary Publishing Group, Inc.
4255 West Touhy Avenue, Lincolnwood (Chicago), Illinois 60712-1975 U.S.A.
International Standard Book Number: 0-8092-2641-3
00 01 02 03 04 05 LB 19 18 17 16 15 14 13 12 11 10 9 8 7 6 5 4 3 2 1

To Janice, who keeps me on course

Contents

Acknowledgments

As always, dozens of hard-working and creative people helped move my words from the keyboard to the book you hold in your hands.

Among the many to thank are Editor Adam Miller of NTC/Contemporary Publishing. Julia Anderson of NTC/Contemporary managed the editorial and production processes with professional courtesy and good nature.

My appreciation extends to the cruise lines and public relations staffs who helped me assemble the massive stack of specifications, itineraries, and prices into manageable shape.

Val Elmore checked facts and edited the manuscript with high skill and good humor.

As always, thanks to Janice Keefe for running the office and putting up with me, a pair of major assignments.

And thanks to you for buying this book. We all hope you find it of value; please let us know how we can improve the book in future editions. (Please enclose a stamped envelope if you'd like a reply; no phone calls, please.)

Corey Sandler
Econoguide Travel Books
P.O. Box 2779
Nantucket, MA 02584

To send electronic mail, use the following address:
info@econoguide.com.

You can also consult our Web page at:
www.econoguide.com.

I hope you'll also consider the other books in the Econoguide series. You can find them at bookstores, or ask your bookseller to order them. All are written by Corey Sandler.

Econoguide: Walt Disney World, Universal Orlando, SeaWorld
Econoguide: Disneyland, Universal Studios Hollywood
Econoguide: Las Vegas

Econoguide: Washington D.C., Williamsburg
Econoguide: Pacific Northwest
Econoguide: Canada
Econoguide: London
Econoguide: Paris (Coming in the spring of 2001)
Econoguide: Miami, Fort Lauderdale, and Key West (Coming in the summer of 2001)
Also by Corey Sandler:
Golf U.S.A.

About the Author

Corey Sandler is a former newsman and editor for the Associated Press, Gannett Newspapers, Ziff-Davis Publishing, and IDG. He has written more than 150 books on travel, video games, and computers; his titles have been translated into French, Spanish, German, Italian, Portuguese, Polish, Bulgarian, Hebrew, and Chinese. When he's not traveling, he hides out with his wife and two children on Nantucket island, 30 miles off the coast of Massachusetts.

Introduction

During the past few years, I've floated from one stunning horizon to the next, a series of journeys that have taken me from my home in one of the rugged harbors of New England to the iridescent waters of the Caribbean, the wondrous ice-carved canyons of Alaska's Inside Passage, the fire-born islands of Hawaii and the South Pacific, and through the manmade wonder of the Panama Canal. I crossed the "pond" from England to the new world, and I played tag with three hurricanes.

Some of the highlights of my recent career at sea:

• A week-long voyage into the wild blue yonder, crossing the Atlantic from Harwich, England to Boston, Massachusetts onboard the elegant *Maasdam*. For the middle five days of the trip we saw nothing but ocean—no ships, no planes, no shoreline. We carried our civilization with us, like atronauts on the way to the moon.

• The wonder in the eyes of a child on a nearly untouched South Pacific atoll where we had been deposited by the elegant *Norwegian Dynasty*; we felt like friendly visitors from another planet.

• A lyrical journey with a grand old lady, in the company of an affable band of jazz lovers on a theme cruise. We were aboard the world's longest passenger ship, and one of the oldest afloat, the *Norway*, a thoroughly updated and maintained ship that travels back to the future in the Caribbean.

• A trip *between* the twin hulls of the *Radisson Diamond* as she lay at anchor off remote San Andres island, a northern outpost of Columbia in the Caribbean Sea. The pilot of our tender drove between the pontoons of the one-of-a-kind, twin-hull luxury cruise ship through a 400-foot-long white tunnel floating on an azure sea.

• A stately procession through the waters at the base of the amazing Titons of St. Lucia on the reflagged, renamed, refurbished *Crown Dynasty*.

• A midnight fireworks salute offshore a Bahamian island as the magnificent *Disney Magic* had a rendezvous with her twin sister *Disney Wonder* on her maiden voyage.

• The unreal baby-blue hues of South Sawyer Glacier at the end of Tracy Arm in Alaska, as the venerable *Universe Explorer* made a slow turnabout in the deep pool at the face of the river of frozen water. We watched squads of seals pass by on ice floes, and were in turn tailed by pods of whales in the Inner Passage.

• The gigantic *Grand Princess,* docked in New York City prior to her maiden voyage, looking like a floating, horizontal version of the Manhattan skyscrapers behind her.

• The rugged *Clipper Adventurer* standing offshore the jetty near my home on Nantucket island unloading its passengers in rubber Zodiac boats, part way on a journey that would take her from Atlantic Canada to the Antarctic.

• A school of flying fish skimming across the bow wake of the *Enchanted Capri* in the iridescent blue Gulf of Mexico. Who needs a floor show in the lounge?

Those were some of the places we went. And then there were the amazing sights onboard the cruise ships that took us there. Things such as:

• The jaw-dropping decadence of an all-chocolate midnight buffet.

• A distant Christmas tree on the horizon at dawn that slowly revealed itself to be an oil rig standing in the icy Atlantic a few hundred miles off the coast of Newfoundland, after nearly a week on a transatlantic crossing the first sign of human civilization other than our own ship.

• A full-scale musical production on a stage that had more technical facilities than many a Broadway theater. And we were moving at 23 knots, 100 miles off the coast of Florida at the time!

• Day after day of gourmet food, presented with artistry and attentive service at breakfast, brunch, lunch, mid-afternoon snack, dinner, and midnight. My children, on the other hand, loved the all-hours room service, ice cream stand, and pizza parlor.

• The incomparable beauty of a Caribbean sunset, glimpsed from a deck chair on the private veranda outside our stateroom.

• The unimaginable heat and bone-rattling rumble of the engine room of a cruise ship moving at full speed through the Pacific. Up above, guests were pampered in air conditioned, elegant luxury, completely insulated and hidden from the stygian scene way down below.

• The calming vista of endless sea—with no signs of land or life for nearly three days south from Honolulu into the South Pacific.

Dear Reader: A Confession

As a travel writer, I love the excitement of an expedition off the beaten tracks in an unusual place. I like nothing better than "going native" anywhere I visit: renting a car to drive on the wrong side of the road in the United Kingdom or Tortola; riding the subways of Seoul or Tokyo; heading out with a guide across the top of a mountain in Vermont or Utah, and generally choosing my own schedule and itinerary.

Put another way, there is nothing I dislike more than a regimented trip where everything is arranged: when and where to eat, entertainment, and minute-by-minute calendars of activities.

Before I began writing guidebooks, I was a voracious consumer of many I found on the bookshelves. I want to know everything there is to know about the places I visit—before I go there, and then I want to wander off.

And so, I fully expected that I would find cruising an intolerably confining and over-organized experience. What if I didn't like the ship? What if the cabin was unappealing? What if the food was awful? What if I didn't like the other people on the ship?

Well, with a bit of careful research before I booked passage, I was able to choose ships that ranged from well-kept old dowagers to a brand-new classic in the making. I knew more about the cabin I had booked than any travel agent. I knew the details of the ship's cuisine in gourmet detail. And I found ways to shield myself from unwanted company when it suited me.

To my surprise, I found I greatly enjoyed going on a cruise. During my seasons at sea, I learned the wonderful sense of peace and relaxation that comes from putting yourself in the hands of a capable cruise staff on a well-run cruise ship.

The Cruising Life

I discovered that I truly enjoyed staying put while the ship kept moving.

My "hotel" traveled with me from port to port, along with a cabin steward and restaurant staff who—at least for the week or so I spent with them—treated me as if I was a combination of their benevolent employer and a best friend.

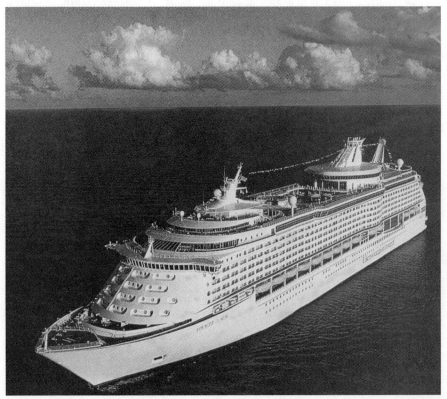

Royal Caribbean's Voyager of the Seas, *the world's largest cruise ship*
Courtesy of Royal Caribbean International

I found that, for a change, I enjoyed leaving the driving and the scheduling to someone else. I concentrated on relaxing.

And then, each day the ship arrived in a new port, I was among the first to clamber into the tender or charge down the gangplank. Based on research I had done before the trip, my wife and I took an occasional organized shore excursion, rented a car and headed away from the tourist section of the port and explored for the day, or embarked on our own shore parties, far from the cruise crowd.

I always intend to do more than my share of off-the-cuff, unplanned travel at almost every opportunity. And I still chafe at any suggestion that someone else plan my trips.

We Are Not Alone

I suppose I should not have been surprised to find myself becoming a cruise convert. It turns out that I'm in very good company. In 1970, approximately 500,000 Americans took cruises; in 1999, nearly 6 million went to sea.

As this book goes to press, the U.S. cruise industry is growing at nearly 10 percent per year, booking close to $9 billion in business in 1999.

According to the Cruise Lines International Association (CLIA), the industry's marketing organization, the average duration of a cruise is about 6.7 days; itineraries are growing at both ends of the spectrum, with an increase in short three- and four-day trips, as well as voyages of 10 days or more in exotic places around the world. Even with the tremendous increase in capacity in recent years, many cruise lines are operating at greater than 100 percent capacity on many trips. (A ship's capacity is calculated on the basis of

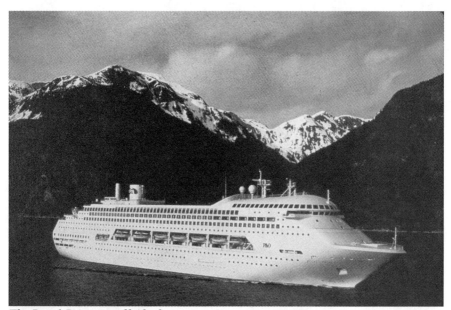

The Regal Princess *off Alaska*
Courtesy of Princess Cruises

double occupancy; a full ship with children or other family members in extra bunks brings a ship beyond its full load.)

During the past decade, cruising has also begun to shed its image as a vacation choice of seniors; although millions of older persons enjoy the stress-free pampered life aboard ship, the average age of cruise passengers has dropped from 56 to 44, according to industry figures.

As popular as cruise vacations have become, according to the CLIA, only about 11 percent of the U.S. population has taken a cruise. But that percentage has more than doubled in a decade.

In 1999, the Caribbean and the Bahamas was the leading destination for cruises. Here are the CLIA estimates:

• Caribbean and Bahamas: 42 percent
• Europe: 20 percent
• Alaska: 9 percent
• Panama Canal and Panama: 7 percent
• Pacific Mexico: 6 percent
• Bermuda: 3 percent
• Other areas, including New England: 3 percent

And cruising continues as mainly an American product, with more than 70 percent of cruisegoers hailing from the United States. The next most popular market is the United Kingdom, representing approximately 10 percent of cruise passengers. The percentage of British and European travelers, though, is expected to rise in coming years as some of the Megaships expand their presence in the Mediterranean and Asian areas.

About This Book

The main purpose of this book is to help you choose the right ship, the right itinerary, the right cabin, and even the right dining options. And I'll also tell you how to find ways to be alone amongst a few thousand other passengers, or how to pick and choose your activities to make the cruise ship meet *your* expectations—and not the other way around.

My staff and I have collected information on the best cruises at any price, along with details of how to get the most for your money—no matter how much you spend—on your voyage, as well as advice on how to travel in economic style from coast to coast.

And we offer a selection of money-saving coupons from a wide range of cruise travel packagers as well as respected sources of clothing and other necessities. There is no connection between the information in this book and the coupons we publish, except that everything between the covers is intended to save you money.

Pardon us for saying so, but we think the cost-effectiveness of this book will speak for itself. With its assistance, you should easily be able to save many times its price while enjoying your cruise.

Chapter 1
How to Choose a Cruise

The first decision is the easy one: resolve to check yourself into a fine hotel and sit back and relax as that luxurious resort floats you from one interesting part of the world to another, plying you with gourmet food (and lots of it), entertaining you with music, comedy, and theater, all the while presenting an ever-changing tableau of ocean, spectacular shorelines, and river canyons.

Now come the more difficult questions:

• Would you prefer a gigantic floating city with a population of a few thousand and dozens of dining and entertainment options, or would you instead choose a well-equipped but small, intimate vessel more like a semi-private yacht?

• Do you want to laze your way through the blue Caribbean, be thrilled by the Inner Passage of Alaska, venture way out to sea on a transatlantic or transpacific crossing, explore the remains of the ancient civilizations of Central America, or cruise the Mississippi on a paddlewheeler?

• Are you looking for a cruise with several consecutive days at sea, or would you prefer a new port every morning: go to sleep in Aruba and awake in Curaçao; lights out in Boston, daybreak in Nova Scotia?

• Does the stateroom of your dreams include a sitting room, bedroom, private balcony with hot tub, and a butler? Or do you just need a place to store your stuff and lay your head when you're not out at the pool, in the dining room, the casino, the barbecue, the theater, or the midnight buffet?

• Are you a blue jeans and T-shirt kind of person, or are you looking for a place to break out the tuxedo or cocktail gown?

• Are you looking for particular sports and health club facilities, such as a golf simulator (or a miniature golf course), a luxurious spa, an indoor swimming pool, or (really!) an ice skating rink out at sea? Or are you more interested in the thickness of the cushions in the lounge?

• And for some people this is the killer question: How much are you willing to pay? Are you looking for a bargain price for good value, or is money no object to your pursuit of pleasure?

The simplest answer to all these questions, and more, is this: before you sign on the bottom line for a seaborne vacation, make yourself an expert on the world of cruising.

Together, in this book, we'll explore ships from massive Megaships that would have dwarfed the *Titanic* to luxurious super-yachts and intimate adventure boats. We'll look at the latest and greatest, and we'll examine a few floating antiques, stylish reminders of the days of the great ocean liners.

The List Price and the Real Price

Cruise and new car brochures have a lot in common: gorgeous pictures of the hardware, photo spreads of handsome models having a great time in exotic places, and a price list that could stop a heart.

But in cars and cruises, only a few unfortunate and generally uninformed people actually pay the sticker price.

In many instances, there's the list price and there's the *real* price. There are many ways to save. In fact, with some cruise lines, you may find it hard to pay the list price—there are sales to be found almost all the time. If you choose cruises and the time of year carefully, discounts of 50 percent or more off the brochure rate are quite ordinary.

Start out with a determination not to pay the prices you see quoted. Contact a travel agent or cruise specialist who has some expertise in cruises, or check with the cruise line directly for special rates.

Be direct and to the point: Ask the agent or reservationist to save you money off the published list price. This accomplishes two goals. First, it announces right at the start that you're aware the list price is often a starting point in a sales negotiation. And it also puts the agent on notice that you expect a close eye on the bottom line.

Tricks to Getting the Best Rate

Here are some of the best ways to pay less than the list price:
- Book early.
- Book late.
- Cruise in off-season.
- Choose a repositioning cruise.
- Cruise a new itinerary.
- Extend a cruise with back-to-back trips.
- Take advantage of special offers for frequent cruisers.
- Take advantage of special discounts.
- Be flexible on the ship's itinerary or date of departure.
- Upgrade your cabin onboard.

Or, if you insist, here's how to end up paying top dollar for a cruise:
- Choose a hot new ship in its inaugural season.
- Insist on sailing during a holiday period.
- Be rigid in your sailing date or itinerary.

- Insist on a particular class of cabin.
- Require a particular bed configuration—especially for a cabin for more than two persons.

Book Early

Many cruise lines offer discounts of as much as 50 percent off bookings made six months to a year in advance. If you sign up for such a deal, be sure you understand your rights in case of an unexpected need to cancel; you might also want to include trip cancellation insurance in your purchase.

If you are planning a major celebration—a wedding or anniversary—or hope to travel on a special occasion such as New Year's Eve or a solar eclipse, you may have no choice but to commit to a cruise six months to a year in advance.

Book Late

If you are flexible on departure date and itinerary, you can really clean up with a last-minute deal. Cruise lines just hate to sail with an unused cabin, and they'll carve deeply into list prices to fill those empty berths.

The downside is that in some cases, cruise lines will upgrade their customers who paid full- or near-full rates. This leaves last-minute cruisers the least attractive cabins, albeit at a deeply discounted rate.

In general, the first cabins to sell out on a cruise ship are those at each end of the spectrum—the lowest-priced staterooms and the most spectacular (and relatively scarce) suites.

Register with a cruise agency or in some cases directly with a cruise line and indicate your willingness to take whatever is available on a particular date or itinerary, and be ready to make a last-minute dash to the airport.

If ever there were an example of this principle at work, consider the last-minute scramble among cruise lines to fill cabins on millennium sailings at the end of 1999. Very few ships sold out at the greedy premium prices many companies asked at the beginning of the year. Rates dropped sharply in the final weeks of the year.

One disadvantage to last-minute booking: You may have to pay top dollar for last-minute air travel to the port unless it is within reasonable driving distance. Be sure to figure in airfare costs to see if the bottom line for a spur-of-the-moment cruise still makes sense.

Cruise in Off-Season

As with most everything you buy, you can expect a better price when there are more sellers than buyers.

In many cases, you'll find cruising in the off-season just as attractive as in the heart of the season; happily, you'll have less company and pay less for the privilege. You may, though, run into problems caused by the weather—late-season hurricanes or unusually rough seas. Do the research and know your preferences before you book off-season—or any other time of the year, for that matter.

Here are a few off-season times for cruising:

- Caribbean and Mexican Riviera. After Labor Day to pre-Christmas, early January, and April through Memorial Day.
- Panama Canal. January and February, and repositioning cruises in spring and fall.
- Alaska. Beginning and end of the season—May and September.
- Bermuda. Beginning and end of the season—May and September.

And there are usually a few dead periods, even in what might otherwise be considered prime season. In most markets, for example, the period between Thanksgiving and Christmas is relatively quiet, as is the period immediately after New Year's Day.

Choose a Repositioning Cruise

There is nothing scarier to a cruise line bean counter than a $150 million ship with nowhere to go and no incoming payments to apply to the mortgage. The Caribbean is pretty much a year-round destination, but most other areas of the world are more seasonal in their draw.

One example of a seasonal schedule puts a ship in Alaska for the summer, then down the West Coast to the Panama Canal in the fall and through to the Caribbean for the winter. The process is reversed in late spring. Or the ship may make a wide detour to Hawaii on its way south to the canal.

These repositioning cruises are sometimes less popular than regular itineraries for a particular ship or cruise line. They may call at unusual ports or spend several days out to sea instead of in port; to some, these are the very things that make repositioning cruises so attractive.

In this book you can read a cruise diary of a week-long repositioning cruise from Harwich, England to Boston, Massachusetts on the *Maasdam*.

Prime Travel Seasons

	Jan	Feb	Mar	Apr	May	Jun	Jul	Aug	Sep	Oct	Nov	Dec
Alaska						★★	★★★★	★★★★	★★★			
Bahamas	★★★★	★★★★	★★★★	★★★★	★★★★	★★★★	★★★↑	★★★↑	★★★↑	★★★	★★★	★★★★
Bermuda					★★★★	★★★★	★★★★	★★★★	★★★★	★★★★		
Caribbean	★★★★	★★★★	★★★★	★★★★	★★★★	★★★★	★★★↑	★★★↑	★★★↑	★★★↑	★★★↑	★★★★
West U.S.	★★★★	★★★★	★★★★								★★★★	★★★★
Mexico	★★★★	★★★★	★★★★								★★★★	★★★★
New England							★★★	★★★★	★★★★			
Canada						★★★	★★★★	★★★★				
East U.S.					★★★★	★★★★	★★★★	★★★★	★★★★	★★★		
World Cruise	★★★★	★★★★	★★★★	★★★★								★★★★

★★ Low   ★★★ Good   ★★★★ Prime   ★★★↑ Prime . . . but hurricane season

Cruise a New Itinerary

A careful shopper may be able to find a bargain fare on a cruise ship pioneering a new port or a new itinerary.

In some cases, the cruise line may be testing the appeal of a new schedule. Or the line may be just beginning to build its business in a new area.

Once again, try to take advantage of any situation where there may be more cabins than passengers.

Extend a Cruise with Back-to-Back Trips

Many cruise lines will offer significant discounts to travelers who book more than one trip in a row. For example, many ships offer alternating east and west Caribbean itineraries and will reward passengers who hire a cabin for both legs.

You may also be able to receive a discount for booking multiple legs of a round-the-world cruise or other long-term cruises.

Take Advantage of Special Offers for Frequent Cruisers

Keep your eyes open for special deals offered directly by the cruise line as well as those offered in conjunction with associations, credit card companies, and other groups.

For example, some cruise lines offer special rates to AARP or AAA members. With my monthly credit card bills, I have often received discount coupons for cruise vacations.

Many cruise lines also make special offers to members of their own clubs of former passengers. Companies may maintain a more formal "club" of passengers with newsletters and get-togethers or they may merely send offers to former clients.

Typical offers range from discounts to upgrades. Some companies offer special discounts to travelers who make a booking for another cruise while onboard ship.

Take Advantage of Special Discounts

Be on the lookout—and don't be afraid to ask—for special programs that offer reduced rates for third and fourth passengers in a room, for single passengers willing to be matched in a double cabin, and other such deals.

Some cruise lines also offer a "guaranteed outside cabin" deal priced at or below the lowest specific outside cabin class. In other words, you won't be choosing a particular deck or type of room, but are willing to accept whatever outside stateroom is available. You just might be lucky enought to get a better accommodation than you would receive by specifying a particular class.

Be Flexible on the Ship's Itinerary or Date of Departure

If you can adjust your travel plans to take advantage of the best available offerings, you are sure to save money.

Let's say you are able to tell a travel agent or cruise line you are interested

Maiden voyages. Do you dream of being first to sleep in a new cabin, first to belly up to the buffet, and first to a new port? There'll be grand speeches, free-flowing champagne and a sky filled with fireworks . . . kind of like the S.S. *Titanic,* presumably without the icebergs.

With a dozen or so major new cruise ships being launched each year, your chances of getting on a maiden voyage are better than ever. You'll find information about many of the upcoming launches in this book.

Many cruise lines will accept reservations for maiden voyages as much as a year ahead of scheduled dates; in some cases, first choice is offered to preferred customers.

The bad news, though, is that as ships become larger and more complex, the chances of delays in announced maiden voyage dates are also better than ever.

If a cruise ship is not available for her scheduled maiden voyage, you may be offered a trip on another ship, or a high-priority reservation on the actual first sailing. Some lines offer discounts or upgrades to soothe

in cruising sometime in February or March, are willing to consider a wide range of ports of embarkation and itineraries, and are willing to travel on any of a wide range of available ships.

In a way, you are putting your business out for sale to the lowest bidder. Of course, you do need to look closely at any offers. And, your agent should be able to give you a full and honest answer about why a particular cruise is being discounted.

Upgrade Your Cabin Onboard

Another strategy is to search for upgrades to cabins once you're onboard the ship. Visit the reception or purser's desk once the ship sets sail and ask about any available cabins. Nearly all cruise lines offer reduced rates on staterooms once there is very little chance of selling that cabin to a last-minute arrival. This scheme will not work, of course, if the ship is fully booked.

Single Cruisers

Like it or not, cruise lines base their fares around double occupancy, building in the costs of meals, entertainment and other services. For that reason, single travelers face "premiums" or "supplements" of as much as 200 percent if they choose to reserve a cabin for themselves.

Some cruise lines are a bit more reasonable, charging only 110 percent to 150 percent of ordinary rates.

Here are some money-saving options:

1. Ask if the cruise line has a singles-matching program. The company will pair you with another single traveler of the same sex, and you will each pay the standard double-occupancy rate. In many cases, if the cruise line is unable to pair you with another single you will end up with a cabin to yourself at half the double rate. Some cruise lines offer to fill up a triple or quad cabin with singles, reducing the cost markedly for all travelers.

2. Look for a cruise line that offers cabins

specifically designed for singles. There are not all that many of these staterooms available; and they are generally found on the older ships. They are often the least-impressive inside cabins, but they do save a bit of money. (Among the vessels with single cabins is the still-impressive QE2.)

3. If the cruise line is going to charge you 200 percent and you don't want to travel with a stranger, why not invite a friend or relative to join you? For the cost of an airline ticket to the port, you'll have comfortable company.

Comparing the Cost of a Cruise to Another Vacation

Cruises sound expensive, and indeed, the most luxurious suites onboard a modern ship can cost several hundred dollars or more per person per night. But the middle range of cabins and the relatively limited number of economy-rate rooms compare well with other types of vacations when you look at the entire picture.

customers made unhappy by delays.

By the way, "maiden" voyages are not always the true first trip for a new ship. Modern cruise ships are generally built at yards in Europe or Scandinavia and go through several "shakedown" cruises near the yards before making a transoceanic crossing; some cruise lines schedule several weeks or months of trips before the formal start of service. Contact the cruise line to see if space is available on these pre-maiden voyages.

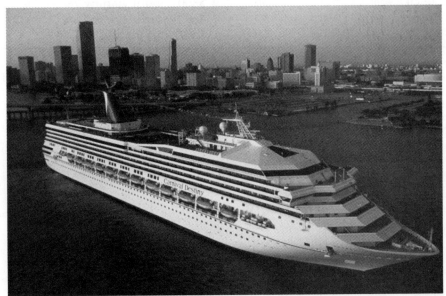

The Carnival Destiny *sets sail*

Photo by Andy Newman/CCL

Think of the cruise equation as:

Cruise Ticket =
    Transportation + Room + Meals + Entertainment + Sports Activities

Of course, the more cruise amenities you use, the better the deal. If you're planning to stay in your room and skip the sumptuous meals, the midnight buffet, and the nightly theatrical shows, perhaps you should stay in a room at a motel on the shore.

Here's an example. It's based on a middle-of-the-market, seven-day cruise in a midrange cabin on a premium carrier such as Holland America or Norwegian Cruise Line, compared to a week's stay at a good-quality resort in Florida or the Caribbean.

	On a Cruise	On a Land Vacation For Two	
Cruise fare for two	$2,000	$0	
Room	$0	$875	7 nights hotel
Transportation	$0	$300	7 days car rental
Entertainment	$0	$500	7 nights
Sports activities	$0	$280	7 days
Breakfast	$0	$200	With gratuity
Lunch	$0	$300	With gratuity
Dinner	$0	$600	With gratuity
Snacks	$0	$200	With gratuity
Drinks	$150	$150	
Other gratuities	$210	$50	Hotel
Total	**$2,360**	**$3,455**	

Not included in either package are airline transportation and airport transfers. Note that some cruise packages include transportation.

Chapter 2
How Big Is BIG?

How big is big enough? Everyone has their own answer. Some people want a floating city, with theaters, nightclubs, ice rinks, climbing walls, shopping malls, and a different restaurant for each night of the cruise. Others prefer a small but safe and comfortable raft in the vastness of the open ocean, their entertainment coming from a connection to the sea.

Today's biggest ships are 100,000 or more tons in size, a Brobdingnagian stature that was considered unrealistic a few years ago. Royal Caribbean's *Voyager of the Seas*, a gargantuan 142,000 tons, nearly overshadowed the skyscrapers of Miami when she arrived at her home port in late 1999. During the holiday season a few weeks later, she set an all-time record for the most guests on a single cruise, carrying 3,537 souls. And Royal Caribbean has plans for at least two more of the Colossus ships in years to come.

Royal Caribbean's modest little boats are three times the size of the *Titanic* and more than double the magnitude of one of the "Megaships" that were the harbingers of the cruising boom of the 1990s.

Many cruise lines have chosen to limit their ships to stay within the "Panamax" specifications, the maximum width and length for a ship to be able to pass through the Panama Canal between the Atlantic and Pacific oceans. The locks of the canal are 110 feet wide and 1,000 feet long; any ship wider or longer than that must go the long way around the tip of South America if she is to be repositioned from one ocean to another.

And how big is too big? Some dreamers—and a few planners—envision a future floating resort that will be a palatial Waterworld.

One such possibility is the American Flagship Project for the *America World City*, a floating hotel offering 2,800 cabins that have a total capacity of 6,200 guests, a convention and meeting space on the seas.

And work has begun on *The World* of ResidenSea, a waterborne condo of 110 luxurious privately owned residences and 88 luxury guest suites. The ship, scheduled to begin service in December, 2001, will be managed by Silversea Cruises. Apartments will sell for $2 million to as much as $6.8 million, some the size of a land-based home.

The concept of economy of scale pushes cruise ships to either end of the spectrum—to small, ultra-luxury (and ultra high-priced) vessels, or to gargantuan ships that have cabins for more than 2,000 guests. On the small luxury ships, cruise lines can charge very high rates per passenger; on huge ships, the costs of the construction of the ship, fuel, showrooms, and other fixed expenses are spread over a large number of guests.

An Econoguide to Small, Medium, and Large

Size *does* matter—in facilities, atmosphere, and the overall experience of a cruise. There are those who prefer citizenship in a city at sea, and others who would rather be in a floating supper club.

I divide cruise ships into classes based on gross registered tons—a measure of capacity I'll define in a moment. Here are the Econoguide size classes:

Colossus	100,000 or more tons
Megaship	70,000 to 100,000 tons
Grand	40,000 to 70,000 tons
Medium	10,000 to 40,000 tons
Small	Less than 10,000 tons

So, how big is big enough? If you have a large cabin, a comfortably uncrowded dining room, and more deck chairs than people, you might consider a Medium 20,000-ton ship big enough. If you're one of 3,000 guests on a 100,000-ton Colossus and find yourself standing in a half-hour line to get to the buffet table, you may decide that ship is not big enough.

And so, let's look at two important measures of size: gross registered tons, and passenger-space ratio. And we'll also define another way to think about quality of service, the passenger-to-crew ratio.

Gross Registered Tons

First of all, tonnage is not a measure of the weight of the ship. A ship of 100,000 tons does not weigh 200 million pounds.

In nautical terms, ton is actually derived from a French measure known as "tonneaux," which referred to a particular size of wine cask.

The concept of **gross registered tons (GRT)** was developed as a means of taxing vessels based on their cargo-carrying capacity. GRT is a measurement of the total permanently enclosed spaces of the ship, excluding certain essential areas such as the bridge and galleys.

In modern terms, one GRT is equal to 100 cubic feet of enclosed, revenue-generating space.

Here are two other ways to think of GRT. A typical four-door compact car occupies roughly 300 cubic feet, or three tons. A basic kitchen refrigerator is between 30 and 40 cubic feet in size, equivalent to three-tenths to four-tenths of one GRT. So, a 100,000-ton Megaship has revenue-generating space equivalent to about 33,333 compact cars or 286,000 kitchen refrigerators.

Passenger-Space Ratio

Another way to look at the size of a ship is to compare the gross tonnage to the number of passengers onboard. The passenger-space ratio, which you'll find listed in the charts of this book, divides gross tonnage by a ship's standard double-occupancy capacity. The higher the space ratio, the less likely you'll find a stranger in a bath towel in your personal space by the pool, or a seat at a dinner table for 12. In this book, the range of space ratios for cruise ships runs from about 19 to about 54, with most ships in the mid-30 range.

Passenger-space ratios are very rough measures. Some ship designers make staterooms large at the expense of public spaces; other ships have sprawling casinos and magnificent open atriums, and offer broom-closet cabins.

As we'll discuss later, some guests are willing to accept a small sleeping room because they don't intend to spend much time behind its closed door.

And the space ratio does not work very well when applied to small adventure ships and sailing vessels that have different designs, including small bridges, galleys, engine rooms and multi-purpose public rooms. This class of ship also typically makes use of open deck space for viewing and dining.

Is Bigger Better?

Sometimes bigger *is* better, if you're looking for a Broadway theater at sea, a waterborne ice skating rink, or a choice of five restaurants for dinner. A bigger ship may also offer larger cabins with more amenities. However, sometimes smaller is better, if you're looking for more personalized service, easier embarkation and debarkation, and calls at less-often visited ports.

Following is a plus-and-minus comparison of large and small cruise ships.

Large Ships
PLUS

+ Generally more stable in rough seas
+ More activities: theaters, showrooms, casinos, ice skating
+ Multiple choices in dining
+ Many newer large ships offer more verandas, larger windows, more cabin choices
+ A larger and more diverse shore excursion program

MINUS

− Deeper draft of larger ships may limit ports or require passengers to use small boats (called tenders) to go to shore
− A small city's worth of people in the showrooms
− Large dining rooms may result in more institutional-style food
− Large passenger capacity may result in long lines for embarkation, disembarkation, and immigration clearance
− 1,000 to 2,000 or more guests will descend upon small ports at once

Small Ships
PLUS

+ Shallower draft may allow visits to smaller ports and require use of tenders less frequently
+ Relatively intimate public rooms
+ More personalized service from cabin and restaurant staff

+ Less structured, sometimes open seating in dining room
+ Quicker embarkation, disembarkation, and immigration clearances
+ May have water-level watersports platform or internal dock
+ Less of an impact on ports of call from smaller passenger loads

MINUS
- Generally less stable in rough seas
- Fewer choices for entertainment
- Fewer verandas and categories of cabins
- Few or no choices for dining

Is a New Ship Better Than an Old Classic?

The only thing you can say for certain about a new ship versus an old one is that a modern ship is, well, newer.

Some spectacular new vessels include amenities and features well beyond the dreams of the most luxurious queens of the sea. But some new ships also have some public rooms that more closely resemble a shopping mall cafeteria than the Palm Court.

Some older vessels are tired relics counting the days until their value at the scrap yard is greater than they can earn carrying passengers. But other veteran ships are handsome classics, offering a sense of elegance and class not duplicated by new construction. Two fine examples: the *Norway*, and the *QE2*.

Nearly every cruise ship is originally built to the specifications of a particular line. A typical life for a cruise ship in the hands of a major cruise line is approximately 10 to 15 years, after which the ships are pushed along to a succession of secondary cruise companies. That doesn't mean there is anything wrong with these older ships, or with the cruise companies. It just means the ships may not match a line's current marketing plan.

There are some areas of concern: A handful of very old ships may not fully meet the current safety regulations, operating under temporary or permanent exemptions. For example, these include old riverboats and antique tall ships, and a few older cruise ships that are due for retrofitting with sprinkler systems. Older ships are also not likely to be very accommodating to persons in wheelchairs and to others who may require an elevator.

New ships include state-of-the-art propulsion, air conditioning, television, telephone, theater, and other facilities. They also are constructed using the latest safety regulations and equipment. Cabins often have internal hallway entrances, permitting portholes, windows, or verandas along the sea.

Many new ships have shallower drafts, which allow visits to smaller ports and less frequently require use of tenders; bow and stern thrusters allow maneuvering in narrow ports. On the minus side, a shallower draft may mean less comfortable cruising in rough weather.

Chapter 3
Where in the World Do You Want to Go?

Where in the world do you want to go? Well, let me refine that a bit: Where in the world's oceans and major rivers do you want to go?

The waters around the United States are the world's most popular for cruising. In this book, we define U.S. waters broadly: We cover any ship that touches an American port or sails nearby. Under that definition we include New England, Canada, the East and West coasts, the Caribbean, Bermuda, the Bahamas, the Mexican Riviera, Hawaii, and Alaska.

I'll discuss many of the most popular cruising destinations a bit later in the chapter. First, though, let's explore the political and economic reasons behind most cruise itineraries.

Oceans Away: International Affairs

Cruising is one of the most international of businesses, and its operations are very much shaped by politics, economics, and protectionism.

I first wrote these words onboard the *Norwegian Dynasty*. At the time she was a Scandinavian-owned vessel built in Spain, registered in Panama, and operated by NCL, a Norwegian company that had its operational headquarters in Miami. We were sailing through the American Hawaiian islands with a 2,400-mile round-trip detour to make a stop at an undeveloped beach on Fanning Island in the Republic of Kiribati in the South Pacific.

Let's deconstruct that global stew.

Today's modern cruise ships are mostly built at a handful of giant shipyards in Italy, France, Germany, and Scandinavia. There is hardly any American shipbuilding industry left, except for smaller vessels and military ships.

The ownership of cruise ships—a new Colossus can cost upwards of $400 million—follows the financing. Many of today's cruise companies are related to major freight shipping lines in Europe, Scandinavia, and Japan.

A ship's registry is for the most part a legal fiction. The great ships of old represented their nation's political and economic strengths, were proud to bear their country's flags and, most important, abided by their home nation's laws, regulations, and customs. The Cunard Line's *Queen Mary* and *Queen Elizabeth*, for example, flew the Union Jack of Great Britain. From the stern of The *France* fluttered the Tricolor. Great American vessels such as the *United States* hoisted Old Glory. Each acted as a floating extension of their homeland.

Today, though, a new cruise ship is most likely to fly the flag of countries such as Panama, Liberia, or The Bahamas. They do so because the accountants and lawyers have determined that the cruise line can save money on construction costs, taxes, and operating expenses by doing so. In addition, if a ship is registered in the United States, labor and immigration laws require that crew members are American citizens or legal aliens.

Many of the vessels flying these exotic flags have never touched the waters of ports in those nations. These are "flags of convenience."

At the start of 2000, there was only one major cruise ship flying the American flag, the elderly *Independence* of American Hawaii Cruises, which is in turn owned by the Delta Queen Steamboat Company. Delta Queen's riverboats are also American-flagged. There are also a number of small American cruise ships on the East Coast and several boats in Alaskan waters.

In the fall of 2000, the new United States Line, another offshoot of Delta Queen, will begin service with the *Patriot*; the company received special dispensation from Congress to reflag a foreign-built ship to carry the Stars and Stripes and an American crew.

Delta Queen may help resurrect a small piece of the American shipbuilding industry with its order for up to five coastal packet ships, the first of which is due to be put into service in 2001.

The Jones Act

Why does a ship sailing from New York on a cruise to New England have to make a port call in Canada? Why does a ship from Honolulu have to steam thousands of miles to Vancouver, Canada or Ensenada, Mexico or a tiny dot of a Pacific island nation before returning? Why can't you cruise up or down the California coast? Why do most Alaska cruises originate in Canada or make a stop in that country as they go to or come from the 49th state?

The answer comes from a nearly two century-old set of laws intended to protect U.S.-flagged vessels from unfair foreign competition.

The Jones Act requires that cargo moving between U.S. ports be carried in a vessel that was built and maintained in the United States and is at least 75 percent owned by American citizens or corporations. The Jones Act actually refers to Section 27 of the Merchant Marine Act of 1920; prior legislation to accomplish essentially the same thing has been in effect since 1817.

(The act has actually done very little to preserve the U.S. shipping industry, of which there is not much left. The same applies for the American cruise industry, where the bill has had the unintended effect of boosting the economy of some otherwise obscure foreign ports whose main advantage is that they are within a reasonable cruising distance of a U.S. port. Witness the Republic of Kiribati I mentioned earlier.)

Nearly 50 countries around the world have laws similar to the Jones Act. The U.S. is especially tough in its ban against flying an American flag on a foreign-built vessel; Canada permits importing ships but requires payment of a tariff equal to 25 percent of the vessel's value, which all but makes foreign vessels economically infeasible.

While the Jones Act applies to cargo, the Passenger Vessel Act of 1886 declares that "no foreign vessel shall transport passengers between ports or places in the United States." Cruise companies face a substantial fine for violating the law.

Railroads, airlines, bus lines, and trucking companies in the United States must follow similar rules of ownership and operation.

Strange Itineraries

Until and unless changes are made to the Jones Act, cruise vacationers have options like these:

• Take a cruise from a U.S. port in Florida or a Gulf of Mexico port (including New Orleans and Galveston) that makes a visit to a Caribbean nation or Mexico.

• Leave from a Canadian port on the East or West Coast and sail to an American destination such as Boston, New York, or Alaska, or the reverse.

• Follow an unusual itinerary on a repositioning cruise, such as a trip from Vancouver to Hawaii, Hawaii to Mexico, or Florida through the Panama Canal to California.

As more and more ships are launched, and more and more ports are opened to welcome their business, cruise lines are on the lookout for new places to visit. A number of new destinations have been developed in the Mexican Riviera, and some U.S. ports have made major improvements to their facilities as a point of embarkation.

Here's just one example: for the past few years, Norwegian Cruise Line has operated cruises among the Hawaiian islands in the spring and fall in between winter assignments in the Caribbean and summers in Alaska. To sail from Hawaii and meet the requirements of the Jones Act, the vessels had to sail a 1,200-mile side trip to an island in the Republic of Kiribati near the equator.

NCL has also decided that its new *Norwegian Sky* will be based in Seattle beginning in summer 2000 for a series of Alaska cruises to Alaska; the ship will make a call at Vancouver, Canada to comply with the law.

The Battle for Repeal

In recent years, there have been several attempts to repeal or modify the Jones Act, led in one way or another by cruise lines or their American representatives and supporters. Opposition to change has come from what remains of the U.S. shipping industry and from American unions. It is unclear whether the U.S. Congress can pass a bill.

One bill would have removed most restrictions, allowing foreign-flag ships to cruise between U.S. ports. A more modest version would create waivers to permit ships that are repositioned from the Caribbean to Alaska and the Mediterranean to make multiple U.S. port stops along the West and East Coasts and grant a limited number of 30-day permits for foreign-flagged ships to sail between U.S. ports. It would also permit U.S. companies to re-flag foreign ships.

According to its supporters, the removal of the Jones Act could virtually destroy the U.S. domestic shipping industry and its 124,000 jobs. According to an industry association, owners and builders of U.S.-flagged vessels pay approximately $300 million annually in federal taxes, and $55 million annually in state taxes. The foreign-ship cruise industry operating out of U.S. ports earns hundreds of millions of dollars a year from American consumers, yet pays no taxes on that income.

American employees pay some $1.1 billion in federal income taxes and $272 million in state taxes; again, foreign workers on foreign-flagged ships do not pay taxes.

And foreign operators are also exempt from minimum wage laws, the provisions of the National Labor Relations Act, the Occupational Safety and Health Act, and some safety regulations applied to U.S. ships and industries.

It is important to note, though, that foreign-owned cruise lines nevertheless contribute to employment of port personnel, they purchase supplies from domestic sources, and support American travel agencies, airlines, hotels, and other elements of vacation travel.

In any case, at least one American company has applied more than a bit of political muscle to gain an exemption to the law. American Classic Voyages, part of Delta Queen and parent company to American Hawaii Cruises (operator of the only remaining major American-flagged cruiseship, the *Independence*), was the only beneficiary of the U.S. Flag Cruise Ship Pilot Project Statute, passed by Congress in 1997. That law allowed the company to purchase a foreign-flagged vessel and reflag it as an American vessel; in 1999, the company signed the papers to acquire the *Nieuw Amsterdam* from Holland America Line. The ship, to be renamed as the *Patriot*, begins service in the Hawaiian Islands at the end of 2000.

Part of the deal also called for the company to contract with Ingalls Shipbuilding in Pascagoula, Miss. for the construction of a pair of 1,900-passenger cruise ships, the first major cruise ship projects at an American shipyard in more than 30 years. The fact that Pascagoula is in the backyard of one of the more powerful Republicans in the U.S. Senate did not hurt the package.

Ports of Call

The Caribbean and Bermuda

The Caribbean basin is the most popular cruising area in the world, and for good reason. There are dozens of attractive and interesting small island nations, with lovely beaches, and easygoing and friendly cultures that have their roots in Africa and Europe.

The Caribbean islands are made up of the Greater Antilles and the Lesser Antilles. The first group is closest to the United States and includes the large islands of Cuba, Jamaica, Hispaniola (which includes Haiti and the Dominican Republic), the U.S. territory of Puerto Rico, as well as the Cayman Islands.

The Lesser Antilles includes the southern portion of the Caribbean, including the Virgin, Windward, and Leeward islands. Included here are the U.S. Virgin Islands of St. John, St. Thomas, and St. Croix, as well as St. Maarten, St. Eustasius, Tortola, Virgin Gorda, Anguilla, St. Barthélemy, Saba, St. Kitts, Nevis, Montserrat, Antigua, Guadeloupe, Dominica, Martinique, St. Lucia, St. Vincent, Barbados, The Grenadines, Grenada, Trinidad and Tobago. Just off the coast of Venezuela are the ABCs: Aruba, Bonaire, and Curaçao.

(By the way, the generally preferred pronunciation is kar-ih-BEE-en, as opposed to kah-RIB-ee-en. The name is derived from Caribs, the indigenous people of the area who were mostly killed by imperial explorers or died as the result of diseases brought to the islands by outsiders.)

Cruises to the Caribbean leave from Florida ports including Tampa, Miami, and Port Canaveral; and from Gulf of Mexico ports including Galveston, Houston, and New Orleans. Other major ports of embarkation located in the islands themselves are San Juan in Puerto Rico, Santo Domingo in the Dominican Republic, and Montego Bay, Jamaica.

Caribbean cruising is typically a series of short island hops. A typical schedule has a ship arriving in port (or off-shore for transfer by ship's tender) in the early morning, and departing in the evening. This is enough time to get a brief taste of the islands—a shopping expedition, a visit to a beach or historical site, a jaunt to an island casino, but not much else. And there may be relatively little pure cruising, days when the ship is out to sea.

Another feature of some Caribbean cruises is a visit to a private island, an extension of the sealed world of the ship. Just as the cruise ship is a city unto its own, a private island is a way to spend some time ashore without the hassles of tourist traps or other tourists for that matter (other than the few thousand or so close friends traveling with you). To some, that's a real appeal; to others, it's an unreal way to travel.

Among the private islands:

- Blue Lagoon Island: Dolphin Cruise line.
- Castaway Cay in the Bahamas near Nassau: Disney Cruise Line.
- Catalina Island off the coast of the Dominican Republic: Costa Cruise Lines.
- Coco Cay in the Bahamas; Labadee off Haiti: Royal Caribbean International.
- Great Stirrup Cay in the Bahamas: Norwegian Cruise Line.
- Half Moon Cay: Holland America Line.
- Princess Cay: Princess Cruises.

In most cases, the cruise ships will anchor offshore and guests will have to transfer to the island by tender, which can result in delays and a shorter visit. (And in rough seas, the tenders may not run, or may be uncomfortable for some guests.) Disney Cruise Line was the first company to construct a pier to tie up its ships at its private island.

If you are booked for a visit to a private island, be sure to inquire about what is included in your cruise package. Some of the private islands are clearly profit centers for the cruise lines, with extra charges levied for water sports and other services.

June through November is hurricane season; August is generally the most active month. That does not mean there are constant storms in the area; in some seasons hurricanes miss the area, and even when they do arrive, the storms can hit one area and miss another and ships can alter course.

You can count on cruise operators to exercise due caution with their expensive ships and litigious passengers. They reserve the right to re-route ships, cancel port calls, and in rare circumstances, cancel an entire trip. It's all spelled out in the fine print in cruise brochures and contracts, along with policies on refunds and credits due that result from cruise changes.

Selected Caribbean Ports of Call

Basseterre, St. Kitts. The island was the first English settlement in the Leeward Islands. Today, it has moved from a sleepy sugar cane economy to an increasingly upscale tourist industry, including quite a few restored plantation houses. Across the sound is the sister island of Nevis, a near-perfect volcano cone that still belches sulphur. Together, the two islands are now an independent nation.

Bridgetown, Barbados. A bit of Britain, with its own Trafalgar Square complete with a statue of Lord Nelson; out of town, the island is a sea of green sugarcanes that stretch to the white granulated beaches. Bridgetown is a lively commercial center that has a distinctly British flavor; out in the countryside are forests of flowers, caverns, and beaches. The island sits on the line between the Atlantic and the Caribbean, approximately 100 miles east of the Lesser Antilles.

Castries, St. Lucia. A lush port on the northwest coast of the island, not far from the twin peaks of Les Pitons at Soufrière Bay and La Soufrière herself, sometimes referred to as the "drive-in volcano." St. Lucia, an independent member of the British Commonwealth, had a small coal mining industry until early in the twentieth century; a sugar cane economy continued until later in the century, supplanted by bananas, and relatively recently—by crops of tourists.

Charlotte Amalie, St. Thomas. The capital of the U.S. Virgin Islands, but its roots as a Dutch port are very much evident in the architecture. The port, pronounced "Charlotte A-mahl-ya," is one of the busiest cruise ports in the world. As such, it is home to a staggering assortment of duty-free shops and other commercial activities aimed at visitors who have dollars to spend. Outside of town is the famed Magen's Bay beach, a white swath of sand that follows the outline of a horseshoe bay.

The islands of St. Thomas, St. Croix, and St. John have been under Spanish, French, English, and Dutch control. St. Croix was at the heart of the slave trade, a way-station from Africa to the West Indies, America, and South America. All three islands were sold by the Dutch to the U.S. government in 1917 during World War I, amidst American fears of the Germans establishing a U-boat base in the area.

Christiansted, St. Croix. Christiansted is the capital of the largest, and one of the more developed, U.S. Virgin Islands. It offers superb golf courses, beaches, and shopping. Another cruise port is located at Frederiksted on the west side of the island.

Cruz Bay, St. John. About three miles east of St. Thomas, this island in the U.S. Virgin Islands is an unusual mix of luxury resorts and a wondrous protected natural park preserve that occupies two-thirds of the island.

Fort-de-France, Martinique. Very French—still a region of France—and very pretty, abloom with orchids, hibiscus, and other tropical flowers. The island is also blooming with expensive shops in Fort-de-France, and it offers a European-tinged nightlife.

Frederiksted, St. Croix. A port on the west side of the large island in the U.S. Virgin Islands, near the popular West End beaches and the island's rain forest.

George Town, Grand Cayman. A former hideout for pirates, today it is legal home to offshore tax shelters and trendy shops. The island's beaches and coral reefs are among the best in the Caribbean. The conservative culture there has banned cruise ship visits on Sundays and taken unfriendly positions against "undesirable" elements.

Great Harbour, Jost Van Dyke. A tiny island northwest of Tortola, renowned as the "party island" of the British Virgin Islands. There are less than 200 permanent residents, a dozen restaurants and bars, and a stunning white sand beach at White Bay.

Gustavia, St. Barthélemy. Just eight square miles, but considered one of the most attractive of the islands. The town of Gustavia, still tinged with Swedish and French designs, is a world-class shopping district. And by the way, everyone calls the place St. Barts.

King's Wharf, Bermuda. King's Wharf is at the tip of Bermuda's West End, home to the Royal Naval Dockyard and the Bermuda Arts Centre and Crafts Market. St. George is another port on Bermuda, known for its narrow, cobblestone streets and the restored 300-year-old King's Square on the waterfront. Bermuda, though discovered by Spanish explorer Juan de Bermúdez in 1515, was first occupied by Sir George Somers and other British colonists who were shipwrecked there in 1609—an event noted by William Shakespeare in "The Tempest." The island was a haven for pirates and privateers and later used as a base for Confederate blockade runners during the U.S. Civil War. The U.S. maintains a large naval base on the island.

La Guaira, Venezuela. A coastal port, offering access to the inland capital city of Caracas.

Marigot, St. Martin. A very French port on the French side of this multinational island. Marigot has a pretty harbor, an old fort, and an attractive shopping district. The beaches on the French side are all lovely; many of the sunbathers seem to have misplaced their suits. The other cruise terminal is at Philipsburg on the Dutch side.

Montego Bay, Jamaica. A resort port on the north shore of Jamaica, home to modern high-rise hotels and all the tourist amenities that go with them. The showplace beach is Doctor's Cave, which stretches for nearly five miles. Cruise ships also call at Ocho Rios.

Nassau, Bahamas. The capital city of the Bahamas. Cruise ships pull up to Prince George Wharf at the foot of town, a short walk to the shops and the famed straw market where native handicrafts and souvenirs are sold.

Ocho Rios, Jamaica. Cruise ships land on the north shore of this large independent island at Ocho Rios or Montego Bay; the bustling capital of Kingston lies on the other side of the Blue Mountains that run down the spine of Jamaica. Kingston, with nearly a million residents, is the largest English-speaking city south of Miami. The rivers of Ocho Rios include the one that tumbles down famed Dunn's River Falls, a 600-foot-high waterfall that has a well-worn set of natural steps, which allow you to climb its wet face.

Oranjestad, Aruba. A mostly independent piece of the Netherlands, the "A" of the "ABC" Islands of Aruba, Bonaire, and Curacao. The desert-like island of cactus, jungles, and shopping lies just off the coast of Venezuela.

Oranjestad, St. Eustatius. A Dutch island with an old history as the merchant center of the Caribbean, at least until the U.S. Revolutionary War when a British fleet destroyed much of the structures on the island because of minor support of the upstart Americans by the local governor. The waters surrounding Statia are cluttered with shipwrecks, coral reefs, and rare fish. Hikers can climb to the rim of an extinct volcano and look into the cone. By the way, anyone with a clue calls the place "Statia," pronounced Stay'-sha.

Philipsburg, St. Maarten. The cosmopolitan port at the capital of the Dutch half of this lovely split-personality island. The Dutch area is more built up, with large hotels and resorts, a few casinos, and a shopping district. The best beaches are at Mullet Bay and Cupecoy and across the unpatrolled border on the French half. Cruise ships also discharge passengers at Marigot on the French side.

Pointe-à-Pitre, Guadeloupe. Two French islands in one: Basse-Terre has volcanic peaks and a mountainous coast; Grande-Terre has beaches and shopping. The two islands are separated by the River Salée. Cruise ships pull into a bay near Pointe-à-Pitre, billed as the "Paris of the Antilles." Guadeloupe is a region of France, along with Martinique, St. Barts, and St. Martin.

Portsmouth, Dominica. One of the most naturally diverse and relatively unspoiled islands of the Caribbean, it is an independent nation. The interior is mostly an inaccessible rainforest; something like 365 rivers cascade down three mountain ranges. The island, whose name is pronounced dom'-in-eek-ah, is also home to one of the last surviving groups of Caribs and a thriving set of folklore and superstitions that have their roots in Africa. Another port is located in Roseau.

Road Town, Tortola. The largest and most populated of the British Virgin Islands and home to the major airport of the area. The best beaches lie on the north side of the island, more-or-less easily reached on a day trip by car on some rather primitive roads.

Roseau, Dominica. A port in the southwest of the island. Another cruise terminal is found at Portsmouth, at the north end.

San Juan, Puerto Rico. The capital of vibrant Puerto Rico, home of ancient forts and cobblestone streets in Old San Juan, as well as some of the liveliest modern nightspots, casinos, and restaurants in the Caribbean. San Juan is also the most active cruise port in the basin. The island itself, a semiautonomous territory of the United States, is 110 miles long and 35 miles wide, home to nearly 4 million residents.

Spanish Town and The Baths, Virgin Gorda. Supposedly named by Columbus because the island's rolling hills somehow reminded him of an overly ample young woman, the island is best known for its interesting beach and rock formation at The Baths, where gigantic boulders form grottos, caves and pools. Its manmade jewels include the opulent Little Dix Bay, Biras Creek, and Bitter End Yacht Club resorts. Roads are very limited; the best way around is by boat.

St. George's Harbour, Grenada. The Spice Island of the Caribbean; it is known for its nutmeg, cinnamon, and cocoa in particular. Formerly a British colony, it had a rocky beginning as an independent nation in the late 1970s and early 1980s, including a questionable U.S. intervention and "rescue" of some medical students. More recently, the island has concentrated on tourism and agriculture. The famed Grand Anse beach is about 10 minutes away by bus or taxi from the cruise dock in St. George's.

St. John's, Antigua. Largest of the British Leeward Islands, it was headquarters to Admiral Horatio Nelson's fleet in the colonial era. Nelson's Dockyard at English Harbour is restored to its Georgian splendor. The island is home to at least 365 beaches—one for each day of the year if you're on a very long shore leave.

Vieques, Puerto Rico. A lovely, lightly developed island off the east coast of Puerto Rico. The island's bays are home to microscopic bioluminescent organisms that put on a light show in the wake of your boat.

Willemstad, Curaçao. A mixture of Dutch, Spanish, English, and native cultures in the Netherlands Antilles, 35 miles off the coast of Venezuela. The famed Queen Emma Floating Bridge will move to the side to permit your cruise ship to enter the harbor. Beaches are more rock and coral than sand and there is a busy refining industry. Willemstad was established by Dutch settlers in the 1630s, about the same time as other Dutch settlers arrived on Manhattan Island; Curaçao has maintained much of its original color, including red-tiled gable roofs.

Bermuda

Britain's oldest colony, dating back to the early seventeenth century and still very much a bit of Old England from High Tea to cricket matches to a good-natured formality in business and social matters. The island was first settled in 1609 by the survivors of the shipwreck of the *Sea Venture*, British colonists who had been heading for Jamestown, Virginia.

Bermuda, about 600 miles east of Cape Hatteras, North Carolina, actually includes some 150 islands, with the six main islands connected by bridges and causeways. The preferred method of transportation is moped or bicycle.

The climate is temperate, but not as hot as the islands of the Caribbean, which lie much further south. The season runs from May through September. The best bargains are often available at the beginning and end of the season—before Memorial Day and after Labor Day.

Cuba on Their Mind

Politics aside, one of the most appealing cruise destinations is the island nation of Cuba. It has beautiful beaches, a lively culture, and ports just 90 miles off the coast of Florida.

Cuba is, of course, off limits to ships sailing from U.S. ports and to most U.S. passport holders. But the political climate could change rapidly.

There are some cruise ships that make visits to Havana from ports including the Dominican Republic, without touching American ports.

All of the major cruise lines have plans on the shelves to bring their ships to Cuba as soon as they are permitted.

Alaska

The hottest waters for cruising in recent years have been in the Inside Passage to Alaska, with nearly half a million passengers visiting coastal towns each year.

Alaska has some magnificent appeals: the spectacular frozen rivers of Glacier Bay and other inlets; the fascinating native, Russian, and American cultures of trading and fishing towns such as Ketchikan and Sitka, and the Gold Rush history of Skagway. Just as appealing: a pod of whales shadowing your ship in a narrow passage between thickly forested slopes and frolicking families of seals on bobbing ice floes.

Alaska is still one of the last great frontiers of the world, and it's certainly among the most remote places in North America. There are almost no roads between towns in the state; residents are served by a fleet of small floatplanes and ferries.

For the cruise passenger, one of the major appeals of an Alaskan visit is that your ship will be within sight of land in

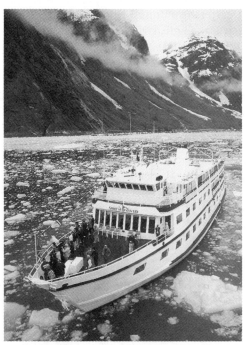

Cruise West's Spirit of Discovery *passes through a glacier-filled fjord in Alaska*
Cruise West

protected waters for most of the cruise. The Inside Passage is sandwiched between the mainland and a series of large and small islands. You can expect generally calm waters in the sheltered arms of the Pacific, with only an occasional jaunt into the open ocean to visit ports such as Sitka.

Many of the cruise ships depart from Vancouver in Canada's British Columbia; Vancouver is one of the most attractive ports I know, combining a thriving cosmopolitan city with mountains and the ocean. It's worth a few days as a stopover at the start or end of a cruise.

Most of the cruises visit the southernmost reaches of Alaska, from Ketchikan to Juneau and Glacier Bay. The more adventurous ships venture further north through the open waters of the Gulf of Alaska and Prince William Sound to Seward.

Many larger ships must anchor offshore because they are unable to come into shallow or narrow harbors.

Holland America Line and Princess Cruises are major players in Alaska and have extensive facilities on shore, including hotels and tours. In fact, Holland America is one of the state's largest private employers.

It's not quite accurate to say that the Alaskan towns visited by cruise ships are untouched. You'll find more than your share of T-shirt and gift shops, tacky tourist bars, and unimpressive bus tours. The appeal of Alaska, instead, lies off the beaten path in the pristine bays and fjords of places such as Glacier Bay, Tracy Arm, and the sprawling Misty Fjords National Park.

Don't go for the weather. It can be cold and rainy most any day of the year, even though you may be blessed with a spectacular, warm day when you least expect it.

Selected Ports of Call in Alaska/Western Canada

College Fjord, Alaska. In Prince William Sound, College Fjord is home to 26 glaciers, each named by an early expedition for one of the Ivy League colleges that funded the Harriman Expedition, which mapped them in 1899.

Haines, Alaska. Home to a rich gold rush history, thousands of bald eagles, and the Tlingit and Chilkat Indian cultures.

Juneau, Alaska. The nation's only state capital with a glacier in its backyard; the Mendenhall Glacier is just outside of town. Also home to the Alaska State Museum and other cultural attractions.

Ketchikan, Alaska. A place that lays claim to the largest collection of totem poles in the world, at Totem Bight and elsewhere around town. Also the gateway to float plane and boat expeditions into the spectacular Misty Fjord National Park, which spreads over more than two million acres and includes sheer granite cliffs that rise thousands of feet out of the water; the area has countless lakes and ponds, and sprawling forests that are home to bear, deer, mountain goat, and other wildlife.

Prince William Sound, Alaska. A large saltwater bay northwest of Juneau, some 15,000 square miles in size and as much as 2,850 feet deep, it contains more glaciers than any other single area in Alaska.

Seward, Alaska. A tiny fishing village that is gateway to some of America's natural jewels: the Chugach National Forest, the Kenai Fjords National Park and Wildlife Refuge, and the Alaska Marite National Refuge.

Sitka, Alaska. The keeper of Alaska's Russian heritage, including an onion-domed cathedral, a restored fort site, and a cultural center. The harbor looks out on a dramatic volcano.

Skagway, Alaska. The northernmost point in the Inside Passage, it was the jumping off point for many Gold Rushers of the 1890s. Its history is saluted by many shops and restaurants. It is also the terminal for the White Pass and Yukon Railroad, which retraces some of the routes taken by the Gold Rushers.

Tracy Arm, Alaska. A fjord that wends its way to the face of two dramatic glaciers, North and South Sawyer.

Valdez, Alaska. It lays claim to the title of the "Switzerland of Alaska" with its perch beneath the snow-capped peaks along Prince William Sound. Valdez is the southern terminus of the 800-mile trans-Alaska oil pipeline.

Vancouver, British Columbia. One of the most cosmopolitan cities of Canada, sharing British, Asian, native, and many other cultures. Home to sprawling Stanley Park with a world-class aquarium, the spectacular Capilano foot bridge that sways over a deep gorge, several significant museums of science, anthropology, and art, and a thriving commercial district and Chinatown.

Victoria, British Columbia. A very English outpost on the far western edge of Canada on Vancouver Island, capital of the province of British Columbia and home to the famed Royal British Columbia Museum and the Empress Hotel. Just outside of town is world-famous Butchart Gardens.

Yakutat Bay, Alaska. Home to Hubbard Glacier, which let loose in 1986 to advance more than 100 feet in a single day, blocking off Russell Fjord. Hubbard is the largest valley glacier in North America, at more than six miles in width and nearly 500 feet in height.

Hawaii

The weather is fine year-round, but the major cruise lines circle the islands mostly as part of repositioning schedules. A typical schedule has ships coming to Hawaii in the fall as they move south from Alaska enroute to the Panama Canal and the Caribbean Sea. The schedule is reversed in the spring.

The complication comes from the provisions of the Jones Act, which require foreign-flagged cruise lines to make a visit to at least one other country after embarkation from a U.S. port. Itineraries sometimes begin in Vancouver or Mexico for repositioning trips. A few lines, including Norwegian Cruise Lines, have extended their Hawaiian seasons with long detours to obscure island nations such as the Republic of Kiribati.

American Hawaii Cruise Line's *Independence* circles the Hawaiian islands year round; she will be joined by the United States Line's *Patriot* in late 2000.

Selected Ports of Call in Hawaii

Hilo, Hawaii. Hilo is a commercial center on the east coast of the Big Island of Hawaii; the island is nearly twice the size of all of the other Hawaiian Islands together, and still growing as the result of slow but steady lava flows into the sea from several active volcanoes. A visit to the Volcanoes National Park by vehicle, or overhead by helicopter or plane, is a tourist highlight.

Honolulu, Oahu. The best-known city of Hawaii is located on the island of Oahu. Nearby to the port is the famed beach at Waikiki, as well as the U.S. Naval base at Pearl Harbor.

Kona, Hawaii. The second port on the Big Island, on the west side, is a quiet backwater. Expeditions leave to tourist destinations and several nearby golf courses and resorts.

Lahaina, Maui. Lahaina has some touches of an old New England fishing port, a remembrance of its days as an important Pacific port for the whaling ships of Nantucket and eastern America. The whale ships are gone, but the whales are still there in the winter. The island is also home to some of the best beaches in the Hawaiian chain. Another port on the island is Kahului.

Nawilwili, Kauai. The very lush and mountainous island of Kauai includes the colorful Waimea Canyon, a small-scale geological feature somewhat grandly billed as the "Grand Canyon of the Pacific" as well as some spectacular waterfalls that are like a scene from "Shangri-la."

New England and Canada

New York and Boston were once among the great transatlantic ports; today they are busy in season with cruise ships to Atlantic Canada, Bermuda, and the occasional crossing of the pond to Europe.

A typical cruise heads north from New York along the coast—sometimes through the Cape Cod canal—to Boston and on to Nova Scotia and sometimes Montreal. Some ships leave from Boston and head north to Canada.

The season for cruises runs from May to October, with the best bargains available before Memorial Day. Weather in New England and Atlantic Canada can be very capricious, especially in the spring and fall. There can be some spectacular October days and ferocious Nor'easter storms.

Selected Ports in New England and Eastern Canada

Boston. A modern metropolis with a great Colonial and Revolutionary War history.

Halifax, Nova Scotia. An historic fishing town of Maritime Canada. Many of the victims of the sinking of the *Titanic* were buried in Fairview Cemetery where rows of headstones form the shape of a ship's hull. Nearby is the picturesque Peggy's Cove, a romantic New England village.

Martha's Vineyard, Massachusetts. The tony resort island off the coast of Cape Cod, Massachusetts. Home to artists, musicians, and fine Atlantic Ocean beaches.

Montreal. The largest French-speaking city outside of France and one of the most cosmopolitan cities anywhere.

Nantucket, Massachusetts. A one-time whaling island 30 miles south of Cape Cod, now primarily a tourist community of galleries, shops, museums, beaches, and home to the author of this book. The narrow and shallow harbor does not permit large ships to enter; smaller ships set anchor well outside of the harbor and send guests ashore by tender.

New York. The Big Apple was once one of the most important ports for transatlantic ocean liners; today the port is home to seasonal service to Bermuda and to maritime Canada, as well as transatlantic crossings.

Quebec City, Quebec. Cruise ships dock on the river below the famed Chateau Frontenac Hotel.

St. Pierre et Miquelon. A pair of tiny fishing outposts of France, south of Newfoundland, Canada.

Mexican Riviera and Central America

The sunny ports of upper Mexico are becoming more popular year-by-year with ships making calls at port cities on the Pacific side, including Ensenada near the U.S. border with California and further south at Cabo San Lucas at the tip of Baja California. On the Pacific mainland are ports including Mazatlán, Puerto Vallarta, and Acapulco.

On the Caribbean side are ports including Calica, Cancun, and Cozumel.

Some cruise ships heading through the Panama Canal make port calls in Caldera, Costa Rica and points off the eastern coast of Panama, including San Andres Island, a northern outpost of Colombia.

The Mexican Riviera has generally fine weather year-round, with high season in the winter.

Selected Ports in the Mexican Riviera and Central America

Acapulco, Mexico. The most famous, and most developed, port in the Mexican Riviera; it has grown from a sleepy fishing village to a world-class resort during the past few decades. Among the best-known sights of the area are the cliff divers of La Quebrada, who plunge more than 100 feet into the waters below.

Cabo San Lucas, Mexico. At the extreme southern tip of Baja California, between the Pacific Ocean and the Sea of Cortez. The bay once sheltered treasure ships from the Orient, and pirate ships waiting in prey. The pounding surf has carved some spectacular sea arches and rock formations.

Calica, Mexico. A recently developed port on Mexico's Quintana Roo coast on the Yucatan Peninsula on the Caribbean Sea, with access to the Mayan ruins at Tulum and the lagoons of Xel-Há.

Cartagena, Columbia. At the top of South America on the Caribbean Sea. In the days of colonial control, Cartagena was one of the principal ports from which the riches of the New World were sent back to the Old. The walled city on Colombia's northern coast was built centuries ago to protect against pirate raids. Today, the port is famed as a shopping mecca, especially for emeralds.

Cozumel, Mexico. Just off the coast of the Yucatan Peninsula in Mexico, and nearby to the Mayan ruins at Chichen Itza and San Gervasio. Palancar Reef, at Cozumel, was discovered by Jacques Cousteau about 30 years ago; it is the second-largest known reef in the world.

Huatulco, Mexico. On Mexico's Oaxaca coast, set against the dramatic backdrop of the Sierra Madre mountains. The area's resorts lie along Tangolunda Bay.

Manzanillo, Mexico. A small but very stylish port of call built around the Las Hadas resort and its dreamscape of a beach.

Mazatlan, Mexico. Mexico's largest Pacific port.

Puerto Caldera, Costa Rica. A commercial port near the tropical paradise of the Pacific coast of Central America, home to exotic birds, butterflies, and tourists enjoying its white- and black-sand beaches. The port lies below San Jose, Costa Rica's capital.

Puerto Vallarta, Mexico. A small fishing village on the Bay of Banderas that has embraced visitors and has become a world-class resort.

San Andres Island, Colombia. A small island off the eastern coast of Panama that is home to a Colombian naval base and not much else. The island is a reminder of the fact that Panama was once part of Colombia before a U.S.-backed revolution, which helped pave the way to American development of the Panama Canal.

San Blas Islands, Panama. A group of 360 lush, low-lying isles off the East coast of Panama that are little changed from the way they were when Columbus visited 500 years ago. The San Blas are home to the Cuna Indians.

Panama Canal

The Panama Canal was built to speed transit of ships from the East Coast of the United States to the West Coast, allowing vessels to avoid the lengthy and sometimes dangerous trip around the Cape of Good Hope at the bottom of South America. The canal still serves that purpose, but its extraordinary man-made and natural wonders are today a tourist draw of their own.

From the Caribbean to the Pacific, ships are lifted 85 feet in three steps at Gatun Locks to Gatun Lake. They cross Gatun Lake to Gaillard Cut where it passes the Continental Divide. From there, ships are lowered 31 feet to Miraflores Lake and then proceed through two more locks at Miraflores Lock before entering the Pacific Ocean.

A 50-mile transit takes approximately nine hours; the alternative to the canal is an 8,000-mile passage below South America.

Until recent years, cruise ships passed through the canal only on repositioning itineraries, usually on journeys from Alaska or Hawaii to the Caribbean and returning. Now you'll find some cruise ships that pass back and forth from the Pacific to the Caribbean for much of the year. Another group of ships make a partial transit, entering from the Caribbean side and going as far as Gatun Lake midway across; there they turn around and exit.

The United States completed the turnover of the canal to Panama at the end of 1999. Most experts expect little or no change in its operations, although the possibility of political instability worries some.

Europe and Mediterranean

Europe is one of the fastest-growing cruise markets, and will continue to expand as a number of cruise companies position their ships there for the summer.

Many of the finest cities of Europe are ocean harbors, including Amsterdam, Barcelona, Copenhagen, Genoa, Helsinki, Lisbon, Monte Carlo, Nice, Oslo, St. Petersburg, Stockholm, and Venice. London is up the Thames River from the sea.

Repositioning Cruises

Many cruise ships follow a seasonal schedule, matching the changing interests of travelers. Here are a few typical cycles:

Alaska/Caribbean. Ships may spend the summer in Alaska, then move south through Hawaii or Mexican Riviera in the fall, passing through the Panama Canal before winter, and finishing out the season in the Caribbean. In the spring, the migration is reversed.

New England/Bermuda/Caribbean. Some ships finish up their winters in the Caribbean and head north to New York or Boston and serve Bermuda in the spring; they then cruise New England and Atlantic Canada in the summer and early fall.

Caribbean/Europe. Some cruise ships finish up Caribbean winter runs and then sail across the Atlantic to the Mediterranean for the summer.

The cruise companies have to move their ships from place to place to accommodate these changing itineraries; the trips between ports of embarkation are known as repositioning cruises. Many cruise veterans seek out these trips because they often offer unusual ports of call, extra days out to sea, and generally lower prices.

Chapter 4
How to Buy a Cruise

Although some cruise lines sell a portion of their available space directly, the vast majority of cruise bookings are made through travel agents.

In theory, it shouldn't matter to you as a buyer. Most travel agents do not charge customers a fee; instead they make their income from commissions received from cruise lines, airlines, hotels, car rental agencies, and nearly every other element of a travel package they put together.

Most larger travel agencies are members of or associated with one or another national association, such as ASTA (American Society of Travel Agents), the CLIA (Cruise Line Industry Association) or NACOA (National Association of Cruise-Oriented Agencies.) If you see one of these logos on the door of an agency or on a brochure or posted on a web page, you have some assurance the agency meets some level of industry standard. Among other things, the company may have posted a bond to protect deposits and advance payments made by clients; and you may be able to enlist the association in any dispute you may have with the agency.

Some industry groups offer training for members, awarding "master" and other titles to agents with particular expertise on cruises or other specialties.

No matter what the string of letters after a travel agency's or agent's name, you should closely judge the quality of service you receive from any travel agency.

My recommendation is that you begin with research of your own, starting with this book, before you speak with a travel agent. Understand the industry, learn about the cruise lines and their ships, and find out about destinations. Check prices in newspaper and magazine ads.

Then make a phone call to the cruise line or check its web page on the Internet, or both. Some cruise lines have begun accepting direct bookings from their website, and it is reasonable to expect special deals, especially on unsold cabins close to the sailing date.

Armed with all of that information, judge the quality of service you receive from the agent or agents you contact.

How to Choose a Travel Agent

Good travel agents remember who they work for—you. There is, though, a built-in conflict of interest here because the agent is—in most cases—paid by someone other than you. Agents receive a commission from the sellers on airline tickets, hotel reservations, car rentals, and many other services. The more they sell (or the higher the price), the more they earn.

I would recommend you start the planning for any trip by calling the cruise lines and airlines, and even a few hotels if you'll need to stay over at a port. Find the best package you can put together for yourself, then call a travel agency and ask them to do better.

If your agent contributes knowledge or experience, comes up with dollar-saving alternatives to your own package, or offers some other kind of convenience, then go ahead and book through the agency. If, as I often find, you know a lot more about your destination and are willing to spend a lot more time to save money than will the agent, you can choose to do some or all of the booking yourself.

You'll have to make a judgment whether an agent is looking out for your best interests—the best cruise line, vessel, and itinerary for you—or whether the promise of a higher commission is clouding your agent's judgment.

My best advice: Interview a travel agent carefully, and don't be afraid to ask questions about commissions and special promotions they receive from the cruise lines. If the agent refuses to discuss the matter or does so in a rude manner, take your business elsewhere. Remember that this is a business transaction, and it is your money—and your vacation—that is at stake.

If you go to a travel agency with one cruise line in mind and are steered toward a different line, make sure the switch makes sense to you. Ask yourself: Who gets a better deal because of the switch—you or the travel agent?

Bids and Rebates

And if you are booking an expensive cruise, don't be afraid to devote a little time and effort to saving some money:

1. Put your business out to bid. There is nothing that says you cannot call two or three agencies and ask for a price on a particular cruise. Some agencies may have better pricing than others or may be receiving a bonus from the cruise line, and they may be willing to share some of that money with you to get your business.

2. Ask for a rebate from your agent. If you're booking a $10,000 two-week luxury cruise, the agency stands to earn a $1,500 commission for perhaps an hour's work. Ask for a reduction in price, or a free room upgrade, or first-class air tickets, or something else back from the travel agency. It's not an unreasonable thing to do, and it's common practice in dealings between agencies and business clients.

Unbundling the Package

You might want to consider "unbundling" a vacation, giving your cruise business to a travel agency or consolidator, your airline reservations directly to the air carrier or a consolidator of tickets, and so on.

Your goal, of course, is to compare the bottom line of a mixed purchase to the all-inclusive package put together by a travel agent.

In some cases, a cruise line may have negotiated special prices for airline tickets from many major gateway airports. Some cruise packages include airfare from these cities. Either way, you should compare the airfare price you could obtain by directly booking a flight to the cost in the package. Find out from the cruise line the credit you would receive if you were to opt to make your own arrangements.

All this said, consider the fact that if you provide your own transportation to the ship, the cruise line is not likely to be very accommodating to you if your flight is late or canceled. In general, if you purchase a package that includes airfare, the cruise line will take responsibility for getting you and your baggage to the ship, from the moment your journey begins. You'll read more about this in Chapter 11 about embarkation.

Travel Agent Rebates

There is one special type of travel agency worth considering. A number of large agencies offer travelers rebates on part of their commissions. Some of these companies cater only to frequent flyers who will bring in a lot of business; other rebate agencies offer only limited services to clients.

You can find discount travel agencies through many major credit card companies (Citibank and American Express among them) or through associations and clubs. Some warehouse shopping clubs have rebate travel agencies.

And if you establish a regular relationship with your local travel agency and bring them enough business to make them glad to see you walk through their door, don't be afraid to ask them for a discount equal to a few percentage points.

One other important new tool for travelers is the Internet. Here, you'll find computerized travel agencies that offer airline, hotel, car, cruise, and package reservations. You won't receive personalized assistance, but you will be able to make as many price checks and itinerary routings as you'd like without apology. Several of the services feature special deals, including companion fares and rebates you won't find offered elsewhere.

Some of the best Internet agencies include:

Atevo	www.atevo.com/
1Travel	www.1travel.com
Microsoft Expedia	www.expedia.com
Preview	www.previewtravel.com.

You can also book directly with a number of major airlines, sometimes taking advantage of special Internet prices, or bonus frequent flyer mileage. Among the airlines that offer online booking are:

American Airlines   www.aa.com
Continental Airlines   www.continental.com
Delta Airlines   www.deltaairlines.com
Northwest Airlines   www.nwa.com
Southwest   www.iflyswa.com
United Airlines   www.ual.com
US Airways   www.usairways.com.

Don't be afraid to do your business over the phone or over the Internet. You should expect the same sort of personalized attention and service; in many instances, I have found I have received better service over the phone than I would receive if I walked into a travel agency.

You'll find a sampling of some capable travel agencies listed in the coupon section of this book. Others can be found in travel sections of newspapers, in travel magazines, and on the Internet.

Understanding Cancellation Policies

One of the problems with booking a cruise is that you are paying in advance for a product not yet delivered. And if you take advantage of some discount programs, you may be laying out thousands of dollars—as much as a year before your cruise date.

In theory, that's OK. You're reaping the benefits of a discount for advance payment or securing a reservation for a commodity that's in very limited supply. There is a value that can be assigned to either situation, and if it makes sense to you, making an advance deposit and payment is acceptable behavior.

But, what happens if your vacation schedule changes? What if there is an illness in your family? What if the cruise line changes the itinerary or substitutes a different ship?

In general, if the cruise line makes a substantial change, you don't have to accept the new deal and can ask for your money back.

But if you are unable to show up at the appointed time, the cruise line has the right to keep some or all of your deposit or advance payment.

Some lines are more accommodating than others. The careful buyer spends the time to closely read the small print at the back of the cruise brochure.

Enlist the assistance of your travel agency, the cruise line, and experienced travelers. But remember this: Put no trust in anything you are told verbally. The only thing that really matters is the written contract. If the cruise line or a travel agent tells you something different from what you see in the brochure or on the booking papers, ask them to put it in writing and sign it and make it part of the contract.

Sample Cancellation Policy

Here's an example of one policy from a major cruise line.

All cancellations and requests for refunds must be submitted in writing to the cruise company. All documents (deposit receipt or tickets) must be returned before the refund can be processed.

The cruise company will assess cancellation charges as follows:

- 76 or more days prior to sailing: Full refund
- 75–46 days prior to sailing: Loss of deposit of $100 per person
- 45–15 days prior to sailing: 50 percent of cruise/package price per person
- 14–3 days prior to sailing: 75 percent of cruise/package price per person
- Less than 3 days prior to sailing: No refund, 100 percent cancellation charge per person.

These charges are just for the cruise portion of the trip, and do not include cancellation or change fees that may be applied by air carriers, hotels, shore excursion suppliers, and others.

And just to add insult to injury, some cruise lines will add an "administrative fee" for changes to bookings after cruise documents have been issued.

Trip Cancellation Insurance

So, what is there to do about the not-insignificant risk to your pocketbook from cancellations?

You might want to consider buying trip cancellation insurance. These policies will pay the penalties caused by any cancellation or interruption due to unforeseen, non pre-existing medical conditions to travelers, their immediate family members, or traveling companions.

Cancellation insurance will also often add coverage for illness or injury while on the cruise, including emergency evacuation, as well as damage, loss, delay, or theft of baggage.

As with any other form of insurance, the higher the potential payout—or the more likely the insurance company will have to pay it—the higher the premium.

Spend the time to read the insurance offering carefully. Pay special attention to the sections that cover pre-existing conditions, generally excluded from coverage.

Unforeseen circumstances might include a traffic accident while en route to the port of departure, jury duty or subpoena, quarantine, a hijacking, or a home rendered uninhabitable by natural disaster. In all of these cases, you'll have to provide legal proof.

If your trip is interrupted midway through the trip because of illness, the refund will be for the unused, nonrefundable portion of your cruise payment, plus the cost of returning home. For example, if you must leave the ship eight days into a 10-day trip, the insurance policy may only pay 20 percent of the cruise cost.

Take care not to purchase more coverage than you need. If you have a $5,000 prepayment on a cruise but the cruise line's cancellation policy says you will lose 50 percent of your advance payment in the case of a late cancellation, you need $2,500 in coverage, not $5,000. Be sure to include in your calculations all the elements of the package, such as airfare, non-cancelable hotel reservations, and other bills explicitly covered by the insurance policy.

All-Encompassing Cancellation Insurance

Although it is understandable that cruise lines don't want to lose money on a stateroom they could have sold to another customer given enough time, that doesn't make it easier on travelers who end up losing money on a cancellation. Some cruise lines have made attempts to soften the blow.

Holland America Line was among the first to offer an enhanced travel insurance policy that permits guests to cancel cruises for any reason up to 24 hours prior to commencement of travel without penalty. The "Platinum" policy is not cheap, but does offer a greatly enhanced sense of well-being, especially if you are booking a cruise for six months or a year off.

Holland America's plan was priced at 5.25 percent to 6 percent of the cruise price for longer trips, and $105 to $170 for one- to two-week Caribbean cruises.

Costa and Carnival and a few others have offered a plan that says should your trip cancellation claim be denied as a result of a pre-existing condition, the cruise line will provide a future cruise credit equal to the value of your cancellation penalty.

Accident and Sickness Insurance

The idea of falling ill or suffering an injury while hundreds or thousands of miles away from home and your family doctor can be a terrifying thought. Although nearly all cruise ships have a medical doctor and small infirmary aboard ship, in the event of serious illness or injury, you'll almost certainly have to be taken to a hospital on shore or even airlifted home.

As we'll discuss in greater detail in Chapter 7, most medical insurance coverage provided by your employer or that you purchase for your family does not cover expenses incurred onboard a cruise ship or in foreign countries.

Some insurance packages sold by cruise companies do include accident and sickness coverage with trip cancellation insurance. The package may provide sufficient coverage.

But before you sign on the bottom line, be sure to consult with your own insurance agent or your company's personnel office to see how far your personal medical insurance policy will reach. Does the policy cover vacation trips and exclude business travel? Are all international locations excluded? Can you purchase a "rider," or extension, to your personal policy to cover travel?

The only reason to purchase an accident and sickness policy is to fill in any gaps in the coverage you already have. If you don't have health insurance of any kind, a travel policy is certainly valuable, but you might want to consider whether you should spend the money on a year-round policy instead of taking a vacation in the first place.

Also be aware that nearly every kind of health insurance has an exclusionary period for pre-existing conditions. If you are sick before you set out on a trip, you may find that the policy will not pay for treating the problem.

How to Pay for Your Cruise Vacation

In general, the best way to pay the fare for your cruise vacation is with a major credit card.

This also applies to all of the other elements involved, including airfare to the port and any necessary hotels and car rental.

I am not endorsing paying high credit card interest rates on loans; in fact, I would recommend instead that you try to pay for vacations from savings. Instead, I am suggesting you take advantage of the card's built-in protection against fraud and other problems.

Here are some reasons to use your credit card:

• You can enlist the bank or card issuer in any dispute with the seller. Although you have authorized a charge to be put on your account, you hold onto your money for the moment. If the seller does not deliver the goods, or if whatever you bought is not what you contracted for, you can withhold payment and enlist the assistance of the company that issued the credit card.

• You'll have the federal Fair Credit Billing Act on your side of the table, which allows you to refuse to pay for a purchase and any finance charges while you make good-faith efforts to resolve a dispute. And your credit card company can apply pressure on the merchant on your behalf, too.

Be sure to follow the rules for disputing a credit card bill. They're generally listed on the back of your monthly statement; you can also discuss them with the customer service department of the credit card company.

• When you are traveling abroad and are paying local currency. Your credit card company will convert the bill to dollars at the bank rate, almost always lower than the rate charged by local merchants or money-changing outlets.

It's fun to go "native" when you travel in a foreign land, paying for your meals and souvenirs with francs in France, pounds in England, krone in Denmark, and shekels in Israel. But you may end up losing 10 percent to 20 per-

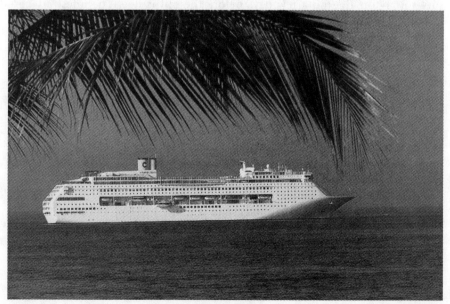

Costa Victoria
Costa Cruise Lines

cent or more of your purchasing power by cashing in your dollars at a money-changing counter at the airport or a hotel where you may have to pay a service charge and almost certainly will receive less than the best rate. You'll get a better exchange rate at a major bank and an even squarer deal by using your credit card.

• When you want to use your credit card's automobile insurance coverage when you rent a car. Many credit cards, especially "gold" and "platinum" cards, offer special automobile insurance coverage for rentals made using the card. Be sure to read the fine print from the credit card company, and don't hesitate to call customer service for clarification before you use the card to rent a car. The insurance coverage usually has exceptions that exclude luxury cars and also withhold payment if it is deemed that an accident was due to negligence by the driver. Finally, some credit card companies do not extend coverage to international rentals.

• When you want to obtain free airline accident insurance on tickets purchased with your credit card. Special insurance coverage for airline flights, purchased from an airport kiosk or machine or directly from an insurance company, is generally not a good deal; you're better off buying and maintaining a good life insurance policy. But if your credit card company offers free coverage for tickets purchased with its card, go ahead and take advantage of the offer.

• When you want an interest-free loan from your credit card company from the time you make your purchase until the due date on your statement. Here's one of the best uses of a credit card, but only for the financially well-disciplined: Make as many purchases as you can on your credit card and then be sure to pay off the bill a few days before the bill is due. The finest art here involves making major purchases just after the closing day of one billing period, which can give you 30 days until the next bill and up to 30 more days beyond then until the statement must be paid.

Paying for a Vacation on the Installment Plan

Do you really want to be paying for your vacation memories for years after you're back home?

That's what you'll be doing if you put your cruise on an installment plan, credit card, or other loan arrangement. What's even worse is taking out a home equity loan (also called a second mortgage) for a vacation. In this case, you could be putting the roof over your head at risk.

All that said, if you do use a loan or credit card, be sure to pay close attention to the APR (annual percentage rate) for the interest charged. Don't be shy about changing credit cards to get a lower rate, or asking your present card issuer to reduce the APR to match another offer you have received.

One plan I cautiously endorse is a pay-in-advance installment plan, sort of a layaway plan for a cruise. Here you put away money before you travel. The sponsor of the plan should pay you interest on your money or offer some other enticement to you. Be sure to understand your rights to receive a full or partial refund if you must cancel your plans before you travel.

Chapter 5
Your Home on the Water

I don't know about you, but my idea of the perfect ship's cabin (and hotel room) is a comfortable, clean, and quiet home away from home.

Cruise line brochures show glorious color photos of spectacular suites and glimpses of the better-looking portions of the smaller outside cabins. If they show one of the lowest-priced, inside cabins at all, it is usually with a wide-angle view that rarely hints at just how minimal the accommodation is.

Then again, some travelers use their rooms as a place to sleep and hang their clothes. If you spend all of your waking time outside on the pool deck, you may not want to spend any money on a veranda or panoramic window; if you don't expect to make it down to your room until way after dark, you might be perfectly happy with a windowless, inside stateroom.

Think about the nature of the cruise itself. If you're on a Caribbean island-hopper, the ship will travel by night and tie up or set anchor in a new port each morning. On this sort of cruise, you might be willing to accept a lesser cabin than you would prefer on an itinerary with several days between ports.

Once you're out of your room, there's no class distinction on nearly all modern ships—all guests eat in the same restaurants, swim in the same pools, traverse the same promenades and lobbies, and participate in the same onboard and shore excursions. (The only exception: On some very luxurious cruises, a few suites have their own pool or deck area and a concierge area.

What You Need to Know About Booking a Cabin

Are you the sort of person who wants to spend time lounging around your luxurious cabin, or would you rather spend time (and the money you've saved) in luxurious public spaces and on-shore shopping expeditions? This is not to say you should seek out (or accept) substandard accommodations, but there have been many times when I've checked into a first-class hotel room at midnight and left at 6 A.M. the next morning for a business appointment; the sitting room was unsat in, the luxurious bath robe un-lounged in, and the spectacular view unviewed.

The same goes for cabins on a ship. Ask yourself how important it is to you to have a window. Are you willing to accept an obstructed view or an inside cabin with no view at all? You can save big bucks if you choose to spend most of your time up on deck or in one of the public rooms of the ship.

One step deeper into the budget section are especially small inside cabins, or staterooms in a particularly unappealing location such as the very bottom of the ship or next door to the disco or the laundry room. If you can put up with living in the low rent district, you can expect to pay a lower rent.

Study the cabin diagrams and ship layouts carefully before booking passage, and have all your questions answered before you commit to a cruise. Although it is sometimes possible to upgrade to a better class of cabin after you are onboard the ship, you cannot rely on that on all cruises, especially those taken during peak seasons when cruise ships may be completely booked.

Cabin size can vary from a tiny closet to a penthouse-like suite. In recent years the trend has been toward smaller cabins on modern ships, for no other reason than to maximize income for the owners. But that trend has reversed lately with the largest Megaships and luxury liners.

Suites offer superior accommodations, and some of the most expensive come equipped with concierge or butler service, and a few may have access to a private swimming pool or lounge.

Inside and Out

The most important distinction between cabins is that of "inside" and "outside" locations.

An outside cabin, as the name suggests, includes at least one wall that is part of the exterior of the ship—usually one of the sides but sometimes overlooking the bow or stern. You can expect at least one porthole or window;

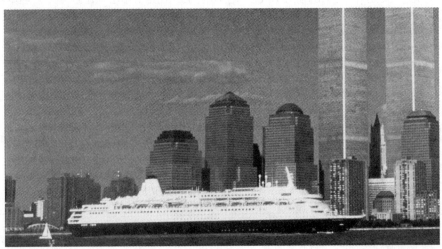

Holland America's Westerdam *in New York*
Holland America Line

on many of the trendiest new ships, some outside cabins include a veranda with a glass door.

A balcony or veranda is a lovely extra, especially on a warm-water cruise. They're a great place to salute the sunset or the sunrise, or to conduct a romantic interlude. (Be aware, though, that not all balconies are all that private—there may be a view from above, or there may not be full partitions on the sides.) And the veranda may be a concern to families that have young children.

A handful of ships include forward-facing balconies at the bow. This affords a great view, but in most conditions, you'll also be facing a 20-knot wind in your face anytime the ship is moving.

Be sure to study the ship's diagrams and check with the cruise line or a trusted travel agent to learn if your chosen cabin has an obstructed or partial view. What does that mean? On many ships, the lifeboats and other necessary equipment are mounted on the side of the ship or on an exterior deck. Try to get as much information as you can from the cruise line: A small winch in a corner of your view is very different from the broadside of a lifeboat completely filling your window.

Is there a promenade deck outside your cabin window or porthole? If so, you cannot count on much or any privacy when the curtain is open.

By the way, on most ships the windows or portholes cannot be opened. The exceptions: suites on upper decks and cabins that have verandas.

An inside cabin is one that has no windows or portholes; on many ships these are also the smallest accommodations onboard. Some passengers will find them unbearably claustrophobic, while others will see them as a comfortable den to sleep between times when they are moving about the ship's public places.

There's one other class of inside cabins on the newest and grandest of ships: an inside balcony with a view of the ship's interior atrium. The first major ship with this sort of accommodation is Royal Caribbean's *Voyager of the Seas,* which has a set of "Atrium Staterooms." (This strikes me as a wholly unappealing veranda in a shopping mall. But then again, this may match some travelers' concept of nirvana.)

Making Your Bed

Many cabins are equipped with twin beds, even on the "Love Boats." It may be possible to have the beds moved together to create a double bed, albeit one with a small gap between the mattresses.

In some especially small cabins, the beds may be arranged in an L-shape. Some older boats use upper and lower berths with twin mattresses on each level. A few cabins have "Pullman" beds that fold up against the wall when they are not used.

If you have any particular requirements or desires, study the ship diagrams before you book a cabin; you may also want to call the cruise line and discuss specific staterooms.

By the way, don't move furniture in your cabin; ask the stateroom attendant whether beds can be rearranged, and allow them to make changes and add appropriate bed linens.

Where on the Ship?

The better and higher-priced cabins are generally on the upper decks, because these afford better views and larger windows or even verandas. The lower down in the ship, the smaller the windows or portholes, and the greater the chance you will feel vibrations or hear noise from the engines and other machinery.

On some older vessels, elevators do not reach all the way to the lower levels, requiring use of stairs for the final approach.

Cabins at the front of the ship may have an angular outer wall because of the shape of the bow. More importantly, these cabins may be noisier during the time when the ship is departing or arriving in a port because of the location of the anchor chain or docking ropes.

Cabins at the stern, especially those on low decks, may be more susceptible to engine noises and heat.

An outside cabin offers views, light, and sometimes air. Watch out for obstructed views—usually lifeboats or docking winches on the outside decks.

The middle of the ship is usually less likely to carry engine noise and vibration. And cabins amidship (the middle of the ship in nautical terms) are affected less by the up and down pitching of the ship.

Avoid rooms that are located near nightclubs, lobbies, elevators, and other locations likely to have late-night noise.

Left or Right?

You might also want to pay attention to whether your room is on the port (left) or starboard (right) side of the vessel. Depending on the direction of the travel, only one side of the ship will be facing the sunrise or sunset, or will receive direct sunlight during the course of the day. Just as on land, the southern exposure receives more sun than east, west, and especially northern exposures. If your vessel is heading west, the port side faces south; heading east, the starboard side will receive more sun.

According to some maritime historians, the preference for location on the ship is the source of the term "posh." British travelers heading out on grand expeditions on P&O ships to India and Asia would specify "port outbound, starboard home" to seek shelter from the sun.

Some travelers also pay attention to the orientation of their beds in relation to the ship. If the berths are parallel with the sides of the vessel, your head and feet will rise and fall with the pitch of the ship; if the berths lie across the stern, your head and feet will rise and fall with the ship's roll.

Which is better? Beats me. I sleep like a bobbing log either way.

Your Floor, Please?

One way to think of a cruise ship is as a skyscraper lying on its side. The "floors" of the ship—known as decks in marine parlance—run down the length of the ship and are stacked from the keel to the topmost sun deck.

The lowest level decks are used for the ship's mechanical rooms, including the engines, fuel tanks, saltwater desalination machinery and freshwater storage, and some of the refrigerators, freezers, and larders for the galley. The lowest decks are below the water level and there are no windows. It's a dark, sometimes noisy, underworld.

On a ship of any significant size, the next few decks are given over to the galley or food preparation areas as well as cabins for most of the crew. On many ships, the lower decks may also be the home of a movie theater or showroom where the absence of windows is not a problem.

The restaurant deck or a combined stateroom and restaurant level is typically three or four decks up from the bottom. On many modern ships, the dining room is at the stern, allowing a wall of windows.

The main deck is the central deck of the ship, usually the home of the purser's office and the reception desk. On many ships, this is the level where you will board the ship at the port of embarkation.

On many ships, a level is denoted as the boat deck, because that is the location of the boarding areas for most or all of the lifeboats. Some modern ships hang their lifeboats way up high to avoid blocking the views from staterooms. The lifeboats would be lowered to a boarding platform if needed.

The promenade deck offers an open or enclosed walkway down one or both sides of the ship. An open walkway is pleasant for strolls or power walks in good weather, although high winds or rain can make the promenade disagreeable. On older vessels the promenade deck was often up high, between the main deck and boat deck; on more modern ships the promenade deck may be the same as the boat deck. On some ships the promenade has been shortened at the bow or stern or both by placement of luxury suites; walkers will have to reverse course for longer walks.

Cabin Locations to Avoid

Here are locations on the ship to avoid:

1. Near the disco, or near the gathering place for a public area such as the theater or dining room.

2. Below the jogging track or the exercise room.

3. All things being equal, the quietest rooms are amidships (the middle of the vessel), away from the propeller at the stern, and the anchor and winch mechanisms at the bow and stern. The midship area may also be less susceptible to roll and pitch.

4. Read the plan carefully to understand whether an available room has a veranda, a full window, or a large or small porthole. (Inside cabins, of course, have no windows or portholes.) Then check to see if the view out the window is obstructed by a lifeboat. Note that some "outside" cabins may lie across from an open promenade instead of being directly over the water. It's still a view, but you may have less privacy than you'd like.

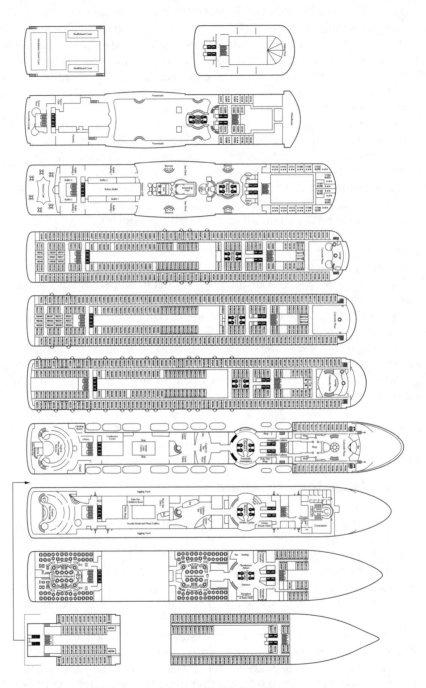

The deck plan for the CostaVictoria, *a modern 76,000-ton megaship that has 964 cabins, nine decks, and an Econoguide rating of ★★★★★*
Courtesy of Costa Cruises

Chapter 6
Expenses Onboard the Ship

One of the appeals of a cruise vacation is the fact that your fare includes all expenses: There are no separate charges for transportation, meals, a hotel room, and entertainment.

Does that mean you can leave your wallet behind? No way.

There are many, many ways to spend money aboard ship and in ports of call. That doesn't mean you have to run up a bill, but let me count some of the ways you can:

Alcoholic Drinks and Soda
Shore Excursions
Ship-to-Shore Telephones
Ship's Photographer
Gift Shops
Art Auctions and Galleries
Health Spa and Beauty Salon
Sports Afloat
Babysitting and Medical Services
Gratuities
Port Charges
Floating Craps Games and Slot Machines
The Bingo Parlor

The truth is, most cruise lines realize a great deal of their profit from shipboard activities. You can run from their entreaties, but I'm afraid you can't completely hide.

Alcoholic Drinks and Soda

On most cruise ships, you'll have to pay for drinks from the bar as well as wine at the table or drinks in your room. You can expect to find waiters hovering over you any time you sit down by the pool, in one of the lounges, and at your dining table. You may also find waiters standing by with a tray of welcome-aboard concoctions as your ship prepares to depart the terminal.

On all but the topmost ranks of cruise ships, the drinks are on you.

But it's perfectly fine to just say no. You also don't have to order a drink to visit any part of the ship, including lounges and showrooms.

The waiters quickly learn to distinguish their best customers from those who don't indulge. By the end of a weeklong cruise you may find you'll have to wave very insistently at a waiter to order a farewell drink if they're not used to standing by.

As with most other expenses onboard ship, if you do order a drink, you'll likely be asked to sign a receipt and the charge will appear on your final bill for the trip.

Drink prices onboard ship are usually comparably priced with what you'll find in an upscale bar on land, approximately $3 to $5 for most selections. Most cruise lines feature a drink of the day at a reduced price; you'll often find the specialty listed in the daily onboard newsletter.

Watch out, too, for bottles of water, soda, or wine on the dresser in your room or in a mini-bar in some cabins. Find out from your cabin attendant whether there is a charge for opening one of the bottles—there usually is.

Here are some ways to save: First of all, juice, ice tea, and water are free, usually available in cafes and lounges onboard.

Most ships have rules against guests bringing their own alcohol aboard. Just between you and me: I have been known to bring a few bottles of wine from home or from a shoreside liquor store, keeping the bottle discreetly out of sight in a drawer or a closet. I can't imagine that a room steward is going to risk a gratuity by turning me in to the purser.

Speaking for myself, I can accept the exclusion of alcohol—I don't want to subsidize someone else's binges—but I do think that paying for soda is a bit of an imposition, especially when I travel with my kids. They are, alas, used to traveling by airplane where the soda flows free and freely. On a weeklong cruise, it's easy to run up a bill of $50 per kid for a few $2.50 Cokes a day. (A few lines, including Disney, offer all-you-can-drink soda cards for kids.)

If you want to be really tight—and I'm willing to include myself in that category when appropriate—bring a few six-packs of soda in your luggage or buy them from a store in port, and keep them cool with a free bucket of ice or the refrigerator found in some cabins.

Shore Excursions

Within hours of departure at the start of a cruise, you can expect to hear the persistent drumbeats of the shore excursion staff. You'll be invited to a meeting where you will hear about the wondrous excitement of a guided tour to Mayan ruins or the Alaskan bush or a Hawaiian volcano.

And the shore excursion host or hostess may tell you, in a hushed, conspiratorial tone, about the fabulous bargains available at a particular shop in an upcoming port. The deals get even better, you're told, if you flash your cabin key or wear a cruise line sticker.

In a phrase: *Caveat emptor . . . let the buyer beware.* Though the shore excursions offered by most cruise ships may well be worthy of your time, they are almost always significantly marked up in price. And the stores touted by the staff are often advertised for a reason—they may pay the cruise line to be included in the excursion spiel or in some way make the ship or the cruise director's staff happy for delivering a boatload of tourists.

One advantage of booking a tour through the shore excursion desk is that the cruise line will then know where a group of its passengers are for the day, and will generally promise to hold the ship if an excursion is delayed.

Be aware that in most ports, operators of excursions have booths on shore offering tours. These may be the same companies and same tours sold by the cruise line, or they may be similar trips offered by independent operators. If you haven't made arrangements in advance, be one of the first passengers off your ship when it docks and look for the booths; ask for a discount.

My recommendation for shore expeditions: Research the ports of call before you set out on your cruise.

Buy a good travel book and learn about the best sights to see, and the recommended shops as laid out by a writer who has no vested interest in anyone but you.

Make a few phone calls to the visitors bureaus for the ports before you travel, and ask about places to go on your own. The Internet is a wonderful source of information, with many visitors bureaus maintaining web pages with links to individual tour operators.

Some cruise lines will send you a brochure of shore excursions a few weeks before you leave for your trip to the port, to whet your appetite for their offerings. I use that brochure as the basis for my own research.

One word of warning: In some cases, a major cruise line may have locked up a particular excursion for its passengers, booking the only floatplane, for example, or arranging for the best seats at a particular show or event.

But before you pay top dollar in the face of that sort of argument, make that phone call and see what you can arrange for yourself. In my experience, there's almost always something you can do for yourself.

I consulted some web pages and made a few phone calls before I embarked on an Alaskan cruise and found that I could save $50 per person on a seaplane tour of the bush by booking it myself instead of paying the price asked by the shore excursion desk onboard the cruise.

Here are further savings opportunities:

• A submarine voyage to the floor of the harbor in several Hawaiian ports is $20 to $30 cheaper when you buy a ticket onshore instead of from the excursion desk onboard the ship.

• You should be able to negotiate a better price for a private guided tour by taxi, Jeep, or limousine by contacting ahead of time tourist agencies in the ports you will visit. Split the fare with someone else you meet on board the ship to save even more.

• Floatplanes for visits to the Alaskan bush—an experience I recommend very highly—can be reserved ahead of time by calling directly to operators or by calling tourism agencies in the ports. The same goes for helicopter trips to the volcanoes of Hawaii.

Too good to be true.
In some locations you'll also see booths touting "free" or deeply discounted tours with deals that seem too good to be true. In many cases, that's exactly what they are. These are come-ons for timeshare vacation offers, and the price for the free helicopter tour or luau or submarine trip is that you'll have to sit through several hours of a high-pressure sales presentation.

First, a real estate or timeshare presentation is not a very good use of your precious shore time; you may not have enough time for the sales pitch *and* the "free" excursion, anyhow. Secondly, in my opinion, timeshares are not a good investment nor a rational way to plan future vacations.

And finally, these presentations can be pretty high-pressure. Just say no.

- If you are planning to make a shopping expedition to a specific store and are reasonably certain you will be making a purchase there, why not call ahead to the store and make an appointment to come in? You can hope for more personalized attention, and the shop may even arrange to pick you up at the dock.
- You can often catch a water taxi to a Caribbean beach at a much lower price than you'd pay to take a party boat.
- When it comes to bus tours to tourist attractions and natural wonders: I figure that if the bus can drive there, so can I.
- And it is almost always much more satisfying to rent a car in port and drive wherever you want, whenever, and with whomever; sometimes it's even considerably less expensive. You can set your own itinerary, and stop at any shop or attraction. And best of all, at least for me: You're not a sardine on a bus.

Start out by calling major car rental agencies. You'll generally find rental companies at airports of most any size, and in many important towns and cities. Bear in mind, the port where your ship may dock or drop anchor may be some distance away from an airport. Call directly to a rental counter to arrange for shuttle service. If the car company wants to charge for a pickup and delivery, try another agency.

You should be able to save $20 or more per day on a car rental in port if you make a few phone calls to rental agencies ahead of time instead of relying on the excursion desk to make arrangements for you.

Car rental rates in obscure locations may be slightly higher than you would find at home, and gasoline rates are almost certainly more expensive on distant islands and ports. But I have yet to see a case where renting a car is not less expensive or comparable in price to a prepackaged tour for two to four travelers.

Check with your insurance agent about your liability and collision coverage, and make sure you make the agent aware of your itinerary if it includes a stop in a foreign country.

Some insurance companies will not extend coverage to you for rental of four-wheel-drive, off-road vehicles. And in any case, you probably should not use your vacation as the place to learn to drive off-road.

Be aware, too, that islands with a British heritage, including a number of ports in the Caribbean, put cars on the left side of the road. For some drivers, the changeover to the "wrong" side of the road is a simple adjustment; for others, it is an exercise in terror.

Finally, a word of warning about going it alone on shore. When you do so, you assume the responsibility for getting back to your ship before it leaves port at the end of the day. If you drive too far away from port, your car suffers a flat tire, your fishing expedition makes a wrong turn, or you simply make a mistake in your own planning, you could end up with the extra expense of catching up with your ship at its next stop.

If you're driving, discuss local road conditions and travel times with the rental company and carry a good map. Ask about how they handle breakdowns and bring with you the phone number for the local office, *not* the toll-free number for reservations. And plan your trip to give yourself at least an hour's cushion at the end of the day.

If you're taking a tour, make sure the operator knows when you need to be back onboard the ship. Again, leave yourself an extra cushion of time.

Ship-to-Shore Telephones

One of the reasons to travel by cruise ship is to cut the cord to the "real world." But, alas, there is always the tug to stay in touch with the family and the office. In today's world of cellular and digital communication, it is relatively easy to make phone calls as you travel. You will, though, have to pay a premium rate to use the ship's long distance services.

Until fairly recently, communications from a ship were exclusively by radio. The ship's radio officer could patch a cabin telephone or a phone on the bridge into a radio signal to shore where it could be tied into a land-based telephone system. You may still find radio-based telephone service on some older vessels. Typical charges range from $10 to $15 per minute.

The state-of-the-art in shipboard telecommunications, though, is the satellite phone. On most ships, passengers can place calls from their cabins directly to a phone located anywhere on the planet. Typical charges range from about $6 to $10 per minute.

One or the other telephone system will work quite well in the most popular cruising areas, including the Caribbean. However, there are still places where even satellites don't cover.

On one cruise I found myself at Fanning Island, which lies just above the equator, nearly 2,000 miles west of South America and 1,000 miles south of Hawaii. The standard satellite links for the ship, including telephone and television, were useless in the vast emptiness of that part of the South Pacific. I was able, though, to visit the radio officer on the bridge and place a call that bounced off a satellite somewhere over Japan and then back to my home in Massachusetts; I've got the bill to prove it.

Here are some ways to save on phone calls:

• Make your phone calls from land at ports of call. Use a telephone credit card with a reasonable per-minute charge. If you are going to be calling to or from a foreign country, call your long distance credit card provider before you set out on your cruise and inquire about the most economical way to place the call.

• Make your phone calls from the ship as short as possible. Pre-arrange with family or the office to set a particular time for your call—you don't want to be put on hold at $15 per minute—and keep the calls businesslike. You can always discuss the weather when you return.

• If you have a cellular or digital phone with a reasonable roaming charge, or no roaming charge (my preference), check with your provider to find out the coverage you can expect when you travel. Don't plan on making cell phone calls from the middle of the Atlantic or from a remote Pacific island. You may, though, be able to place and receive calls if your ship is passing just off shore from a major city or when it is in port.

• Look into computer e-mail services available from your ship, a service being offered by a number of cruise lines. You will be able to send and receive messages to family, friends, and your office—provided they have e-mail accounts—typically for a small fraction of telephone costs.

Ship's Photographer

On some cruise lines they'll be on you like flies on jam: The ship's photographers will be happy to document your every moment on film. They'll be there as you come onboard for the first time; they'll be there at the Captain's Welcome Aboard Dinner; and they'll be there at most every onboard activity.

If you'd like to come home from your trip with pictures to prove you've really been on a cruise, or to show yourself stuffed into a tuxedo and cummerbund or a cocktail dress at the Captain's Dinner, the photographers will be happy to oblige.

On some of the most spectacular of the Megaships and Colossuses, you'll even find a state-of-the-art "blue screen" studio where a bit of electronic magic can place you against most any backdrop. Didn't quite make it to the lip of the volcano? Who's to know? Even stranger: How about a picture of you in front of an Alaskan glacier, taken onboard your Caribbean cruise?

Photographs are not cheap—on most ships a 5 x 7 picture costs $5 to $10. Multiple copies of the same picture should be priced at a lower rate; ask for a discount if one is not offered. Formal studio portraits cost more.

There is no obligation that you make a purchase. If you don't like the picture, don't buy it. And there is nothing wrong with waving off the photographer if you're not interested in posing; tell them to save their film for someone else. As with waiters in the bars, by a few days into the cruise, the ship's photographers will have a pretty good idea of which passengers were going to be their customers and which ones would be a waste of film.

On many cruises you can also sit for a formal family portrait in a studio setting; in this instance there may be an obligation to make a purchase. Be sure you understand the terms before saying "Cheese."

One deal you might want to consider: On the most modern of ships you can arrange to have your own film developed and printed and delivered to you within a day or so. Compare the prices to what you would pay on shore and add in the convenience and amazement factor: You can show off your pictures on the plane ride home.

Gift Shops

You can find just about anything you'd care to spend money on in a shipboard gift shop. That's not to say that you should.

Typical items include costume jewelry, cruise clothing, pharmaceuticals, cosmetics, liquor, perfume, and all manner of souvenirs. The shops seem to be constantly offering some sort of a "once in a lifetime" sale.

My opinion, since you asked, is that you should consider these shops as emergency resources, kind of a floating 7-Eleven for things you need in a hurry and can't wait to purchase in the next port of call.

The shops may be of value if you are unexpectedly invited to sit at the Captain's Table and your most formal outfit is a T-shirt that proclaims, "I'm with stupid." Many shops sell or rent formal wear, albeit at premium prices.

Another reason to visit the ship's gift shop is if you absolutely must own a T-shirt or a jacket emblazoned with the name of the ship or cruise line.

Remember that on most ships, you can obtain free aspirin, Band-Aids, shampoo, and other sundries from your cabin attendant or from the purser's office. You should also be able to obtain seasickness pills and aspirin from the office of the ship's doctor.

Art Auctions and Galleries

We all know the official slogan of the amateur art collector: "I don't know much about art, but I know what I like."

That's all very well and good, but do you also know how much the art you like is worth? On some cruise lines, especially those in the mid- to upper-price range, you'll find an onboard art gallery or auction.

On one cruise I took, an earnest young man was passing himself off as an expert in "fine art" and conducting several auctions of paintings and sculptures that he declared at various times to be priced at either "80 percent off retail" or "80 percent of retail." There's a huge difference between those two discounts, and even more scary is the fact that I have absolutely no idea what the true "retail" price for a piece of art should be.

The auctions he conducted were also not pure exercises in capitalism. The seller had a reserve price—a minimum price—for each piece and though the bidding might start low, the painting or sculpture was not going anywhere until someone offered at least that minimum amount.

So, is an onboard art auction a fraud? I have absolutely no idea, because as I said I have no idea of the true value of the items.

My advice: If you know the value of art, go forth and drink the free champagne and hunt for a bargain. If you don't know the value of art, but find something you really like, decide for yourself what the item is worth to *you* and see if you can buy it for that price.

But don't try to make an "investment" in art unless you do know the value of the items for sale.

Oh, and be sure you understand any shipping costs, duties, and other charges that might be assessed on your purchase before you make a bid.

Health Spa and Beauty Salon

If the rockabye motion of the ocean, lying by the pool, and the overall cruise experience are not quite relaxing enough, or you feel the urge to beautify yourself or undertake a new course of exercise, most ships offer an onboard Health Spa that is fully prepared to coddle you in luxury. The spa is also ready to give your credit card a serious workout.

Basic facilities include beauty parlors and barbers to manicures, massage rooms, saunas, and steam rooms. But on many ships, that's just the starting point. On a typical voyage you might find offerings such as a full body massage with aromatic oils and therapeutic heat for about $90, a reflexology consultation and analysis for about $70, and something called an onithermie superdetoxification treatment for about $120.

That last is described as a regime in which lotions rich in kelp, ivy, and seaweed are placed on the body and covered with a blue clay and then excited with electrodes. The treatment is supposed to reduce cellulite and remove toxins in the body that contribute to cellulite and reduce energy.

Sports Afloat

Swimming in the pool, working out in the gym, playing basketball on the sun deck or shuffleboard alongside the pool, hiking around the promenade deck, and repeated trips to and from the buffet line are all included in your fare.

But you'll also find some additional sports facilities that are offered at an extra cost. These include:

• **Golf.** The offerings here include driving ranges and golf simulators that allow you to step up to the tee with a real club and drive a ball into a screen that carries the image of a famous fairway. On some cruises, you'll also find a PGA-certified instructor who can help you with your game. Some of the golf programs are tied into shore excursions to courses in ports of call.

• **Water sports.** In warm waters, you may be able to rent snorkel or scuba diving equipment, sailboats, or arrange for water skiing and other activities in port. (You'll need to be certified to use scuba devices; some cruises can arrange for the training onboard the ship.)

• **Skeet shooting.** This holdover from the glory days of the transatlantic liner is available on a few ships. The modernized version uses biodegradeable targets and quieter guns.

Some of the smaller, luxury ships make their advanced sports part of the basic package. For example, the *Radisson Diamond* includes a marina at the stern used to launch watercraft available to all guests in certain ports.

Babysitting and Medical Services

Many cruise lines offer free activities for children. You'll likely have to pay for private babysitting in your room, or for special group babysitting activities.

You'll also have to pay for video arcades. Some companies, including

Disney Cruise Line, make it very easy to run up a bill. Kids (if you give the cruise line permission) have their own credit card they can use to purchase arcade time, as well as soda and gifts from the stores.

In Chapter 7, I also discuss how medical services on ship are your own responsibility, and not often covered by your basic medical insurance policy.

Gratuities

Like it or not, nearly all the service staff onboard most cruise ships receive very little in the way of salary, sometimes the equivalent of only a few dollars a day. They make their income from gratuities offered by guests.

There is no requirement you give a tip; but the fact is, this is considered part of today's cruise environment.

Most cruise lines will helpfully provide passengers with a "suggested" schedule of tips. On most ships, the amount ranges from $7.50 to $12 per person per day.

Here's a typical breakdown:

Cabin attendant	$3.50 per person per day
Waiter	$3.50 per person per day
Busboy	$1.50 per person per day

It may also be recommended you tip the head waiter and/or maitre d' another $1.50 per person per day. Those tips are truly voluntary. If the managers of the restaurant have performed some especially notable service to you, go ahead and remember them with a gratuity. If not, take solace in the fact that the managers are paid a reasonable salary while the cabin attendants and waiters are not.

(Want some scary math? Multiply 1,000 passengers times $1.50 per day for the head waiter and maitre d' and ask yourself if you're in the wrong business.)

Drinks from the bar and many other special services—such as the health spa and special-order room service deliveries—will typically have a 15 percent tip added to the bill.

As I have noted earlier, on many ships you can charge the gratuities to your shipboard account and hand your servers a card indicating that. You can also give cash.

The traditional time to extend gratuities is at the final dinner before disembarkation. You can expect all of the service staff to be especially attentive to your needs that evening.

There are a handful of cruise lines that charge their passengers enough of a premium to allow a "No Tipping Permitted" or a "No Tipping Required" policy. Among lines that say tipping is not required are Cunard, Holland America Line, Radisson, and Windstar.

The lines that completely prohibit tipping include Seabourn and Silversea.

Port Charges

Many cruise lines advertise their rates without including port charges and fees. These can easily add $100 or more to each ticket. Be sure you know whether these fees are included in the price of your cruise.

Floating Craps Games and Slot Machines

If you want to gamble, many cruise ship companies are perfectly happy to take your money. Onboard casinos range from a few slot machines in a bar to glitzy miniatures of Las Vegas.

You won't find casinos on many smaller ships and adventure cruises; the Disney Cruise Line decided to forgo gambling on its family-oriented vessels.

In most cases, the casinos do not operate when the ship is in port.

Let's get a few things straight right away: First of all, the fancy casino onboard your ship, just like the fabulous resorts of Las Vegas, Reno, Lake Tahoe, Laughlin, and everywhere in between was not built as entertainment but as a place of business. That business is the extraction of cash from your wallet or purse.

Secondly, the success of that business is based on the fact that nearly every visitor can be counted on to *lose* money at gambling tables and slot machines. Some will lose more than others, and a few will even come away with an occasional small or large or huge win; but always remember that the pockets of the casino operators are lined with the money left behind by the losers.

And third, if you are a serious gambler, shipboard casinos may not be the best place to invest your capital. Passengers on a ship are a captive audience.

I'm not going to offer lessons on gambling here. If you're going to bet serious money, I'd suggest you buy a book or two about gambling.

I will, though, offer my Three Econoguide Rules of Gambling:

• **Rule Number One of Gambling.** Don't bet more than you can afford to lose.

• **Corollary to Rule Number One of Gambling.** Don't bring with you to the table (or with you onboard the ship) more money than you can afford to lose.

• **Second Corollary to Rule Number One of Gambling.** Don't beg, borrow, or steal more money than you can afford to lose. The casinos will make it very easy for you to tap into credit cards or savings accounts, and they may even offer unsecured loans. Whatever the source, it will still be a debt and probably will include an unpleasant interest rate.

Slot Machines

At one time, the conventional wisdom may have been that table games—from roulette to 21 to baccarat—were where the real action was at a casino. The slot machines were looked down upon as the province of the low roller.

Today, the average bet in a casino is still considerably higher at the tables, but don't believe for a moment that casinos look down on slot machines as being less interesting than the table games. At most casinos, slots deliver about half the revenues. That percentage is even higher on most cruise ships.

Here's the rap on slots: They are dumb, require no skill, and provide no human interaction. They are pure exercises in luck, and like other casino bets, they ask the player to put aside the knowledge that the casino is almost sure to win over time. They don't call them "one-armed bandits" for nothing.

The odds against winning are based on the number of reels (rolling sets of symbols), the number of symbols on each reel, and the computer settings made by the casino operator. The highest payoff five-reel machines may work out to a chance of something like 1 in 3.2 million pulls for the jackpot.

Most slot machines pay better jackpots to bettors who play the maximum number of coins on a pull. So, if you are willing to bet about $1 per pull, you generally would be better off at a quarter machine putting in five coins at a time ($1.25 per pull) than putting in a single dollar token at a dollar machine.

Video Poker

Video poker machines are very popular, offering the chances for a bit of reward to players who have a bit of skill. There are dozens of different formats, but most of them come down to versions of Stud Poker. The machine will deal you five cards and you can choose to hold any or all of them or draw from one to five new cards. After the second round of cards, the hand is evaluated and winning hands are paid off.

Most machines pay off only on a pair of jacks or better. In addition, the relative payoffs are much higher for the best hands. Therefore, professional video poker players generally recommend throwing away any low hands and always making a play for the high-payoff hands. For example, in standard poker you would almost never draw to an inside straight (seeking to fill out a straight with a gap in the middle, as in 9-10-Q-K), but in video poker it might be worth a chance.

The Roulette Wheel

Round and round she goes, where she stops nobody knows. Some historians track the roulette wheel back to the ancient Chinese or Tibetans of 1,000 years ago; the famous French scientist and mathematician Blaise Pascal is credited with adapting the wheel to a casino game in 1655.

Of the four major table games (roulette, craps, blackjack, and baccarat), roulette offers the poorest odds to the player.

It is, though, one of the simplest of games to play. In the standard game as played in Nevada and onboard most ships, the wheel is divided into alternating red and black compartments that are numbered from 1 to 36; in addition, one compartment is numbered 0 and another 00. A player can bet on any of the 38 numbers directly, and is paid off at 35:1. (Here is the House Advantage presented about as clearly as possible: there is a 1 in 38 chance of a particular number coming up, and the winning payoff is 35:1.

The 0 and 00 are excluded from the payoffs on red/black, odd/even, columns, or rows. In other words, the casino wins all bets on color, odd/even, or groups of numbers if 0 or 00 comes up.

The American game with the 0 and 00 numbers added to the layout gives the house a 5.26 percent advantage on most bets; the worst gamble for the player is the five-number bet, which gives the house an advantage of more than 7 percent.

Blackjack (21)

Blackjack, also known as 21, is one of the more popular casino games and—on one level—one of the easiest to play. All you have to do is request cards from the dealer, one at a time, until you get as close to a card value of 21 as you can. If you get closer to 21 than the dealer, you win; if you go over 21 or if the dealer is closer to that magic number, you lose. If you and the dealer tie, your bet is returned to you.

Betting is relatively simple, too. You are always betting against the dealer that your card value will be better than the dealer's.

But, as I've said, although blackjack is easy to play, it is not easy to win. It is, though, one of the few games at the casino that can be consistently beaten, or at least fought to a draw, by a well-educated and careful player.

A player who understands the basic strategy and bets conservatively can expect to win about 1 percent of total action over the course of time, which doesn't sound like much but can quickly mount up into serious money. Players who can count cards and adjust the levels of betting and strategies based on the current condition of the deck can expect to win much more.

The line between winning and losing is always slim, and the casino always stands to benefit from a mistake by the player.

Watch the players at the table, or ask the dealer about the protocol for indicating whether you want to hit or stand. Some casinos are more picky than others about hand signs used at the table. In most casinos, you indicate you want another card by scratching your current cards toward you on the felt or by waving at the dealer with a "come to me" gesture. (Looser dealers will permit you to nod your head "yes" or perform some other positive signal.) To indicate you want to stand, you can slip your cards, face down, under your bet or give some sort of a "wave off" signal.

The reason casinos are sometimes picky about the signals used is they don't want a bettor to ask for his money back on a losing bet because of any ambiguity about betting intentions.

Other casino protocol: Handle the cards with one hand only; don't take the cards off the table, and don't touch your bet once cards have been dealt. If you are busted, turn over all your cards and watch the dealer take away your bet.

Craps: A Flurry of Action

Craps is one of the more exciting games at the casino, one where the players and even the various casino employees are encouraged to yell, shout, and otherwise encourage the little cubes of plastic to come up properly.

The thrower (called the shooter) makes a money bet, covered by one or more opponents. The shooter throws the two dice against the far wall of the craps table. (This is an important rule of the casino; the boxman or pit boss may halt the game if they don't feel you are throwing the dice with enough force to ensure an honest tumble.) If the first throw totals 7 or 11, the player wins; but if 2, 3, or 12 is thrown, the player loses. In any of these cases, betting and throwing are repeated.

If the throw totals 4, 5, 6, 8, 9, or 10, that number becomes the player's point, and throwing is continued until the same point is made again or a 7 is thrown. If the point is made, the player wins, but if a 7 is thrown, the player loses both the bet and the right to throw again.

Even more complex is the betting protocol for craps. If you're going to be risking your capital at the craps table, pick up a specialized book on gaming or ask the casino management for a lesson.

The Bingo Parlor

Your grandma may not refer to Bingo as gambling, but that's what it is, and on many ships this is where you'll find the big action.

Every ship has its own prices and special promotions, but in general, Bingo is Bingo. You'll find traditional games where the goal is to fill in a straight or diagonal line as well as "coverall" versions where the winner must fill in all the numbers to win.

There are basic prizes of $25 to $100 per game, and there are jackpot and progressive rounds where the prize rises with each unsuccessful game until one player takes home a large payment.

And then there are lotteries intended to keep you coming back for more Bingo games. One of the better payouts was onboard a Norwegian Cruise Line voyage; near the end of the trip, one player was awarded a free cruise for two passengers of up to two weeks on any NCL ship.

Bingo cards typically cost several dollars per game. Less expensive cards and two-fer promotions are offered on most cruises, too, although the prize payout for lower-priced cards is usually concomitantly lower.

Don't look to finance your kids' college education, or even your next cruise vacation on the basis of your Bingo winnings. The careful player performs a rough calculation of the odds of winning based on the number of players, and then looks at the price to play and the possible prize. If you go to all of that trouble, you'll probably decide the game is a pretty poor bet. Instead, if you think of an hour of Bingo as fun, pay the price as entertainment.

A Cashless Society

On most cruise ships, cash is not expected or not accepted. Instead, you'll be asked to establish a credit account with the purser's office when you board. From that point on, you'll be able to sign for all expenses onboard the ship.

Some ships issue a magnetically encoded charge card for use aboard. Others give you a printed card with your name and cabin number on it, while on some cruises all you need to do is announce your stateroom number.

(On the most modern of ships, your cabin key is also your personal credit card as well as your embarkation and disembarkation pass.)

On many ships you can also charge gratuities to your charge account. You should receive a receipt for the tips and a card to give to your room attendant, waiter, and busboy to inform them you have paid for a tip that should be credited to their account.

On some ships you will receive a preliminary accounting of your bill a few

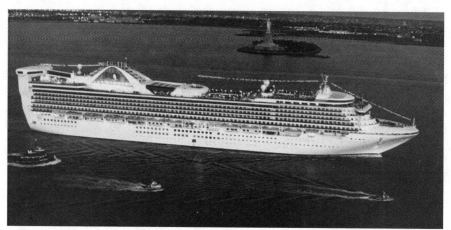

The Grand Princess *arrives in New York*
Princess Cruises

days before the end of the trip; take the time then to check over the statement and bring any errors to the attention of the purser's office.

You'll receive a final itemized bill early on the morning of disembarkation. If the bill is correct, on most ships you're set to leave; on some ships you'll have to visit the purser's office to check out.

If there are errors on the bill, head for the purser early. It is not unheard of for someone else's charges to be applied to your account, or for accidental double billing. Stand your ground and politely demand that the purser show you the signed receipts for all of the charges posted to your account.

If you do not have a credit card or choose not to use one, you will likely be asked to make a cash deposit to open an account.

On most ships, the one place where the onboard charge card is not valid is at the casino. Here they expect visitors to use (and lose) cash or travelers checks. You can, though, arrange for a separate line of credit with the casino manager. And some shipboard casinos also have credit card cash-advance ATMs, a convenience I find fiscally appalling.

Chapter 7
Safety at Sea

No one who reads this book hasn't heard of the *Titanic*, and there are precious few cruise goers who don't make nervous jokes about the famous marine disaster when they put on their life vests for lifeboat drills.

Safety at sea is not a joking matter. In a real disaster, passengers and crew can find themselves with nowhere to go but into the water—hundreds or even thousands of miles away from the security of dry land and shelter.

In 1999, there were about ten significant accidents involving cruise ships: one liner sank off Malaysia, a classic 83-year-old tall ship was blown from her moorage and lost at sea in a hurricane in the Caribbean, another lost power in the Gulf of Mexico as a tropical storm bore down on her, three small vessels ran aground in Alaska, one megaship on her maiden voyage washed up on the rocks in the St. Lawrence River, and another large cruise ship had a middle-of-the-night collision with a freighter in the English Channel. That sounds scary, but consider this: in all of these accidents, not a single person was killed, and only a handful of injuries were sustained.

Today, the biggest fear is not striking an iceberg in the North Atlantic. Radar, satellite navigation systems, and improved construction have pretty much solved that problem. Instead, the real threats to travelers are fire at sea, contagious diseases, or contaminated food.

Modern Safety: After the *Titanic*

For the record: the "unsinkable" RMS *Titanic* struck a glancing blow against a large iceberg some 400 miles from Newfoundland in the cold North Atlantic on April 14, 1912 at 11:40 P.M. The ship sank two hours and 40 minutes later.

Although the ship went down quickly, that would still seem to be more than enough time to evacuate the 2,200 passengers and crew. However, the designers of the *Titanic* trusted too much in the promises of technology; the supposedly unsinkable ship did not have enough seats in the lifeboats for all aboard, and the lifeboats themselves were not designed well enough to overcome the severe list of the sinking ship. Only about 700 survived.

SOLAS: The Legacy of the *Titanic*

From the *Titanic* disaster, though, came one positive development: the convening in 1914 of the first International Convention for the Safety of Life at Sea, which became known by its comforting acronym, SOLAS. The agreement among shipping nations has been updated and expanded several times since.

Today, most of the world's nearly 140 seagoing nations are parties to the agreement. The countries that subscribe promise to apply the regulations of SOLAS to any ships that fly their flag. (Panama, The Bahamas, and Liberia, common "flags of convenience" for cruise lines, are signatories.)

In North American waters, the cruise industry cooperates with the U.S. Coast Guard, which inspects all foreign-flag vessels operating from North American ports and issues certification that is required before U.S. passengers can embark. Coast Guard certification also includes quarterly lifeboat and firefighting inspections.

The original SOLAS convention set rules that ships have enough lifeboat seats for every person aboard and also required there be a lifeboat drill on each voyage. And ships were required to staff their radio rooms at all times.

The SOLAS regulations have been improved over the years. Modern ships now must have partially or totally enclosed lifeboats.

In recent years, much attention has been shifted to fire safety at sea. Nearly all older vessels are now under orders to be refitted to add fire sprinklers and automatic controls of fire doors.

Save Our Ship!

With the advent of satellite navigation, improved radar and radio systems, and computers, the chances of collisions between ships or accidents involving obstacles in the water has become more and more remote. This is especially true for modern cruise ships. The owners of your basic $300 million megaship that has a few thousand vacationers aboard have what lawyers would call a huge liability exposure; most cruise lines are extremely conservative in their operations. That doesn't mean, though, that accidents don't happen.

Royal Caribbean's *Monarch of the Seas* struck a rock off the coast of St. Maarten just after midnight on December 15, 1998; three of her 18 watertight compartments began taking on water. Her captain was able to steer the ship back to port where it was intentionally beached on a bed of sand. Meanwhile, all 2,557 passengers were called from their cabins and sent to their muster stations. By 4:15 A.M., all had been evacuated from the ship in tender boats, without injury.

In May of 1999, the 30,000-ton *Sun Vista* suffered a fire in its engine room and all 1,104 passengers and crew were forced to take to lifeboats off the coast of Malaysia in the middle of the night where they watched the ship go down.

In September of the same year, a fire on board Carnival's *Tropicale* disabled its engines, leaving it to drift in the Gulf of Mexico as Tropical Storm Harvey approached it. The ship, with 1,700 passengers and crew aboard, drifted for nearly a day in rough seas before the crew was able to restart one of the engines and move slowly out of the way of the storm and then eventually head back to port in Tampa. Passengers complained of lack of air conditioning, faulty toilets, and other issues of comfort, but there were no injuries.

In the summer of 1999, three small ships had problems in Alaska's Inside Passage. The *Spirit of '98* struck a shoal in Tracy Arm, a narrow fjord that leads to a pair of spectacular glaciers, about 40 miles southeast of Juneau. All 93 passengers were transferred by raft to another ship. Earlier, the *Wilderness Adventurer* ran aground in Glacier Bay National Park, and a sister ship, the *Wilderness Explorer* ran aground in an inlet 70 miles west of Juneau.

In August and September of 1999, Norwegian Cruise Line suffered a pair of costly mishaps. First, the *Norwegian Dream* inexplicably collided with a large freighter in the English Channel; passengers were able to stay onboard as the ship continued to port in England, but the ship was disabled for more than a month for repairs. And then the line's brand new *Norwegian Sky,* on its first official cruise after arriving from the shipyard in Europe, ran aground in the upper St. Lawrence River at the mouth of the Saguenay River in Quebec. Ferries, whale-watching vessels, and private boats were mobilized to help evacuate passengers, but the ship eventually floated free and was brought into Quebec City for repairs to its hull, rudder, and one of its propellers. NCL was forced to cancel the next six weeks of sailings for the much-anticipated ship.

Fire! A Remaining Threat

In 1996, five crewmembers of the *Universe Explorer* were killed in a laundry room fire as the ship sailed near Admiralty Island, west of Juneau, Alaska. Seventy-three passengers were hospitalized, mostly for smoke inhalation.

The ship, built in 1958, had passed its quarterly Coast Guard fire inspection the week before. But it was operating under an exemption from fire regulations that required refitting to install a fire sprinkler system.

As this book went to press, some dozen older ships had been given until the year 2005 to fully comply with fire safety regulations.

Commodore, which owns the *Universe Explorer* and charters her to other operators, refitted the ship during the winter of 1998–99 to add sprinklers and other controls and firefighting equipment.

In the summer of 1998, the decades-younger *Ecstasy* caught fire just off the port of Miami. That blaze, blamed by the cruise company on sparks from welding that was going on even while the ship was at sea, caused significant damage to some of the work areas on the ship. But there were no fatalities; some passengers were treated for smoke inhalation. The ship returned to port and the cruise was canceled.

Hurricanes and Bad Weather

Cruises are rarely canceled because of storms, but the weather can result in a choppy ride, a rerouting that may include cancellation of a port visit or substitution of a destination out of the way of the storm. In some extreme cases the ship may be unable to return to its planned port of debarkation and passengers may have to travel by bus or other conveyance to their intended destination.

All that said, it would take one heck of a storm to threaten a large cruise ship. But cruise companies don't want to risk their customers falling or having a ship full of vacationers too green to come out of their cabins.

Modern weather equipment, including satellite receivers aboard ship, permit captains to outrun a hurricane or steer around massive storms.

In late October of 1998, disaster struck the venerable S.V. *Fantome*, the flagship of the Windjammer fleet. The *Fantome*, a 282-foot-long, four-masted schooner built in 1927, apparently broke up and sank when it was overtaken by Hurricane Mitch off the coast of Honduras.

As the storm approached Central America, the ship was ordered to stop at Belize City to drop off its passengers so they could be flown back to Miami. The ship then headed out to sea with its crew of 31 to avoid the storm, but the hurricane kept changing its path and eventually overtook the ship. The *Fantome's* last radio message said it was experiencing 100-knot winds and the ship was rolling 40 degrees. After more than a week, the search for the ship and its crew was abandoned.

And then in late November of 1999, the cruise world lost another classic when the 83-year-old S.V. *Sir Francis Drake* apparently broke free of her mooring in a hurricane and was swept out to sea and lost. Hurricane Lenny, one of the most severe storms of the twentieth century, parked off the Caribbean island of St. Martin for several days.

The *Sir Francis Drake* was in port at Marigot for repairs on her auxiliary engine. As the storm approached, all passengers and crew were disembarked to shore. The ship was secured with 15 lines and both anchors at a huge commercial-ship mooring buoy in Marigot Harbor. When visibility returned after three days, the ship and another tall ship were gone. An intensive search with private aircraft and ships, aided by U.S. Coast Guard satellite data, was unsuccessful. No trace was found of either vessel, except for a floating life raft, later identified as being from the *Sir Francis Drake*.

The 165-foot-long ship had been built in Germany in 1917 and in recent years had sailed throughout the British Virgin Islands.

See the Cruise Diary in this book for stories of two cruises I took in 1999 that were forced to make changes because of nearby hurricanes.

Doctors Onboard

Cruise ships carrying more than 50 passengers will have a doctor onboard; some smaller luxury ships, especially those that venture to remote corners of the world, also carry a doctor. Most ships also have an infirmary or hospital and nursing staff. Few on-ship facilities are suitable for surgery, though.

That said, there is no guarantee that a ship's doctor will be especially well qualified or that the ship's hospital well-equipped for critical emergencies such as heart attacks. The goals of most medical facilities are to treat any minor illnesses or injuries, and stabilize seriously injured patients until they can be transferred to a full-service hospital. If you have any particular medical concerns, be sure to discuss your travel plans with your own physician and with the cruise line.

Medical services aboard ship are not free; consultation fees and charges must be paid for by passengers. Most health plans, including Medicare, do not cover the costs of medical care at sea and in foreign ports. You might want to consider purchasing supplemental health and emergency evacuation insurance; this coverage may be included as part of a cancellation policy offered by many cruise lines or available separately from the cruise line or through your own insurance agent.

In recent years, some cruise lines have upgraded their medical facilities as ships have grown into small floating cities. As an example, most Holland America Line ships have an infirmary equipped with much of the emergency equipment used in emergency departments, including an X-ray machine, defibrillator, electrocardiogram machine, and an intensive care unit.

The *Grand Princess* includes SeaMed, a telemedicine program that links the ship's medical staff with the Emergency Department physicians and specialists at Cedars-Sinai Medical Center in Los Angeles. This "virtual ER" allows X-rays, electrocardiograms, and other monitoring signals to be transmitted from the ship to the hospital by satellite.

Travelers with Medical Conditions

Most cruise lines will not book passage to a woman in the third trimester of pregnancy. Beyond that, most companies require that passengers must notify the line at the time of booking of any physical or mental illness, disability, or other condition for which special accommodations or the use of a wheelchair may be necessary.

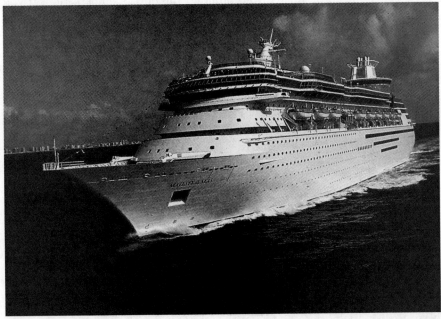

Royal Caribbean's Majesty of the Seas
Royal Caribbean International

Cruise lines reserve the right to refuse passage or terminate a vacation if the ship's doctor determines travel may pose a risk to the passenger or others.

A Pre-Cruise Medical Checklist

There are few of us who don't have a health or diet concern of some sort. Consider the fact that soon after you embark on a cruise you will find yourself hundreds or even thousands of miles away from the nearest full-service pharmacy and potentially in the hands of a doctor and clinic that has no record of your medical history.

Here are some ways to protect yourself; these suggestions are adapted from Holland America's excellent pre-cruise brochure.

1. Gather a supply of all prescription drugs and medications sufficient to cover your trip from home to the port of embarkation, the entire cruise, your return home, plus a few extra days in case of delay. Most major cruise ships have a supply of common medications onboard; but they may not have your precise prescription.

2. Place all medications in a carry-on bag that is not checked on your airplane flight and not given to the stevedores at the cruise port. In other words, carry your medications with you from home to your stateroom.

3. Carry a written list of all medications with the brand names and generic equivalents and the dosage you take. Put the list in a separate place from the carry-on bag with the medications.

4. Bring with you the names and phone numbers of your doctors at home.

5. If you have a medical condition, consult with your doctor about your cruise plans, including flights from home to the port of embarkation. If you have a significant medical condition, bring a copy of your medical records. If you have a heart condition, bring a copy of your most recent EKG.

6. Make sure you or your travel agent convey all special needs to the cruise company before you travel. Inform the company about the need for a wheelchair, oxygen, or other equipment.

7. Consider the purchase of travel insurance to cover cancellations due to medical conditions. If you have a medical condition that is of concern, look for a policy—more expensive, but more valuable—that does not exclude pre-existing conditions from coverage.

8. Consider purchase of supplemental insurance to cover medical expenses at shipboard infirmaries or in foreign ports. This sort of coverage may be included with trip cancellation policies. But again, pay attention to exclusions of pre-existing conditions.

9. If you require a special meal, such as low-sodium, low-cholesterol, low-fat, or other arrangements, be sure to inform the cruise line several weeks in advance of your visit.

Travelers Who Have Disabilities

Although most cruise lines can be counted on to be accommodating to persons with disabilities, the fact of the matter is not all ships are appropriate for persons in wheelchairs or those who have significant medical problems.

To begin with, many older ships were designed before consideration was given to persons with special needs. Only a handful of rooms and few, if any, public restrooms may be accessible to guests in wheelchairs.

And antique ships, such as tall ships and windjammers, do not have elevators and are otherwise difficult for persons with disabilities.

If you do book passage on a ship that claims wheelchair accessibility, be aware that not all areas of the vessel may be served by elevators. And you may also find that some ports of call are not equipped to handle all visitors. You should also be aware that in some ports the cruise ship may not tie up at a dock, instead transferring guests to shore by tender boats, which may not be easily navigated by all guests.

Seasickness

Could there be anything worse than spending thousands of dollars, traveling thousands of miles to a port, setting sail on a fabulous cruise ship—and then finding yourself so awfully seasick you cannot leave your bed?

That's the scary thought that keeps many travelers away from cruises, and causes more than a bit of concern among those who do go down to the sea in ships.

The good news, though, is that modern ships are pretty stable. And there are a number of things you can do, from common sense to common medication that can help you ignore the rolling and pitching of a cruise ship. (Rolling is the side to side motion caused by seas that move across the beam of the ship; pitching is the up and down movement of the ship as the bow rides waves coming at the ship or a following sea that attacks from the stern.)

Modern ships use one or more forms of stabilizers to reduce roll. These devices are like underwater wings that work against the motion of the ship in rough water. The size and length of larger ships goes a long way toward reducing pitch; and sailing ships are relatively less likely to roll because they are held to an angle of heel by the pressure of the wind on the sails.

Here are some things you can do to reduce your chances of seasickness:

• Give some thought to the waters your ship will travel. The Caribbean and the inside passage of Alaska are usually calmer than the waters of the Pacific and the North Atlantic.

• Choose the time of year you cruise. June through late fall is hurricane season along the East Coast and sometimes the Gulf of Mexico. That doesn't mean the seas are always stormy at that time of the year, but on average, one or two hurricanes a year disrupt the cruise calendar.

• Pay attention to the cruise itinerary. Some ships spend one or more days out to sea without making a port call; most cruisegoers relish the calming effects of nothing but ocean. But if you do suffer from occasional seasickness, you might want to seek out an itinerary that allows you to set foot on land every eight or 12 hours or so.

• Select a more stable cabin. Most cruisegoers find that a cabin amidships (in the middle of the ship) and on a lower deck will roll and pitch less than a cabin that is up high and at the stern or bow.

• Reduce your alcohol intake. Alcohol can make you dizzy and disoriented and upset your stomach. Need I say more?

• Consider taking a seasickness medication such as Dramamine or Bonine before the ship gets underway. In my experience, both work quite well, although they may make you drowsy. (Be sure to consult with your physician if you have any other medical conditions that might complicate use of such medication.) Many cruise ships have stocks of seasickness pills available for guests; check with the purser's office or the medical office. Some travelers find relief with the use of accupressure wristbands and other devices.

Epidemics Onboard

Cruise ships are, alas, a near-perfect environment for the transmission and spread of disease. You have passengers gathering from all over the world, then mingling in enclosed dining rooms, theaters, and showrooms. Add to the equation, the large central kitchens and the tons of food that must be stored onboard the ship and prepared for the near-continuous round of meals, snacks, and buffets.

Finally, consider the fact that passengers are visiting remote ports where the sanitation may not be as advanced as onboard ship or at home.

In recent years there have been several outbreaks of diarrhea, influenza, and food poisoning onboard cruise ships.

All that said, most cruise ships visiting American ports do a good job of maintaining proper hygiene, under the watchful eye of the U.S. Centers for Disease Control and Prevention. Every vessel that has 13 or more passengers is subject to inspections at least twice a year by the CDC. The resulting scores are published every two weeks in the Summary of Sanitation Inspections of International Cruise Ships, known in the industry as the Green Sheet.

A ship must receive a score of 86 percent or higher to be acceptable; ships that fail are subject to re-inspections and could eventually be prevented from sailing from a U.S. port if problems are not fixed. The CDC also distributes the list of inspections to travel agents and the press.

You can look at a list of recent inspections of cruise ships on the Internet, at the following address:

www.cdc.gov/nceh/programs/sanit/vsp/scores/scores.htm.

You can also contact the CDC by phone at (888) 232-6789 and request a copy of the most recent Green Sheet, although I was warned that the agency is understaffed and may not be able to respond quickly over the phone.

And you should use good judgment. Don't eat foods onboard you wouldn't have at home; make sure hamburgers and seafood are fully cooked, for example. And take special care with anything you eat or drink in foreign ports.

Security Onboard Ship

In recent years, several newspapers and television shows have made a big deal about a supposed "crime wave" aboard cruise ships.

Here are the facts: Cruise ships are a relatively safe environment, less dangerous than most any other small town.

Onboard, there are two sources of threat to your possessions and personal safety: The crew, and the passengers. A third danger lies in some ports of call.

The fact is that cruise ships draw their crews from all over the world, often from areas of relative poverty. And the crew is often out to sea for six months or longer, without return visits to their homes. Add to all this the fact that some travelers, including single women, may be overly relaxed on their sea vacations.

Most cruise lines are very specific in their instructions to crew members regarding prohibitions on fraternization with passengers outside of their official duties in the dining room, bar, or elsewhere.

But that does not mean you should totally abandon any concern for safety: Lock your door when you are in your cabin, keep valuables in the safe (or at home), and take the same sort of care with strangers you meet on ship that you would with someone you met in a bar in your town.

Finally, there is this: When you are in international waters in a vessel that (like nearly all cruise ships) flies a foreign flag, you are outside the reach of U.S. laws and enforcement agencies. Theoretically, the laws of the nation of registry apply while on the seas. How much do you know about the legal code of Liberia, Panama, or The Bahamas? For most intents and purposes, a cruise ship is like an independent floating nation.

If a crime or incident does occur while you are at sea, though, be sure to document every detail with the ship's officers, as well as for yourself. Then do the same when the ship reaches its next port of call, and again with the U.S. Coast Guard if the ship touches an American port.

Most cruise lines do not permit visitors onboard ship without pre-arrangements through the purser or other officer. Hand-carried luggage is X-rayed and passengers go through a metal detector prior to boarding.

The most modern of ships include a passenger cruise card ID with a magnetic strip. The card is used as an identity instrument to disembark or re-board the ship at port calls (allowing the purser to know if all of the guests have returned at the end of the visit), and also as a shipboard charge card, and as an electronic key to the stateroom.

On newer ships in the Princess fleet, the card is linked to a color photograph of the guest, which can be displayed on a monitor at the gangway.

Chapter 8
Dining on the High Seas

Sometimes it seems as if the logic of many cruise vacationers is this: "I paid $250 a night for this cruise, and by God, I'm going to eat $250 worth of food every day."

Not that most cruise lines don't go out of their way to encourage you to eat. In fact, there's a bit of a war of the restaurants and buffets amongst most of the major cruise lines: Call it the Floating Battle of the Bulge.

The staff is going to be pushing food at you at most every turn, and in most cases the food is pretty good. And when you sit down to dinner, your waiter is going to encourage you to sample anything and everything on the menu: Look twice at the dessert offerings and he is likely to bring you both the cheesecake *and* the double dark chocolate dream cake.

I am particularly partial to salad, and I enjoy freshly grated pepper on most everything; my wife's secret indulgences are a piece of blue cheese as an intermezzo before the main course, and a cup of cappuccino at the end of the meal. We can judge the quality of the service we receive onboard a ship by how long it takes before our waiter and assistant learn to automatically stand by with extra salads, pepper, cheese, and coffee at the appropriate times in the meal.

Eat Until You Drop

There's a lot of eating onboard a cruise ship. In fact, on some ships you could just about go from meal to snack to meal, from dawn until after midnight. And then you could probably order room service to get you past the munchies at 3 A.M.

Here's a typical meal lineup, in this case from the *Norway,* the classic, older flagship of the NCL fleet:

    6–8:30 A.M. Eye Opener, Great Outdoor Restaurant
    7:30–10 A.M. Breakfast service, Windward and Leeward dining rooms
    8:30–11 A.M. Late breakfast, Great Outdoor Restaurant
    Noon. Lunch (*first seating*), Windward and Leeward dining rooms

12:30 P.M.–3 P.M. Lunch buffet and barbecue, Great Outdoor Restaurant
1:30 P.M. Lunch (*second seating*), Windward and Leeward dining rooms
4–6 P.M. Coffee and snacks, Great Outdoor Restaurant
6 P.M. Dinner (*main seating*), Windward and Leeward dining rooms
6–11 P.M. Le Bistro Supper Club (*by reservation*), Pool Deck aft.
8:30 P.M. Dinner (*late seating*), Windward and Leeward Dining Rooms
Midnight–1 A.M. Mini-midnight buffet, Casino
Midnight–1 A.M. Chocoholic midnight buffet, Windward and Leeward
dining rooms.

But wait: If you're in one of the suites, your cabin attendant will deliver a small tray of hors d'oeuvres in late afternoon to stave off sudden pangs of hunger. And, oh yes, there is also 24-hour room service if you have a sudden need for a turkey sandwich at 3 A.M.

To me, that late-night buffet, sometimes known as the Midnight Buffet, is the ultimate in wretched excess—and an occasional wicked delight. Typical offerings range from crab legs to Steamship Rounds of Beef to gourmet pizza. On all Norwegian Cruise Line ships, one night of each cruise is given over to the aptly named Chocoholic Buffet: an absolutely sybaritic exercise in late-night gluttony. Oh, yes, we gave in to our baser instincts, too.

Dinner Seatings

On most larger ships, the dining rooms have two seatings: a "main" or "first" seating, and a "second" or "late" seating. On many ships, breakfast is open to all from about 7 to 9 A.M.; lunch may have a first seating at noon and a second seating at 1:30 P.M. or may be open seating. Dinner is usually served at 6 or 6:30 P.M. and again at about 8 P.M.

For most Americans, an 8 P.M. dining time is a bit later than we're used to. You'll waddle out of the dining room close to 10 P.M., perhaps to catch a show, and then be well situated for the midnight buffet. Still, it can be gotten used to.

However, if you are flying from the East to the West Coast, factor in the time change. When we flew from Massachusetts to Honolulu to pick up a cruise there, we lost six hours. Our internal clocks were set at 2 A.M. for the 8 P.M. seating for the first few days of the cruise; we quickly changed to the 6 P.M. main seating. The same would apply for Europeans flying to Florida or the Caribbean to pick up a cruise. Coming from the West Coast to Florida, the late seating will be more comfortable, at least for the start of the trip.

If you have a strong preference for a particular seating, make your wishes known early and often—enlist your travel agent on your side if necessary. In some cases, you may find that your preference is not available; some cruisers don't accept no for an answer and take up their wishes with the maitre d' on arrival. Remember: Most cruise crew members depend on tips for much of their income, and a subtle reminder of this may grease the way to the dining time or table you want.

On many ships you can expect to find yourself assigned to a table with others. A typical dining room has tables for four, six, eight, and occasionally even more. You should also be able to find a two-seat hideaway, although the "deuces" are often tucked away in corners.

My wife and I are quiet and private by nature and we always push for a table for two; one way or another, we always get one.

You can expect that the occupants of your cabin will be seated together; you may have to wave the flag to bring together friends or family members in other cabins.

Can you change your table assignment once you are onboard? Perhaps. A lot depends on how full the vessel is, and the reasonableness of your request.

If you cannot stand your tablemates, take the subject up quietly and in privacy with the maitre d' or the cruise director.

About Cruise Cuisine

Start with this: imagine the challenge of every day preparing 2,000 breakfasts, 2,000 lunches, 2,000 dinners, plus breakfast, brunch, lunch, afternoon, and midnight buffets. Then add in the fact that you must carry nearly all your food supplies with you, reprovisioning once a week or every 10 days.

And, oh yes: Your cramped kitchen is in a pitching, rolling ship. You cannot use an open flame because of safety concerns. And your crew is a mini–United Nations.

Then there are the passengers, many of whom look at their all-inclusive cruise fare as a license to make demands of waiters and the chef they would never attempt at home or at a restaurant where they were paying a la carte.

All that said, it is nevertheless true that most cruise cuisine is pretty good. In general, the budget end of the cruise market delivers decent institutional-

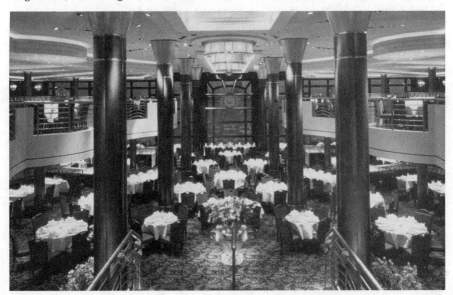

The Grand Restaurant on the Century
Celebrity Cruises

quality food. The vast group of top-of-the-line ships offers quality approaching that of a first-class restaurant on land. And the ultra-luxury ships add caviar, champagne, and an extra level of personal attention.

The most luxurious of ships will sometimes offer to prepare any special request the galley can possibly accommodate; don't assume they'll be able to rustle up some fresh venison in the middle of a transatlantic crossing. But if you give the chef enough advanced notice, he may be able to find some at an upcoming port of call.

Most cruise lines offer vegetarian and low-calorie alternatives on every menu. If you require a special diet beyond that, such as kosher, low-sodium, or gluten-free, be sure to advise the cruise line several weeks before sailing. In some cases, the special meals will be prepared and frozen off the ship and prepared as needed.

Room Service

Most cruise ships offer room service food without extra charge. On some lines, you can order from that day's restaurant menu; other ships offer a more limited menu for meals taken in the cabin.

You can also pay for drinks and wine from the bar, and order special canapés—a bucket of shrimp, for example—if you somehow have the appetite for something special.

A Sensible Dining Strategy

Face it: you're going to go off your diet on a cruise vacation. That's one of the appeals of cruising.

But you don't have to overdo it. Here are a few tips:

• Choose your meals. You don't really need to visit every food offering every day. Pick and choose the ones that most appeal to you.

• Eat in moderation. Take smaller portions, or avoid cleaning every morsel off your plate. You might be able to get your waiter to deliver half portions.

• Consider the "spa" low-calorie or heart-healthy dishes offered on most menus. Eat an extra portion of salad, with a fat-free dressing, instead of a cream-based clam chowder.

• Increase your level of exercise, especially on days at sea when you won't be disembarking from the ship. Use the health spa or take a half-dozen laps around the promenade deck. It's romantic, fun, and helps work off the calories.

• Don't be afraid to skip an occasional breakfast or lunch. It won't kill you.

Chapter 9
Get Me to the Port on Time

For most of us, before we get onboard our cruise ship, we have to travel to the port. That may involve a lengthy air flight or a drive.

Among your first decisions as a savvy consumer is whether to book your own transportation from home to the port, or to take advantage of travel packages offered by the cruise companies.

In some cases, the cruise line may be able to offer you a discounted airline ticket because of arrangements with major carriers. You might, though, find you can do better by yourself. In any case, making your own arrangements offers you the greatest flexibility on your schedule, including the ability to stay over en route or before or after your cruise.

The Advantage of Booking a Package

One advantage of booking through the cruise company is that the line may take responsibility for you from your home airport to the ship. Many cruise lines dispatch employees to arrival airports to help with transfers to the ship.

If your flight is delayed, canceled, or diverted, they'll know about the situation, and may help you get to the ship. Be sure you understand the commitment of the cruise line to tracking its incoming passengers.

In some instances, the cruise line may hold the departure of the ship by a few hours to accommodate late arrivals. In other situations, the line may make arrangements to fly passengers to the next port call.

During a "sickout" by American Airlines pilots in early 1999, several major cruise lines chartered planes and made other special arrangements to get their guests to the waiting ships.

The cruise line should also take responsibility for matching you up with misdirected luggage.

On an Alaskan cruise I took, a group of passengers made it to the ship while their baggage took a vacation somewhere else. The cruise line delivered them to their cabin, offered a basic kit of personal supplies, and arranged to have their bags catch up with them two days later at the first port call.

A few weeks later, I was cruising in the South Pacific and met a couple whose clothing was a week behind them. They had to do without their luggage for six days out of a 10-day voyage because the ship was heading out to sea and a stop at a remote island that had no airport. The cruise line chose to offer them a few sets of T-shirts and shorts from the gift shop, outfits that did not work very well on formal nights in the dining room.

Note that I say the cruise line "may" be able to help. Be sure to check with the company and discuss their policies before you book tickets. Then make certain everything you are told verbally is also presented in writing in the cruise line's brochures, contracts, or other confirmations you may receive.

Making Your Own Arrangements

On the other hand, if you make your own arrangements to get to the port, you may end up waving at the stern of your cruise ship as it leaves the pier. And costs of overnight accommodations and transportation to the ship's next port of call will probably be your responsibility. Here are a few tips to reduce the chances of missing your ship:

1. Consider traveling to the port the night before your departure.

2. Notify the cruise line of the flight arrangements you have made. The line may have other passengers on the same plane and may be making special arrangements for them.

3. If you encounter problems with the airline, be sure to inform them you are flying to catch a cruise departure. They may be able to re-book you on another flight or another airline if necessary.

If you do end up missing the ship, immediately call the cruise line's port representative. Most companies have an office at ports of embarkation; if not, call the phone number listed in your cruise confirmation papers.

Arriving Early

There is one other situation where you will likely have to make your own arrangements: if you choose to fly to the port the day before your cruise—my preference—or stay afterwards in the final port.

Why do I prefer to fly to the port a day ahead of departure?

First of all, I don't want the stress of worrying about missing a departure because of a delay while flying to the port. This is especially true in the wintertime, when bad weather can wreak havoc on airports and schedules everywhere in the country.

Secondly, I prefer to spend a day of rest in a port city before getting onboard the ship. Many cruise travelers pass too quickly through some of the most interesting cities in the world, rushing from the airport directly to the ship and missing exciting places such as Vancouver, Miami, Boston, New Orleans, and other points of departure.

This also allows me a day or so to become acclimated to time zone changes in distant ports before I get on the ship. In that way, while the passengers who have been traveling all day to get to the port head for bed, I'm immediately ready to enjoy the cruise.

Getting from the Airport to the Ship

Your cruise company is likely to offer a service to transport guests from the airport to the ship. This may be included in your cruise if you have booked airfare through the cruise line, or you may be able to purchase the transfer service separately.

I can see the advantages of having a prearranged service with a direct connection to the cruise company, but I also know that in general, transfer service is overpriced and may be less convenient than arrangements you can make on your own.

Do a little research and compare the cost and convenience of a taxi from the airport to the pier, or a rental car or limousine service.

Just how overpriced are transfers? On one trip in the Hawaiian islands, the cruise line charged $20 per person for a bus trip a few miles from the pier to the Honolulu airport. Guests had to wait while their bags were collected and loaded onto a huge bus, and then wait again at the airport while the bus was unloaded and bags distributed. Meanwhile, my wife and I got off the ship half an hour later and grabbed a taxi; the fare was $17 for the two of us, including a tip. And we got to the airline counter ahead of the bus-borne horde.

The same applied in Vancouver on the return from a voyage north to Alaska. The cruise company's bus was not only overpriced, it would have delivered us to the airport four hours before we needed to wait in line for our flight. Instead, we arranged for a rental car that was delivered right to the dock and we spent the morning at a museum, had lunch in Chinatown, and drove to the airport on our own schedule.

If you're concerned about making a tight connection, contact a taxi company or a limousine service before you embark and arrange for a pickup at the dock when your ship returns.

Airline Travel

Why is there a section about airline travel in a book about cruising? Simply because the vast majority of cruise passengers begin their vacation by boarding an airplane and flying to a port in Florida, San Juan, Vancouver, New Orleans and other major locations.

Let's start with a *very* real-life scenario.

I'm flying south from Boston to Miami to pick up a cruise from the bustling port there. My ticket, which I bought in advance and includes a Saturday night stayover, cost $217.50 for a round-trip. The businessman across the aisle will suffer through the same mystery meal, watch the same crummy movie, and arrive in Miami at the same millisecond I do. The only difference will be the fact that he paid $909 for his ticket. And in first class, someone who (in my humble opinion) has more money than sense, has paid $1,560.50 for a slightly wider, slightly plusher seat and a relatively better meal. (I'd rather spend some of that money on a better place to sleep and a meal at a restaurant where half the meal doesn't end up in your lap.)

All of those prices are real, as I write these words. Now, consider a few more positive examples.

Somewhere else on this same plane there is a couple who were bumped off a previous flight because of overbooking. They are happily discussing where to use the two free round-trip tickets they received in compensation.

And up front in first class, where you arrive a millisecond earlier, a family of four is traveling on free tickets earned through Mom's frequent flier plan.

Me, I'm perfectly happy with that cut-rate ticket and I'm also due for a 5 percent rebate on airfare, hotel, and car rental, all arranged through my travel agent.

And on my trip back home, I will get on the flight I really wanted to take instead of the less-convenient reservation I was forced to sign up for when I bought that cut-rate ticket. How will I do this? Read on.

Alice in Airlineland

In today's strange world of air travel, there is a lot of room for the dollarwise and clever traveler to wiggle. You can pay an inflated full price, you can take advantage of the lowest fares, or you can play the ultimate game and parlay tickets into free travel.

There are three golden rules when it comes to saving hundreds of dollars on travel—be flexible, be flexible, and be flexible. Here's how to translate that flexibility into extra dollars in your pocket:

• Be flexible about when you choose to travel. Go during the off-season or low-season when airfares, hotel rooms, cruises, and attractions are offered at substantial discounts. Try to avoid school vacations, including the prime summer travel months of July and August, unless you enjoy a lot of company.

• Be flexible about the day of the week you travel. In many cases you can save hundreds of dollars by bumping your departure date one or two days in either direction. Ask your travel agent or airline ticket agent for current fare rules and restrictions. If this puts you into port a day or two ahead of the departure of the ship, use the time to become acclimated to a new time zone and to explore.

The days of lightest air travel are generally midweek, Saturday afternoon, and Sunday morning. The busiest days are Sunday evening, Monday morning, and Friday afternoon and evening.

In general, you will receive the lowest possible fare if your stay includes all day Saturday; this class of ticket is sold as an excursion fare. Airlines use this as a way to exclude business travelers from the cheapest fares, assuming that businesspeople will want to be home by Friday night.

• Be flexible about the hour of your departure. There is generally lower demand—and therefore lower prices—for flights that leave in the middle of the day or very late at night. The highest rates are usually assigned to breakfast-time (7–11 A.M.) and cocktail-hour (4–7 P.M.) departures.

• Be flexible on the route you will take, and be willing to put up with a change of plane or stopover. Once again, you are putting the law of supply and demand in your favor. For example, a non-stop flight from Boston to Tampa for a family of four may cost hundreds more than a flight from Boston that includes a change of planes in Atlanta (a Delta hub) before proceeding on to Florida.

(You should also understand that in airline terminology, a "direct" flight does not mean a "non-stop" flight. Non-stop means the plane goes from Point A to Point B without stopping anywhere else. A direct flight may go from Point A to Point B, but may include a stopover at Point C or at more than one airport along the way. A connecting flight means you must get off the plane at an airport enroute and change to another plane.)

Consider flying on one of the newer, deep-discount airlines, but don't let economy cloud your judgment. Some carriers are simply better run than others. Read the newspapers, check with a trusted travel agent, and use common sense. As far as I'm concerned, the best thing about the cheapo airlines is the pressure they put on the established carriers to lower prices or even to match fares on certain flights. Look for the cheapest fare you can find and then call your favorite big airline and see if it will sell you a ticket at the same price—it just might work.

• Don't overlook the possibility of flying out of a different airport either. For example, metropolitan New Yorkers can find domestic flights from La Guardia, Newark, White Plains, and a developing new discount mecca at Islip. Suburbanites of Boston might want to consider flights from Providence as possibly cheaper alternatives to Logan Airport. Chicago has O'Hare and Midway. From Southern California there are major airports at Los Angeles, Orange County, Burbank, and San Diego.

• Plan way ahead of time and purchase the most deeply discounted advance tickets, which usually are non-cancelable. Most carriers limit the number of discount tickets on any particular flight. Although there may be plenty of seats left on the day you want to travel, they may be offered at higher rates.

• In a significant change during the past few years, most airlines have modified nonrefundable fares to be non-cancelable. What this means is that if your plans change or you are forced to cancel your trip, your tickets retain their value and can be applied against another trip. At the beginning of 2000, most airlines charged a fee of about $75 to reissue a ticket.

• If you're feeling adventurous, you can take a big chance and wait for the last possible moment, keeping in contact with charter tour operators and accepting a bargain price on a leftover seat and hotel reservation. You may also find that some airlines will reduce the prices on leftover seats within a few weeks of your departure date; don't be afraid to check with the airline regularly, or ask your travel agent to do it for you. In fact, some travel agencies have automated computer programs that keep a constant electronic eagle eye on available seats and fares.

• Take advantage of special discount programs such as senior citizens' clubs, military discounts, or offerings from other organizations to which you may belong. If you are in the over-60 category, you may not even have to belong to a group such as AARP; simply ask the airline ticket agent if there is a discount available. You may have to prove your age or show a membership card when you pick up your ticket or boarding pass.

• Consider doing business with discounters, known in the industry as consolidators or, less flatteringly, as bucket shops. These companies buy the airlines' slow-to-sell tickets in volume and resell them to consumers at rock-bottom prices. Look for their ads in the classified listings of many Sunday newspaper travel sections. Be sure to study and understand the restrictions; if they fit your needs and wants, this is a good way to fly.

Standing Up for Standing By

One of the little-known secrets of air travel on most airlines and most types of tickets is the fact that travelers with valid tickets are allowed to stand by for flights other than the ones for which they have reservations; if there are empty seats on the flight, standby ticket holders are permitted to board.

Some airlines are very liberal in their acceptance of standbys within a few days of the reserved flight, while others will charge a fee for changes in itinerary. And some airline personnel are stricter about the regulation than others.

Here's what I do know: If I cannot get the exact flight I want for a trip, I make the closest acceptable reservations available after that flight and then show up early at the airport and head for the check-in counter for the flight I really want to take. Unless you are seeking to travel during an impossibly overbooked holiday period or arrive on a bad weather day when flights have been canceled, your chances of successfully standing by for a flight are usually pretty good.

One trick is to call the airline the day before the flight and check on the availability of seats for the flight you want to try for. Some reservation clerks are very forthcoming with information; many times I have been told something like, "There are 70 seats open on that flight."

Be careful with standby maneuvers if your itinerary requires a change of plane en route; you'll need to check the availability of seats on all of the legs of your journey.

And a final note: Be especially careful about standing by for the very last flight of the night. If you somehow are unable to get on that flight, you're stuck for the night.

Your Consumer Rights

The era of airline deregulation has been a mixed blessing for the industry and the consumer. After an era of wild competition based mostly on price, we now are left with fewer but larger airlines and a dizzying array of confusing rules.

The U.S. Department of Transportation and its Federal Aviation Administration (FAA) still regulate safety issues. Almost everything else is between you and the airline.

Policies on fares, cancellations, reconfirmation, check-in requirements, and compensation for lost or damaged baggage or for delays all vary by airline. Your rights are limited and defined by the terms of the contract you make with an airline when you buy your ticket. You may find the contract included with the ticket you purchase, or the airlines may "incorporate terms by reference" to a separate document that you will have to request to see.

Whether you are buying your ticket through a travel agent or dealing directly with the airline, here are some important questions to ask:

- Is the price guaranteed, or can it change from the time of the reservation until you actually purchase the ticket?
- Can the price change between the time you buy the ticket and the date of departure?
- Is there a penalty for cancellation of the ticket?
- Can the reservation be changed without penalty, or for a reasonable fee? Be sure you understand the sort of service you are buying.
- Is this a nonstop flight, a direct flight (an itinerary where your plane will make one or more stops en route to its destination), or a flight that requires you to change planes one or more times?
- What seat has been issued? Do you really want the center seat in a three-seat row, between two strangers?

You might also want to ask your travel agent:

- Is there anything I should know about the financial health of this airline?
- Are you aware of any threats of work stoppages or legal actions that could ruin my trip?

Overbooking

Overbooking is a polite industry term for the legal business practice of selling more than an airline can deliver. It all stems, alas, from the rudeness of many travelers who neglect to cancel flight reservations that will not be used.

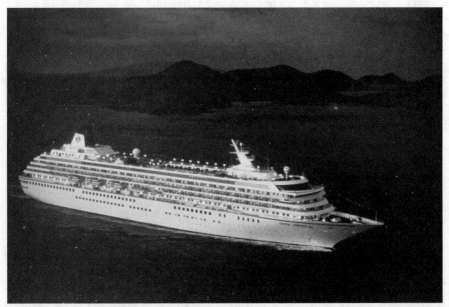

Crystal Symphony
Crystal Cruises

Airlines study the patterns on various flights and city pairs and apply a formula that allows them to sell more tickets than there are seats on the plane in the expectation that a certain percentage of ticket holders will not show up.

But what happens if all passengers holding a reservation do show up? Obviously, the result will be more passengers than seats, and some will have to be left behind.

The involuntary bump list will begin with passengers who check in late. Airlines must ask for volunteers before bumping any passengers who have followed the rules on check-in.

Now, assuming that no one is willing to give up their seat just for the fun of it, the airline will offer some sort of compensation—either a free ticket or cash, or both. It is up to the passenger and the airline to negotiate a deal.

Some air travelers, including this author, look forward to an overbooked flight when their schedules are flexible. My most profitable score: $4,000 in vouchers on a set of four $450 international tickets. The airline was desperate to clear a large block of seats, and it didn't matter to us if we arrived home a few hours late. We received the equivalent of three tickets for the price of one, and you can bet that we'll hope to earn some more free travel on future tickets purchased with those vouchers.

The U.S. Department of Transportation's consumer protection regulations set some minimum levels of compensation for passengers who are bumped from a flight due to overbooking.

If you are bumped involuntarily, the airline must provide a ticket on its next available flight. Unfortunately, there is no guarantee there will be a seat on that plane, or that it will arrive at your destination at a convenient time.

Now if you are traveling to the port on the day your ship is scheduled to depart, you probably do not want to even consider the possibility of being bumped. Let the airline staff know you are flying to a cruise and stand your ground if you feel your vacation is threatened.

If the airline can get you on another flight that will get you to your destination within one hour of the original arrival time, no compensation need be paid. If you are scheduled to get to your destination more than one hour but less than two hours late, you're entitled to receive an amount equal to the one-way fare of the oversold flight, up to $200. If the delay is more than two hours, the bumpee will receive an amount equal to twice the one-way fare of the original flight, up to $400.

It is not considered bumping if a flight is canceled because of weather, equipment problems, or the lack of a flight crew. You are also not eligible for compensation if the airline substitutes a smaller aircraft for operational or safety reasons, or if the flight involves an aircraft with 60 seats or less.

How to Get Bumped

Why in the world would you want to be bumped? Well, perhaps you'd like to look at missing your plane as an opportunity to earn a little money for your time instead of an annoyance. Is a two-hour delay worth $100 an hour to you? For the inconvenience of waiting a few hours on the way home, a family of four might receive a voucher for $800—that could pay for a week's hotel plus a heck of a meal at the airport.

If you're not in a rush to get to your destination—or to get back home—you might want to volunteer to be bumped. We wouldn't recommend doing this on the busiest travel days of the year, or if you are booked on the last flight of the day, unless you are also looking forward to a free night in an airport motel.

Drive?

Everyone's conception of the perfect vacation is different, but for me, I draw a distinction between getting there and being there. I want the getting there part to be as quick and simple as possible, and the being there part to be as long as I can manage and afford. Therefore, I fly to just about any destination that is more than a few hundred miles from my home. The cost of driving, hotels, meals en route, and general physical and mental wear and tear rarely equals a deeply discounted excursion fare.

If you do drive to the port, though, you can save a few dollars by using the services of AAA or another major automobile club. Before you head out, spend a bit of time and money to make certain your vehicle is in traveling shape: A tune-up and fully inflated, fully inspected tires will certainly save gas, money, and headaches.

And if you are taking your own car to the port, be sure to inquire ahead of time about parking facilities. Find out the charges, and determine what level of security is provided. You may want to look into leaving your car at a secured garage, away from the port.

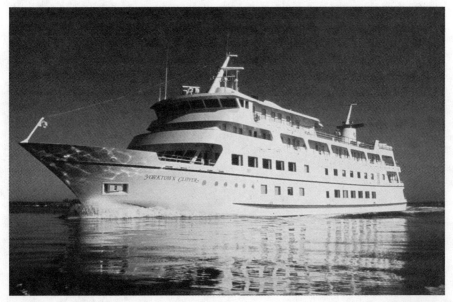

Yorktown Clipper
Clipper Cruise Line

Renting a Car

Your travel agent may be of assistance in finding the best rates; make a few phone calls by yourself too. Sometimes you'll find significant variations in prices from one agency to another.

Car rental companies will try—with varying levels of pressure—to convince you to purchase special insurance coverage. They'll tell you it's "only" $7 or $9 per day. What a deal! That works out to about $2,500 or $3,330 per year for a set of rental wheels. Of course the coverage is intended primarily to protect the rental company, not you.

Before you travel, check with your insurance agent to determine how well your personal automobile policy will cover a rental car and its contents. I strongly recommend you use a credit card that offers rental car insurance; such insurance usually covers the deductible below your personal policy. The extra auto insurance by itself is usually worth an upgrade to a gold card or other extra-service credit card.

The only sticky area comes for those visitors who have a driver's license but no car, and therefore no insurance. Again, consult your credit card company and your insurance agent to see what kind of coverage you have, or what kind you need.

Pay attention, too, when the rental agent explains the gas policy. The most common plan says you must return the car with a full tank; if the agency must refill the tank, you will be billed a service charge plus what is usually a very high per-gallon rate.

Other optional plans include one where the rental agency sells you a full tank when you first drive away and takes no note of how much gas remains when you return the car. Unless you somehow manage to return the car with the engine running on fumes, you are in effect making a gift to the agency with every gallon you bring back.

I prefer the first option, which requires making it a point to refill the tank on the way to the airport on getaway day.

Although it is theoretically possible to rent a car without a credit card, you will find it to be an inconvenient process. If the rental agency cannot hold your credit card account hostage, it will most often require a large cash deposit—perhaps as much as several thousand dollars—before it will give you the keys.

Chapter 10
Packing Your Bags

What kind of weather can you expect at your destination and all your ports of call?

If you're sailing from Vancouver to Alaska, you can expect a wide range of conditions from warm and sunny to cold and drizzly. And if you head to the mountains on a shore excursion, you could find a bit of winter in July on a glacier. In eastern Canada, it can be damp and cool in August.

In Hawaii and the Caribbean, temperatures are generally moderate to hot all the time.

Wherever you go, pack some light sweaters or jackets to wear on deck in the evening when temperatures cool. Your ship will be moving, too, usually adding a 15- to 20-mile-per-hour breeze to whatever wind there is at sea.

Find out from the cruise line about the dress suggestions for dinner. Most ships have one or more "formal" nights, plus a number of theme dinners— Western, '50s, Island, and the like.

Like it or not, the definition of "formal" has loosened up greatly on most ships. Only a few lines request men to wear tuxedos; a conservative suit or a blue blazer and gray slacks will not raise any eyebrows. Women have a range of options from cocktail gowns to pant suits. Put another way, on most ships "formal" means the night when you don't wear a T-shirt and jeans.

What happens if you show up at dinner on a formal night inappropriately dressed? On some ships, the maitre d' may discreetly suggest you return to your cabin and seek new attire. On other ships, he might suggest you visit an alternative casual dining room that night. Or, he might look away, preferring to keep his relations with you—and his potential gratuity—undamaged.

On some ships you can arrange to rent a tuxedo and other formal wear; check before you depart to see if such services are available.

Find out if the ship has an onboard laundromat or a reasonably priced laundry or dry cleaning service. On a longer cruise this can allow you to pack less clothes and obtain a mid-ocean cleaning.

Find out about health club and sports facilities onboard the ship and think about whether you will be visiting any beaches on shore. Pack a bathing suit, sandals, sun hat, sneakers, and any other appropriate articles. The cruise line will provide beach towels and may offer other amenities such as bathrobes and slippers for some or all of its passengers, sometimes discriminating on the basis of your class of cabin.

One other thing: Think twice and even three times about whether you want to bring any valuable jewelry with you. You'll have to worry about its security getting to the ship, onboard the ship, in port, and getting home.

Paperwork and Passports

Almost every cruise visits a foreign port. That's part of the romance of it all—and a legal requirement for any vessel that does not fly a U.S. flag.

Many tourist ports do not require visitors to have a passport to enter, and will accept a birth certificate or a driver's license. The same generally applies for U.S. citizens returning to this country from those destinations.

However: Immigration laws and regulations can change, and you may find some immigration inspectors are more picky than others.

I strongly recommend you bring a passport. If you don't have one, it's not a huge bother to obtain one. Your travel agent, U.S. Post Office, or county clerk can usually help you with the paperwork. The standard process can take a few months, but there are ways to speed it up considerably.

The cruise line will also likely send you some embarkation papers to fill out and bring with you to the port. One form is used for immigration purposes; inspectors at foreign ports and in the U.S. on your return will likely work from a list provided by the cruise company.

Some cruise lines will send passengers a personal questionnaire to be used in producing a shipboard newsletter or registry to allow people to locate guests with similar interests or backgrounds or those from particular locations. You do not have to participate or fill out this sort of form. You may also find an application for an onboard credit account.

The cruise line will likely send you a set of luggage tags. If you have purchased an airport transfer service from the cruise line, these will be used to identify your bags when you arrive at the airport. If you make your own way to the ship, these luggage tags will be used by cabin attendants who deliver bags to staterooms. Fill out the tags, including your cabin number—you should find that number on your cruise contract.

Medical Needs and Personal Supplies

If you are taking any medications or have any significant medical conditions, speak with your doctor before heading out on your trip. Consider bringing a copy of your current medical records in case you need to visit the shipboard clinic or an onshore facility. If you have a heart condition, for example, your doctor might want you to bring a copy of a recent electrocardiogram.

If you are on medication or have a medical condition, ask your doctor whether you can safely take one of several commonly used seasickness preventatives or remedies. (Most are considered quite safe and effective, but the question is worth asking.)

Be sure to pack a full supply of required medicines—bring along a few additional days' worth to deal with possible delays on your return. You might want to ask your doctor for a backup set of prescriptions in case you need to replace bottles during your trip. Pack your medication in a carry-on bag that does *not* get checked at the airport or at the dock.

Although most cruise ships can supply you with seasickness pills, aspirin, and most personal toiletries, you're better off bringing your own supply. Again, pack these in your carry-on bags.

I also recommend you bring a sunscreen that has a high SPF rating, especially on Caribbean and Hawaiian voyages, but also for Alaska and other destinations. It is quite easy to ruin your vacation with a bad sunburn, and overexposure to the sun's rays is a long-term health risk.

Finally, consult with your insurance agent or personnel office to be sure you understand the limits and nature of your health insurance. Most policies do not cover emergency medical treatment onboard a ship, and many exclude coverage for treatment in foreign countries. And policies may also not pay for expensive emergency medical evacuation from a ship or from a foreign port.

You can, though, purchase special medical insurance for your trip. Policies are offered by most cruise lines; some travel agencies or insurance agencies may also sell policies. Be aware that most policies exclude coverage for pre-existing conditions. Be sure you understand all the terms of a policy before you buy one.

If you expect to rent a car in port, be sure your policy gives you proper coverage. Some policies do not cover foreign countries, and some exclude coverage for certain types of vehicles, including luxury cars and off-road vehicles. Consult with your insurance agent for advice, and check with your credit card company to determine the limits of any liability and collision coverage that may be automatically offered with auto rentals that are paid for with the credit card.

Cameras

Almost everyone documents their vacation on film, but not everyone is happy with their results.

If you're strictly an amateur, consider buying one of the new autofocus, autoexposure, zoom lens pocket cameras. They do just about everything but take the picture for you, and the quality is generally quite good. Expect a decent model to be priced in the range of approximately $100 to $200.

A standard lens for 35mm film is about 50mm, while a typical wide angle lens is 35mm and a moderate telephoto focal length is 100mm. Therefore, a zoom lens that runs from 35mm to 100mm covers most situations; even better is a zoom that is slightly wider and longer, say 28mm to 135mm.

When you buy film, pay attention to the speed rating, also called ASA or ISO rating. The higher the number, the "faster" the film. A fast film allows you to shoot in lower-light conditions, or at a higher shutter speed to stop the action, or at a smaller lens aperture, which generally gives you a sharper image with a better depth of field. Professional photographers will tell you that faster film doesn't deliver perfect color or that your photos may be more grainy in appearance when larger prints are made. That is true, but you are taking vacation snapshots, not studio portraits.

I recommend you use film that has a rating of at least 400, which allows picture-taking at the midnight buffet as well as on deck and in port. If you know you're going to be shooting mostly low-light images in museums and onboard, look for film that has an 800 rating.

It's a good idea to buy your film at a reputable dealer before you leave for your trip. You'll certainly save money over a purchase in a tourist port, and you'll have a reasonable expectation that the film is fresh and has not been unnecessarily subjected to heat.

A word of caution: Film can be damaged by exposure to heat. Don't leave your film out in the sun. You'll also get the best results if you have your film processed sooner rather than later. Try to avoid leaving a roll of film in your camera for months just because there are a few unexposed frames.

One other warning: In theory, airport X-ray machines will not harm photographic film. However, faster film such as ASA 800 stock is more susceptible than slower film and there may be a cumulative effect from passing through six or eight machines over the course of changing planes on a trip. You might want to consider carrying a small zipper pouch for your film and asking airport security personnel to hand-inspect the pouch. Return the film to your carry-on bag after you are through the X-ray machine.

It's also a good idea to pack one or more sets of replacement batteries for your camera. You don't want to discover you've run out of juice just at the moment a humpback whale breeches alongside your ship.

If you are traveling with a video camera, be sure to bring the battery charger with you. Most modern cruise ships offer standard 110-volt electrical outlets in the cabins. You may need a voltage adapter on some older ships and certain European cruise ships that supply 220 volts.

Arriving at the Pier

Most ships have a window of several hours for arriving passengers to check in and get onboard. Cruise ships generally depart in the early evening, and may be open for check-in as early as 1 P.M.

When you arrive at the pier you may find a curbside check-in for your bags. Be sure to determine that the persons reaching for your bags are legitimate employees of the cruise line or stevedores from the port; look for an ID badge or card. They may have a list of arriving passengers. Be sure, too, that they are checking in your ship and not another one at the same port.

Your luggage tags should have your name and cabin number clearly marked on them. Double-check to see that the tags have not come off in the airplane or vehicle en route to the pier.

At other ports, you may have to drag your bags into the terminal for check-in. Again, be sure that you deposit your bags with the right cruise line.

Hold onto your overnight bag with a change of clothes, medications, cameras, jewelry, and other valuables. Be sure you also hold onto your cruise documents, including your passport.

On nearly every ship, your bags will be delivered to your cabin. Sometimes they may arrive before you make it to your cabin, while on other ships the bags may not make it to your stateroom until after the ship has sailed from the port. (On most ships, the first night's dinner has a casual dress code.)

You'll probably find that lunch will be served to arriving passengers, sometimes in the dining room, but more often as a casual buffet.

It is not necessary to tip a cabin attendant who brings your bags to your room onboard the ship; protocol calls for a tip to be delivered at the end of the voyage. If your bags are taken at the curb by a stevedore or employee of the port, a tip may be in order; check with the cruise line in advance or ask a representative at the dock whether the service is included in your fare.

Boarding the Ship

When you get onboard, you will likely be escorted to your room by a cabin attendant. (The fancier cruise lines make this into a bit of an event, outfitting the attendants in starched jackets and white gloves.)

Check out your room. Be sure the attendant shows you how to operate the heating and cooling system. Find out if there is a safe in the room. If you're lucky enough to have a veranda, learn how to open and close the door. Locate the life vests. If you want extra pillows or blankets, ask for them. If the cabin has two single beds that can be brought together to serve as a queen-sized bed, ask the attendant to rearrange them.

And of course, if you find that the cabin is not what you thought you had purchased—a porthole instead of a window, upper-and-lower berths instead of a double bed, an inside broom closet rather than the Owner's Suite—now is the time to make a beeline to the reception desk or purser's office onboard the ship. It may be possible to switch to another cabin if the ship is not full.

If no mistake has been made, you may still be able to upgrade your cabin if better accommodations are available. On many ships, this is one way to obtain an upgraded room at a decreased price: The purser or onboard hotel manager may offer deep discounts on any available upgraded cabins once it is absolutely impossible to sell them to someone not already onboard the ship.

Lifeboat Drills

One of the first scheduled events on a cruise is the lifeboat drill, often conducted in port before departure. It's something that could save your life in the extremely unlikely event of an emergency at sea, and it's a requirement of vessels operating throughout most of the world.

When you arrive in your cabin you should find one life vest for each person who will sleep there; ask the cabin attendant for assistance if you cannot locate the vests or if the number is incorrect. On many ships, the vests themselves are marked with a letter or number code for an "assembly station." You'll also find information about your assigned assembly station on a placard near the door of your cabin.

Listen for the instructions that will be announced over the ship's public address system; you'll likely be asked to return to your cabin, pick up your life vest and proceed to the assembly station. When you arrive, a member of the crew will check your name off the list of passengers assigned to that lifeboat; in theory, a crew member may come looking for you if you don't show up.

Finally, you'll be instructed on how to properly put on the vest, shown the location of the emergency whistle and beacon on each vest, and given an explanation of how the lifeboats are lowered into position for boarding.

Pay attention to any instructions about fire safety. As I've already noted, fire is much more of a threat on a modern ship than collision with an iceberg.

Customs and Immigration Information

There are two official steps in the process of entering a foreign country and returning to your home nation—immigration and customs.

Put simply, immigration is the process of clearing you into a country, and customs is the process of allowing your possessions the same privilege.

In this section, I'll concentrate on customs and immigration processes for American citizens leaving and returning to the United States. Similar requirements apply to citizens of other countries; ask the cruise line or your travel agent any specific questions about your situation.

Immigration

The Immigration and Naturalization Service, part of the Department of Justice, is responsible for the movement of people in and out of the United States.

For information on obtaining a passport or other immigration questions, contact the nearest passport agency in person or by mail or phone; you may also be able to obtain assistance from some U.S. post offices and some town or city clerks of court. Your travel agency should also be able to direct you to the nearest and most convenient office.

You can write for information by addressing a letter to the passport agency at the nearest of the following zip codes: Boston 02222-0123; Chicago 60604-1564; Honolulu 96850; Houston 77002-4874; Los Angeles 90024-3614; Miami 33130-1680; New Orleans 70113-1931; New York 10111-0031; Philadelphia 19106-1684; San Francisco 94105-2773; Seattle 98174-1091; Stamford, CT 06901-2767; Washington, D.C. 20524-0002.

The cruise line will ask to see your passport or identification papers before you embark on the ship. This allows the company to certify to foreign destinations that all passengers are legally able to enter; in most cases you will not have to produce your passport to actually enter the country at the port. The next time you will have to produce your passport is likely to be upon your return to the United States.

Customs

On the customs side, administered by the U.S. Customs Service, there are two principal concerns—security and duties.

Obviously, it is not a smart idea to go through an inspection point with illegal drugs or weapons. Also prohibited—lottery tickets, obscene articles and publications, seditious and treasonable materials, and hazardous articles such as fireworks, dangerous toys, and toxic or poisonous substances.

It's a good idea to carry prescription drugs in a pharmacist's bottle or with a copy of the prescription from your doctor. In a pinch, your hometown pharmacy should be able to certify that the pills you carry have been ordered by an accredited physician.

Duties are a special form of taxes levied on certain types or amounts of imported goods. As this book goes to press, each returning U.S. resident is permitted to bring home up to $400 in goods without having to pay duty. Included in that $400 exemption is up to 100 cigars and 200 cigarettes; residents over the age of 21 can also bring back one liter of alcohol. The next $1,000 worth of items is taxed at a flat duty rate of 10 percent.

Traveling with children. If a single parent is traveling with a minor child, the cruise line or immigration authorities may refuse boarding or entry without a legally binding letter from both parents—even if they are divorced—granting permission for the minor to leave the country. Consult an attorney and the cruise line for advice if you fall into this category.

Note that certain items, including Cuban cigars and other products, are generally not allowed into the U.S., even though they are readily available in Canada and some other nearby countries. In 1998, restrictions on travel to Cuba were relaxed slightly, and U.S. residents are now permitted to bring back up to $100 in Cuban goods purchased in Cuba itself.

Other acquisitions may qualify for duty-free treatment under other exemptions, such as the Generalized System of Preferences, which awards duty-free treatment to many goods from developing countries. Fine art (not handicrafts) and antiques older than 100 years are commonly acquired items that also do not require the payment of duty.

And there are all sorts of interesting sidetrips in the regulations. For example, though fine art is exempted for duty, you may be liable for tax on the picture frame that surrounds it.

If your cruise included a visit to one of the U.S. Virgin Islands, the personal exemption is $1,200, although no more than $400 worth of items within that $1,200 exemption can come from foreign nations outside the U.S. Virgin Islands.

If you are returning directly from any of the following countries, your customs exemption is $600; note that if you make an intermediate stop at another country, the exemption drops back to $400: Nevis, Saint Lucia, Saint Vincent and the Grenadines, and Trinidad and Tobago.

Finally, to qualify for an exemption you must be returning from a stay abroad of at least 48 hours and you cannot use more than one exemption within a 30-day period.

Be sure to check with the cruise line or the U.S. Immigration and Customs Service for the latest regulations.

Regulations for returning Canadian citizens are similar, with an exemption of up to $500 (CDN), including up to 40 ounces of alcohol, 200 cigarettes, and 50 cigars.

The "Duty-Free" Confusion

In most seaports and airports, the streets and corridors are chock-a-block with "duty free" stores. If you didn't know better, you could reasonably assume this meant that items for sale there are free from duty when travelers return home. That's not the case.

Articles sold in duty-free shops are free of duty and taxes for the country in which the shop is located, and items sold there are intended for export.

When you arrive in the United States, these items are subject to duty after you exceed your personal exemption.

Registering Foreign-Made Valuables

If you cross through customs with an expensive Japanese camera on your shoulder, an Italian scarf on your neck, and a fancy watch or piece of jewelry on your arm, the inspector can assume that all these items were purchased abroad and not in your neighborhood mall.

To establish that you brought these items from your home, bring proof of purchase, an insurance policy, or jeweler's appraisal. Or, you can register the serial numbers or other marks with Customs before you leave home.

Customs pays particular attention to expensive cameras (including special lenses and video equipment), binoculars, radios, foreign-made watches, and other similar appliances. To register items, take them to the customs office and obtain a validated Certificate of Registration (CF 4457) form; bring the form with you on your travels.

Prohibited Food Products

In general, you can bring home-packaged foods in sealed cans, bottles, and boxes. Baked goods and all cured cheeses are also permitted.

Most fruits and vegetables are either prohibited from entering the country or require an import permit. Every fruit or vegetable must be declared to the customs officer and must be presented for inspection, no matter how free of pests it appears to be.

Note that the states of Hawaii and California also have very strict prohibitions against the import of fruits and vegetables; the regulations are in place to protect against the introduction of pests and diseases that could be damaging to the native crops.

Plants, cuttings, seeds, unprocessed plant products and certain endangered species either require an import permit or are prohibited from entering the United States. Meat, poultry, and processed food products including ham, frankfurters, sausage, and pate are either prohibited or restricted, depending on the animal diseases prevalent in the country of origin. Canned meat is permitted if the inspector can determine it is commercially canned and can be kept without refrigeration.

Transportation of Currency

You may take on your trip as much currency or monetary equivalents as you wish. However, if you take out or bring into the United States more than $10,000, you are required to file a report with the U.S. Customs Service.

Chapter 11

Cruise Diaries: A Season at Sea

Crossing the Pond on Holland America's *Maasdam*

We decided to pop over to London to catch a musical in the West End.

The trip east across the Atlantic began with a hectic trek through steamy Boston to a hellious scene at Logan Airport: a block-long line of passengers waiting to drag their bags to the check-in counter of Virgin Atlantic.

The 747 jumbo jet, crammed with more than 500 passengers, took off late, of course. We spent the night crammed into a narrow seat in the economy section, sandwiched between a very large woman with four bags of oddly configured stuff at her feet and several caterwauling babies across the aisle.

Tossing and turning in our seats, we desperately tried to snatch a few moments of sleep between interruptions: a meal served at 10 P.M. on tiny plastic dishes perched on the uncertain support of a tray table; a forgettable movie on a tiny screen, and the sales pitches for useless trinkets from the onboard duty-free store.

The good news was that we were moving across the Atlantic at about 500 miles per hour. Mercifully, we landed at London's Gatwick Airport at the reasonable hour of 8 A.M., except that it was 3 A.M. to us and we had slept in our clothes all night.

After dragging our bags through customs, we squeezed onto a packed train from Gatwick to downtown London. It was two more hours before we were able to make it to our London hotel, where—miracle of miracles—we were able to check in and go to our room (although most of the others on line were told they would have to wait for the arrival of the cleaning staff.)

The room itself was typical for a European city: very small and relatively expensive—about $200 per night for a view of a back alley in Kensington.

We fortified ourselves with coffee, tea, chocolate, and other forms of caffeine to fight off the effects of the sleepless night and the sudden five-hour change in time zones. Exhausted and jittery, we managed to stay awake through *Miss Saigon* in the West End and stroll the streets of one of our favorite cities.

The bottom line: an overnight flight to Europe is a very efficient way to get from Point A to Point B. It is, in general, not all that pleasant in between.

Coming Home

Two days later, we began our trip home. We floated westward, happily ensconced in an attractive stateroom with a picture window looking out on the ocean–not huge, but larger than our room in London–and waited upon by a cabin attendant, room service, and dining room staff.

As you may have guessed, we were not on a 747 this time. Instead, we crossed the Atlantic on the elegant *Maasdam* of the Holland America Line, a week-long trip at 20 knots that would deposit us back in Boston.

Our voyage was a repositioning cruise, a special trip to move a cruise ship from one part of the world to another. The *Maasdam* had traveled through Europe and the Baltic in the summer, and was being dispatched to the east coast of the United States for a series of trips through New England to the Maritime Provinces of Canada. Later in the fall, she would move south from Boston to Florida for winter cruises in the Caribbean.

Repositioning itineraries can offer some of the best bargains in cruising, with extended periods at sea and unusual ports; however, they're not everyone's cup of tea. A transatlantic cruise is not one I would recommend for first-timers, and certainly not for someone who is apprehensive about the prospect of being cooped up on a ship for a week.

The ship departed from Harwich, about 70 miles east of London. Harwich (pronounced har'-itch) is a busy commercial port on the English Channel, home to cruise ships, freighters from around the world, and passenger and car ferries to the Hook of Holland and other destinations in Europe. The modern cruise terminal is about 50 yards from the train station, about an hour's ride from London's Liverpool Street Station.

For the middle five days of the trip we saw nothing but ocean–no ships, no planes, no shoreline. We carried our civilization with us, like moon explorers.

However, no astronaut has ever lived in the lap of luxury like we did.

Elegance Afloat

Holland America Line is a notch above the middle of the market. It offers much of the refinement and a bit of the service of the luxury lines at a price closer to that of the economy brands. The company was purchased by Carnival Cruise Lines in 1989, but has maintained its own identity and class well in the succeeding decade.

The *Maasdam* is an elegant ship, one of four nearly identical sister ships in the HAL fleet. It's a particularly workable design with lots of attractive public space including a stunning showroom and handsome dining room; hardly a tiny ship at 720 feet long and 55,451 tons, within it feels much larger.

One of the hallmarks of Holland America is the onboard collection of art, spread throughout the ships. At most every turn, you're greeted by paintings, sculptures, and antiques, most with a maritime link or a connection to great Dutch explorations. A large electronic map on the upper promenade charts the ship's progress and can also be programmed to display famous maritime explorations, including those of Columbus, Captain Cook, and others.

One of the prettiest public rooms is CrowsNest up high over the bow with views ahead, to port and starboard, and toward the stern over the Sports Deck.

On this cruise without any port calls, there was something going on almost everywhere most times of the day. In fact, we found it hard to find a place that would remain private and quiet for more than a few hours before another activity or group began. The attractive library on the upper promenade deck, with a wall of windows behind the reading desks, was busy much of the day.

The *Maasdam* is among the few modern ships with a covered promenade that makes a complete circuit of the ship, four laps to the mile. Another nice touch, common to many of the Holland America ships, is a moveable dome over the pool deck. In warm and dry weather, the dome is retracted to leave the pool area open to the sky but still protected from winds; in cool or wet weather, the dome remakes the deck into a large indoor pool and patio area.

On our crossing of the Atlantic, we greatly appreciated both the covered promenade and the dome.

How We Almost Missed the Boat

If I ever needed a reminder of my own advice about confirming departure times (and ports) before the start of a cruise voyage, I received one with the *Maasdam*.

The published departure time—printed right there on our tickets—was 6 P.M. We decided to get to Harwich a few hours early to walk around the port city; we arrived near noon to find a sign announcing that the gangplank would be withdrawn at 1:30 P.M., and the ship would sail an hour later.

Passengers who had purchased transfers from Holland America from the airport or London to the port had been notified on arrival. Those of us who made our own way to Harwich nearly missed the boat; we were among the last to climb aboard.

This is not insignificant on any cruise, but especially so on a transatlantic repositioning cruise like ours. If you miss a cruise ship sailing out of Miami, for example, you should be able to fly on ahead of the vessel to meet up with the rest of your itinerary in Nassau or wherever the ship was headed next. On our cruise, though, there was to be no intermediate port between Harwich and Boston in seven days.

And so, a reminder to you and me: Confirm your departure and arrival times a week before you travel and if you are making your own way to the port, do so again a day before you begin your trip.

Crossing the Pond

We pulled out of Harwich on a Sunday, entering into the English Channel in the company of large freighters and fishing vessels. Monday morning we continued through the channel with the south of England to starboard and France to port. We sailed past Penzance, the Scilly Islands, and the distant, green shores of Ireland. And then we were out in the Atlantic.

It would be the following Friday before we saw another sign of human life–a huge oil rig anchored in the cold waters a few hundred miles out to sea off the coast of Labrador. And it would be Saturday before we saw distant land.

The summer of 1999 was a particularly active season for hurricanes. As we left port on Sunday we were aware of the progress of Hurricanes Cindy and Dennis, both of which were churning off the East Coast of the United States. But our course on the Great Circle Route, an arc to the northwest to above the 50th Latitude, was well north of the storms, or so we thought.

In this modern age of satellites, weather radar, and in-room CNN, it's all but impossible for a ship to be caught unawares by a storm. Two days into our weeklong journey, the captain . . . and most everyone else on the *Maasdam* . . . knew that Cindy had pulled away from the coast and was moving northward toward Iceland. In other words, it was due to cross our path.

On Wednesday, the master of the ship changed our course, heading due south off the Great Circle Route to drop below the storm. And so we did, but not without experiencing a few days of fierce weather in the North Atlantic: gale winds of up to 46 knots and seas to 27 feet. That said, we found the *Maasdam* to be extraordinarily stable in very rough seas; the modern stabilizers countered much of the rolling motion leaving just a bit of end-to-end pitching. Up top, the water in the swimming pool was almost wild enough for a surfing competition; the crew finally had to drain the pool for safety. The mostly experienced passengers handled the weather pretty well, although we noted a few casualties to seasickness, including our waiter in the dining room.

By Friday, the storm was gone and we proceeded down the coast of Labrador and Newfoundland, passing within 200 nautical miles of the location of the resting place of the *Titanic*, a particularly empty stretch of ocean, especially at night.

Entertainment Afloat

The 800 or so guests (out of a possible capacity of about 1,200) represented a more sophisticated than usual group of travelers, aboard for the romance of it all and not for the ports of call.

The card rooms and libraries were packed for most of the trip. By night, the lounges were filled with an unusually diverse crew of entertainers, including a big band, two comedians, an instrumentalist, a pair of tap dancers 40 years too late for the Borscht Belt, a troupe of dancers and singers, and the *Maasdam's* capable house band.

A major lure, for some, was the special presence of the Harry James Orchestra, a big band troupe that carries on the name and arrangements of the famous bandleader; James died in 1983, but the band was continued by a former member of the group, Fred Radke. The orchestra performed half a dozen times on the trip.

Also onboard was comedian Marty Brill, a veteran performer and writer. He tailored his witty shows to the mellow crowd aboard the *Maasdam*; some will remember him for the sharper edge he displayed as a cohort of Lenny Bruce. In fact, Brill portrayed Bruce on Broadway in a one-man show.

The dance troupe put on enthusiastic and capable revues, right up the middle of the road. The dancing was pretty good, especially on the small (and sometimes pitching) stage; the singing was, well, enthusiastic. A Broadway medley was the best offering. Another night we saw a bit of "Personality," an uninspired salute to performers most of whom were dead long before the young dancers first strapped on their shoes: Maurice Chevalier and Jimmy Durante included, plus soulless recountings of Frank Sinatra, The Supremes, Sammy Davis Jr., and Elvis Presley.

And then there was the food, which was somewhat mystifying: the presentation was very good, but the preparation was disappointing. In other words, the food looked great, but tasted rather ordinary. It was a common commentary we heard at most every turn at dinner time.

We found the ship's photographers a bit too much in evidence at boarding, formal dinners, and many other shipboard activities. My wife and I are not at all keen in being interrupted at dinner by a member of the cruise director's staff made up as a pirate, or as a Dutch milkmaid, each accompanied by a cameraman. But they kept coming. If you're not comfortable shooing the photographer away, do remember, though, that you don't have to buy any photos they take.

All in all, though, we found Holland America Line's product to be a very good one. Nice ships, nice appointments, great crew, and a most relaxing crossing.

A Grand Old Lady: The Swinging SS *Norway*

Late October on the *Norway* was a tale of two hurricanes.

It was also a wonderful journey of more than 60 fabulous musicians, and hundreds of dedicated fans, spread nicely down the length of the world's longest cruise ship. Our trip was one of two week-long Jazz Cruises in the Caribbean, a long-standing tradition on NCL that attracts a loyal following each year.

The *Norway* is one of the last of the transatlantic steamships, built as the SS *France* in 1962 and lovingly restored and updated by Norwegian Cruise Line as the *Norway* for modern days and modern cruise passengers.

The Winds of October

The *Norway* was out in the Western Caribbean on a seven-day cruise as Hurricane Irene suddenly arose south of Cuba. On Thursday, the storm passed over Cuba and set its aim on the Florida Keys.

We had arrived in Miami on that same Thursday to spend a few days enjoying the lively culture and scenery of the area. The skies began to darken in the afternoon, though, and by evening the rain began to fall in colossal downpours. We went to bed in our hotel on the water on narrow Miami Beach, secure in the weather forecast that the storm would head into the Gulf of Mexico, missing Miami and making landfall further north around Tampa. We awoke to find that Irene had changed her mind and was making a hook to the east and coming on shore just outside of Miami.

Throughout the day, torrents of rain fell, as much as 15 inches in parts of Miami. In the afternoon, wind gusts of as much as 75 mph raked the area. Funneling through some of the canyons between high-rise hotels on the beach and in downtown, the winds knocked over palm trees and brought down signs and utility poles. Tragically, four people were killed when they stepped into pools of water that contained downed power lines.

We took a midday expedition from our hotel to a shopping mall, crossing one of the sea level causeways between Miami Beach and Miami; the water lapped at the side of the road and our little rental car vibrated wildly in the wind. After a brief and uneasy stay, we crossed back to Miami Beach and buttoned ourselves into the relative security of the hotel.

Until the cable television system at the hotel failed at nightfall, we tracked the storm as best we could. We wondered where the *Norway* had gone to avoid the storm. And, we wondered, where would she be the next morning at 6 A.M. when she was scheduled to arrive in Miami to unload her passengers and pick us up for our voyage?

The *Norway* Is Located

It turned out that the *Norway* had more or less kept to her schedule at sea, heading east to its planned stop at Great Stirrup Cay, NCL's private island in the Bahamas, north of Nassau. Ironically, Stirrup Cay had just been reopened to NCL ships after the repair of damage caused by Hurricane Floyd a few months earlier.

In many ways, if you're going to travel in the company of hurricanes, a large, fast, and well-provisioned cruise ship is a good place to be. Hurricanes, though they are huge weather events, are nevertheless typically only 25 to 50 miles across with strong winds extending out perhaps 100 miles from the eye. They usually move at speeds of about 10 to 15 miles per hour, and forecasters are pretty capable of predicting the general direction of travel.

And so, unless a ship's captain makes a very bad decision and heads directly into the path of an oncoming storm, he can instead take his moving platform away from its path. The *Norway* can make as much as 20 knots in most conditions, about 23 miles per hour, and run ahead of the storm.

The rub, though, comes when the ship has to return to a particular port to unload its passengers and pick up a new group. And in this case, Hurricane Irene lay between Stirrup Cay and Miami.

As prodigious rain and winds pounded Miami Friday night, we heard the news that the Port of Miami–along with the airport through which most of the arriving guests would pass, and most everything else in the area–was officially closed.

NCL's corporate headquarters in Miami was of no use; earlier in the day, the reservations clerks were promising that the *Norway* would sail the next day without any delay. By afternoon when we called again, the main office was closed "because of hurricane conditions." That much we knew; what we didn't know was where the *Norway* would spend the night and where she would be at 6 A.M. the next morning.

The *Norway* ended up circling Stirrup Cay all day Friday, unable to offload its passengers because of rough seas and uncertain about when the U.S. Coast Guard would reopen Miami harbor.

Saturday morning dawned clear and beautiful, the storm moving northeast to Fort Lauderdale and then up the coast. We ventured out onto the streets of Miami, dodging downed palm trees, cautiously creeping through intersections with non-functioning traffic lights, and making our way to the pier. There, as we crossed the causeway from Miami Beach to Miami, we saw in the distance the unmistakable blue hull of the *Norway* just entering the harbor.

It was nearly 11 A.M. before the ship finally tied up at the pier on Dodge Island, and 1 P.M. before the first passengers began to disembark. Buses were waiting to take them to airports in Miami or Fort Lauderdale, where another storm-created mess awaited. Hundreds of flights had been canceled on Friday, and many aircraft were out of position for their Saturday schedule.

When we finally were allowed to embark at nearly 3 P.M., there were only a few hundred of us on board. More than a thousand guests and many of the jazz musicians who were to be the stars of the week-long theme cruise were not expected to arrive until late in the evening, hours after our scheduled 4 P.M. departure.

Moon Over Miami

Captain Geir Lokøen advised passengers he would wait as long as he could for late arrivals; as it turned out that stretched to after 11 P.M. Saturday night. The last baggage loaded by the stevedores were two huge upright basses.

We were happy to be finally at sea. As we went to bed, though, there was vague warning of another tropical disturbance deep in the Caribbean. We put our trust in the advanced technology on the bridge and the many years of experience of the captain and officers, looking forward to our arrival on St. Martin two full days later.

And right on schedule, the *Norway* arrived at Phillipsburg, the Dutch capital of St. Maarten. There is no dock big enough or waters deep enough to permit the *Norway* to tie up at a landing pier; instead, we set anchor in the harbor. We joined a few hundred fellow passengers on the first tender to shore.

St. Maarten has long been one of our favorite islands in the Caribbean, with a bustling commercial center on the Dutch side around Phillipsburg and a very French, relatively quiet other country called St. Martin with its capital at Marigot. (If you're coming to stay, you'll find a wide range of hotels and condominiums on the Dutch side and the best beaches, trendiest shops, and extraordinary small restaurants and patisseries on French territory.)

We picked up a rental car in Phillipsburg and headed out on a circuit of the island on the single road that circles the island–more or less two lanes wide, mostly paved, and possessed of a few relatively gnarly switchbacks as they cross the central spine of hills on the island.

Just over the border between the Dutch and French sides (a simple stone marks the border) are the Terres Basses (Lowlands) that include some of the loveliest beaches in all of the Caribbean: Baie Longue (Long Bay), Baie aux Prunes (Plum Bay), and Baie Rouge (Red Bay). We stopped for a swim at the nearly perfect strand of Baie Longue; at the north end of the beach is the ultra-exclusive resort of La Samana, regular home to Hollywood and rock stars and the otherwise well-possessed; if you have to ask the price for a night's stay, you can't afford to sleep there.

On our visit, though, the beach was all but deserted. Two other couples, dressed only in suntan lotion and sand, occupied blankets 50 yards in each direction. There was, though, plenty of company in the crystal waters; hundreds of iridescent fish accompanied us as we swam.

Next stop was Marigot, where we picked up a peasant lunch worthy of the Provençale: a fresh-baked baguette, a wedge of exquisite Catalane cheese, and a few bottles of Ting, a Caribbean grapefruit soda. (We would have completed the picnic with a jug of wine, but there were those switchbacks ahead of us on the road.)

We continued our tour through the open plain of La Savane and then the small village of Grand Case, a refuge of haute cuisine cafés. Somewhere around the Quartier d'Orleans, we tuned the car radio into a local station to hear the mayor of Phillipsburg declare a state of emergency: Hurricane José was barreling north, heading directly for St. Maarten, and the U.S. Virgin Islands of St. John and St. Thomas.

Returning our rental car, we headed into Phillipsburg to see a sight few tourists have ever experienced in the Caribbean: shopkeepers were turning away visitors with credit cards. The town was shutting down ahead of the storm, and so we took the tender back to the *Norway*.

A Change of Plans

It came as no surprise at dinner to hear Captain Lokøen announce that our plans for the next day had been scrambled by the storm. The port of St. Thomas had been closed by authorities, and instead we would steam north to the Bahamas to stay ahead of Hurricane José.

The next day I met with Lokøen in his spacious office just off the bridge. We began by talking about the weather.

I asked why we had not diverted westward to make an unscheduled stop at Jamaica instead of adding another day at sea to the schedule. Lokøen said he had considered Jamaica, but a visit there would have made it impossible for the ship to make its way to its planned stop at Stirrup Cay three days hence. And, he said, there was no certainty that Hurricane José wouldn't make a swing westward. The safest route was to stay ahead of the storm and be ready to move out of its way if it moved east or westward.

A cruise in hurricane conditions, Lokøen said, is a "search for solutions." In the middle of the week, a change in ports does not matter as much, he said. Some guests may be disappointed because the ship has to skip a port, he said, but more would be upset if the *Norway* was unable to get back to its home port on time.

The *Norway* could dock in Florida at Miami, Fort Lauderdale, or Port Canaveral, Lokøen said. In an emergency, she could offload its passengers in the Bahamas, but the airport there could not easily transport passengers back to Miami, especially if four or five other cruise ships in the area chose to come into Bermuda.

"We have many contingencies," Lokøen said, "but every contingency needs a contingency."

A Man in Love

I left the contingency planning to the captain and his staff. Instead we talked about the ship that would take us out of José's way.

"I have always been in love with this ship. Since I was a boy," Lokøen said. "I went to sea when this ship came out in 1962," he continued. "I was 15 years old. I knew I could not be a captain of this ship as long as I was a Norwegian citizen because it flew a French flag."

Of course all that changed when Norwegian Cruise Line purchased the SS *France*, laid up in a French dock after its career as a transatlantic liner had been ended by the arrival of the jet airplane.

Lokøen has been with NCL for 21 years, including 15 years on the *Norway*. For nine of those years he was master of the *Norway*, making him the longest-serving captain in the history of the ship. Soon after our cruise in late 1999, though, he was due to leave the *Norway* to oversee the construction of the sister ship to the *Norwegian Sky*, scheduled to set sail in late 2000. When the ship goes to sea, Lokøen should be at the helm, moving from the oldest ship in the fleet to the newest.

We talked about the changes NCL has made to the *Norway* over the years. "When she was the *France*, she was perfect," Lokøen said. "She's still very seaworthy and a nice ship to take the elements."

When the ship served as a liner, she had four engines and four propellers. She was converted to two engines and propellers; much of the original equipment remains in place deep down in the hull. Two decks of luxury staterooms were added to the top of the ship in 1990; down below some of the former fuel tanks for the unused engines were filled with permanent ballast to balance the extra weight.

Within the ship, the Windward dining room is essentially unchanged from its days as the first-class restaurant. A sky of electric stars twinkles in a dome over the tables. The Leeward dining room, though it serves the same food, is much less impressive.

Among the unusual features of the *France* were the Provençale Villas, a set of staterooms on the original upper deck that surrounded a small private courtyard. When the ship was converted to cruising, a pool was installed to nearly fill the courtyard. Today, if you can find an obscure doorway on Fjord deck marked "Porthole," you can enter into an unusual world frozen in time. The villas are still there, but instead of a view of the sky, they have a view of a porthole into the swimming pool.

One of the most important modifications to the ship was the addition of a pair of massive tenders mounted on the forward deck. The 71-ton, 86-foot-long vessels can deliver 450 passengers to a dock or pull up on the beach like a landing craft with a ramp that lowers from the front. Instead of soldiers with machine guns, though, defenders on the beach are assaulted by tourists rushing to the barbecue.

The tenders are necessary because the *Norway* is unable to enter many smaller ports around the world; built for stability on transatlantic crossings, she has a deep draft of 34 feet. That puts her in the same class as the *QE2*, which has a draft of 33 feet.

"Without these tenders we would not be able to do what we do with this ship," Lokøen said. "It's the best solution to cruising in the Caribbean.

"The most common complaint is that the ship is difficult to find your way around on," Lokøen said. "This is because it was originally built with two classes, with gates and decks cut off from each other."

That structural problem may also present a limit to the useful life of the *Norway*. International maritime safety regulations that go into effect in 2009 will mandate that all shipboard stair towers go from the lowest deck to the highest. On the *Norway*, many of the stairs serve only portions of the ship, and Lokøen observes that reworking the internals of the stairs would be extremely expensive.

Operationally, the ship can take many more years, Lokøen said. He said it was NCL's goal to keep the *Norway* in service until 2009. I do have to point out that shortly after our cruise, NCL was dragged into a process that ended up with the company losing its independence; in early 2000, the company was taken over by a joint operation owned by Star Cruises of Malaysia and Carnival Cruise Lines. It is uncertain what, if any, changes will be made to NCL's fleet in years to come.

A Floating Jazz Festival

For nearly two decades, NCL has carried jazz fans out to sea with some of their favorite performers for an intense week of concerts and get-togethers.

I have to admit right up front that my wife and I are not serious jazz fans, something that made us a distinct minority among the 1,800 passengers on board the *Norway*. In a way, though, it was a great advantage: we strolled from lounge to showroom to café, sampling musical styles without the baggage of experience.

Among the performers aboard the ship for the week were the Ray Brown Trio, the Freddy Cole Quartet, the Jimmy McGriff Quartet, the Eddie Higgins Trio, Sphere, singer Ernie Andrews, and the 19-piece Frank Foster & His Loud Minority Big Band.

Featured performer in the Saga Theatre was Ernestine Anderson, a classic jazz and soul singer; without a bit of expectation we took a seat. A minute or two later, we were converts and made plans to attend her next three shows. It was only later that we learned her history: a spectacular debut in 1956, performances with the likes of Lionel Hampton, Quincy Jones, and Ray Brown, appearances at Carnegie Hall, Kennedy Center, and the Hollywood Bowl, and more than 30 albums. After a number of years in forced retirement, she has been enjoying something of a revival in recent years. And as she told her audience, she was making her first, somewhat wobbly, appearance on the gently rolling stage of a cruise ship.

One other thing: the crowd onboard the *Norway* for the Jazz Cruise was the happiest group we have ever traveled with. We left Miami seven hours late; we missed our scheduled port call in St. Thomas; the seas were slightly rougher than some would have preferred. We heard nary a word of complaint: the music and the clubs and the parties were just fine, thank you.

In 2000, NCL plans three jazz cruises in October, and a Big Band cruise in November. In September, one cruise specializes in music of the fifties and sixties, and another on country music. Other theme cruises offered by NCL include pro football, hockey, basketball, and baseball.

Onboard the *Norway*

Don't look for a spectacular glass and chrome atrium or flashing neon buffets on the *Norway*. Remember instead this ship's history as the oceangoing expression of French culture. This is classic European elegance afloat.

You can check out a collection of relics from the *France* in a cabinet on International Deck port side forward. International Deck, the covered stroll that connects the shops and clubs was originally the promenade deck of the *France*. The most attractive of the public rooms is Club Internationale, the former first-class smoking lounge of the *France*.

A decidedly modern space on the ship is the Sports Illustrated Café, a sports bar equipped with dozens of television monitors and decorated with memorabilia from many sports–a Nolan Ryan uniform next to a pair of Dan Jansen's ice skates and an autographed picture of Don Larsen.

Alas, the video screens were tuned to just one channel–all-sports ESPN, which is sometimes a good thing but not always. Our cruise on the *Norway* took place during the baseball playoffs; while the rest of the sports world watched classic matchups between the New York Yankees and the Boston Red Sox, and the New York Mets and the Atlanta Braves, ESPN was showing a totally forgettable golf match, and during one memorably poor choice the café's monitors showed a curling match while we strained–unsuccessfully–to pick up a ball game on a portable radio we had brought along.

More so than on most ships, on the *Norway* there is a large difference between the least expensive rooms and the middle of the range. This ship was built as a two-class vessel; more than half of the passengers were looking just for transportation across the Atlantic, and the lowest echelon cabins are just that–basic transportation. The lesser staterooms are very small and the portholes are more like peepholes.

Cabins in Class A and B and suites, on the other hand, were built for cruisers and are quite nice with large windows and sitting areas. A handful of suites include verandas.

There are, also, significant differences between the two dining rooms on the *Norway*. The Leeward Restaurant was built for the second-class patrons, and it can most charitably be described as ordinary; there are no windows and the low ceiling makes it feel more like a college dining hall than an eatery on a luxury cruise ship. The Windward Restaurant, built for first-class diners, is much more attractive, with a central circular dome decorated with a twinkling starfield ceiling; again, though, there are no windows.

The setting aside, the food and service is the same in both dining rooms. And NCL's food is a cut or two above ordinary, among the best menus, presentation, and quality you will find among ships in the middle and upper-middle range of cruise ships.

But the real star is Le Bistro. This small, very elegant restaurant comes equipped with a first-class Continental menu, extremely attentive waiters, and drop dead gorgeous appointments, including a window wall. Le Bistro is open every night for dinner; reservations are available a day in advance. There is no extra charge to dine there, although guests are asked to leave a gratuity of $5 per person per meal. The menu does not change from day to day, although a special chef's recommendation of one or two entrees is added each evening.

Our floating island missed the hurricanes, chauffeuring us on a music-filled, pampered excursion back to the future.

Crown Dynasty: If It's Wednesday, This Must Be Grenada

The *Crown Dynasty* is a well-turned out young lady with an excellent pedigree, despite the fact that she's been through more than a few hands over the years.

She was built in Spain in 1993 as the *Crown Dynasty* for the original Crown Cruise Line; she then went on to the lavish operations of Cunard Line as the *Cunard Dynasty* and then for a short time as the *Crown Majesty* of the Majesty Cruise Line. In 1997, she took on the name of *Norwegian Dynasty* under a two-year lease to Norwegian Cruise Line.

In 1999, she became the first ship of the new Crown Cruise Line, a premium brand that is part of Commodore Cruise Line. And in the process she regained her original name and an end-to-end polishing and refurbishment.

Crown's goal is to offer a "premium" cruise at a less-than-premium price, with prices positioned just above the level you'd pay for most mid-range ships like those in the Carnival fleet, for example. I believe they've succeeded, at least for that portion of the cruise market not looking for a city at sea; the *Crown Dynasty* is more of an elegant little town.

This is a handsome mid-sized ship with more style and class than most mass-market megaships, but with a lot less to do. Don't expect Broadway shows or huge dance floors. Don't look for alternative restaurants. And don't expect a jaw-dropping skyscraper atrium.

Think instead of the *Crown Dynasty* as a comfortable way to float from interesting place to place, all the while cosseted in the lap of near-luxury. This is not the opulent and sybaritic *Seabourn Legend* or the *Crystal Harmony* (but you're not paying the stratospheric prices of those lines, either), but it is also not the pedestrian world of a Carnival party ship, either.

Crown Cruise Line has modeled its operations around the original intention of the builders of the *Crown Dynasty*, a premium cruise a notch above the middle of the market.

We sailed on one of the first cruises after Crown began operations, and though not perfect, the cruise line's intentions were obvious.

The cabins were nicely appointed, with above-average attention from attendants. We stayed in a junior suite, the same size as the best oceanview stateroom but decorated with lovely glass and chrome appointments and located up high above the lifeboats. There are just a dozen deluxe suites, and these include private balconies.

The Hamilton Dining Room is a handsome room at the stern, with three walls of windows. On our shakedown cruise, dinners were well prepared and presented, with excellent beef and seafood offerings. Crown has contracted with the same provisioning company that serves the well-regarded galleys on Celebrity Cruises in the Caribbean.

Lunches and breakfasts, alas, were less impressive. Missing was a midday barbecue or special meal; according to Crown, though, the line has plans to upgrade the other meals to the level of dinner. Guests who cherish tables for two will find doubles very scarce, and we found the dining room staff surprisingly uncooperative when guests asked for special treatment; again, we were told the new staff would be given further training on delivering premium service.

Something we did like was the relatively low-key entertainment programming. The casino was lively deep into the night, you could find a bingo game if you really wanted, and there were the usual art auctions and pitches for photography, but guests who wanted to ignore the sideshows could easily do so. There were very few announcements to the ship at large; instead, the in-room television sets were used to alert guests to activities.

The small Gombey Lounge, forward on the St. George's deck, is used for nightly entertainment. It was basic fare, put on by a troupe of earnest, young dancers and singers. There's no movie theater on the ship, but the televisions in the staterooms offer two channels of current films.

The real star of the Caribbean cruise was the itinerary, with stops at five islands on a seven-day cruise. Departing from Aruba, the ship spent one day at sea and then stopped at St. Lucia, Barbados, Grenada, Bonaire, and Curaçao on succeeding days before returning to Aruba.

Crown Cruise Line has put together a better-than-average collection of shore excursions in each of its port of call.

St. Lucia is among the more interesting islands in the Caribbean; the *Crown Dynasty* made an early morning procession into the small harbor at Soufrière, which sits at the base of the awesome twin mountain spires of Gros Piton and Petit Piton. From there, she proceeded to a pier in the capital of Castries.

We boarded a sailing catamaran at Castries and headed back down the coast to Soufrière; there we clambered into a taxi for a visit to the famed drive-in volcano up the hill above the harbor. Don't expect to see Mount Vesuvius; what we've got here is the collapsed caldera of a long-ago volcano just around the bend from The Pitons. Black mud bubbles up in pools (after a heavy rain you can expect to see geysers) and the air is heavy with the smell of sulphur.

Nearby in Soufrière is the Diamond Botanical Garden, a lush private plantation. Paths lead to gardens and natural stands of many of the fruits and flowers of the island en route to an encounter with a 40-foot waterfall of hot water from a volcanic source.

Back on the catamaran for the cruise back to the ship, the rum punch ran freely, and the enthusiastic young crew helped keep the journey a party at every turn. We anchored at a secluded beach at Anse Cochon and then cruised through the yacht anchorage at Marigot Bay on the way back to the ship at Castries.

Bustling Barbados offers a full range of attractions, including visits to the Mount Gay Rum distillery, Atlantis submarine tours of offshore reefs, and Harrison's Cave, a natural limestone cave with a 40-foot waterfall that cascades into a blue-green lake.

Grenada is a lovely island, with spices and fruit hanging like manna from the trees: bananas, coconuts, nutmeg, cocoa, mangoes, breadfruit, and more. Also sugar cane, cinnamon, ginger.

We put on our hiking boots and headed out on a climb of Morne Gazo, an undisturbed rain forest that rises to 1,140 feet above the harbor; the walkway to the top is paved in fragrant nutmeg shells.

On the way back to St. George's Pier in Grenada, our driver took us through a succession of little towns including the intriguingly named Perdmontemps, something close to French for "waste my time." The settlement is at the site where a French settler thought he saw the glimmer of gold. It turned out to be a waste of time, leaving behind today a simple village on the hillside with a quaint name.

We also visited the Grenada Sugar Factory, better known as the maker of Clarke's Court Rum. The hospitality center offers tastes of the company's wares, better sampled after you've hiked the rain forest than before. Especially tasty and potent is the distillery's Spice Rum.

I crossed the field from the shop to the hulking distillery and asked one of the workers for a tour. We stepped through the gates and back in time nearly a hundred years. Most of the machinery for conveying, chopping, and processing the sugar cane is from the nineteenth century; a furnace burns cane husks to make steam for a 90-year-old Scottish engine with a huge geared wheel.

There's a tourist agency at the cruise dock and from there you can take a ferry for a few dollars to Grand Anse beach, or hook up with a taxi for tours.

Bonaire is famed for its reefs, magnets for snorkelers and scuba divers from around the world. The reefs, alas, had been damaged by a freak hurricane in the fall of 1999, but the waters are still filled with an amazing variety of sea creatures.

We took a tender out to the Samur, a lovely Siamese-style junk that made its way all the way from Bangkok, Thailand to Bonaire. Beneath her teak decks is a lovely set of cabins occupied by some of the young crew.

We sailed out of the harbor and to the isolated "No Name Beach" on Klein Bonaire, a small barrier island offshore from the capital of Kralendijk. Careful snorkelers could find openings in the sharp coral reef just off shore to swim down the length of the beach; I set off alone from the san spit back to the anchored ship a few hundred feet off shore, accompanied all the way by a set of barracuda and an army of neon blue and green fish.

You can also take a water taxi directly from Kralendijk to Klein Bonaire.

Curaçao, the last port of call on the trip proved the most adventurous. We rented a four-wheel-drive jeep for a seven-hour tour of the island in an escorted convoy. Traveling most of the time on steep and narrow paths along the beach and hillsides, stops include Boka Tabla, a sea cave on the rough west side of the island, a real bat cave, and a beach stop.

Crown Cruise Line is off to a good start; industry scuttlebutt says the company plans to add several more smaller, high-end vessels to its fleet. The *Crown Dynasty* is due to sail out of Aruba in the winters of 2000 and 2001, with summer calls to Bermuda from Philadelphia and Baltimore and a two-week fall excursion from Baltimore to Atlantic Canada and Quèbec City.

Ahoy, Mickey! *Disney Magic* and *Disney Wonder* from Port Canaveral to the Bahamas

As we drove north on A1A on the flat barrier island of Cocoa Beach in Florida, traffic suddenly slowed to a near-stop. That seemed perfectly understandable, for none of us was prepared for the sight of a bright and shiny 100-story skyscraper floating on its side at the end of the road.

We were there for the maiden voyage of the *Disney Magic*, the $350 million firstborn of the Disney Cruise Line.

Now let me say right up front that I had my misgivings about the *Disney Magic* before I crossed the gangplank. I spend an inordinate amount of my time with Mickey Mouse and friends each year, keeping my travel books on Orlando and Anaheim up-to-date. It's not that I don't like Disneyland or Walt Disney World, it's just that I had a fear that too many parts of my world were coming together. I wanted the glamour, excitement, and sublime relaxation of a cruise, not the oh-too-popular hubbub of the theme park.

Well, I was 90 percent wrong, and 100 percent satisfied. Disney has done a wonderful job of creating a pair of cruise ships that—like a Disney classic film—bring together our dearest fantasies, an impressive display of artistry, and some welcome touches of the real world.

Disney chose as its initial target the 90 percent or so of travelers who have never taken a cruise before; at the same time, even the most experienced cruise veteran will recognize how Disney has paid loving homage to the great ocean liners of the past.

The fantasy begins with the exterior design of the twin ships, which consciously evoke the memory of the classic transatlantic liners of the pre-jet era, vessels like the *Queen Mary*. Their long, sleek hulls are painted jet black; atop the white upper half sit a pair of bright red smokestacks. It's just about the way a child (of any age) would draw an ocean liner.

The black, white, and red colors of the ships, together with bright yellow lifeboats, not only evoke the colors of the great liners, they also match the color scheme for the admiral of the fleet, Mickey Mouse.

These are true Megaships, more than three football fields long at 964 feet from stem to stern, 11 decks tall, and 85,000 tons in size.

The artistry begins with those two smokestacks. The ultra-modern power plant for the ships requires only one set of pipes and those run through the stack toward the stern. The forward smokestack is there because the ship looks better with one. And as long as you've got this big stack, why not make some use of it: Disney's "Imagineers" installed a funky sports bar way up high and a dream-world club for teenagers (no adults allowed) at its base.

And the Imagineers took hold of the ship's design in a myriad of other wondrous ways—things like a truly spectacular central atrium with glass-walled elevators; a quartet of extraordinary and quirky restaurants that deliver fine food and more than a bit of Disney magic; a Broadway-quality theater that offers a different show every night; and a floor full of nightclubs for adults including a comedy club, a country-western bar, a jazz club; and a sophisticated chrome-and-glass piano bar where Noel Coward would have felt right at home.

The interior design of the *Disney Magic* is based around an Art Deco vocabulary, with rounded chrome and brass, carved wood details, and lovely oversized portholes along some of the interior promenade decks. The *Disney Wonder* is based on slightly different Art Nouveau flourishes.

The real world lies in the modern-day amenities, such as private verandas, relatively spacious family cabins that have nice touches such as privacy curtains to separate the kids from the parents, and an overall sense of elegance. Disney has left neon flash to Royal Caribbean, Carnival, and others; the real competition to these ships, at least in terms of design, are the Queens of Cunard present and past.

And finally, back to the fantasy. What kid wouldn't add a spiraling waterslide to the top-deck, kids-only swimming pool (adults have their own pond and there's also a third pool for families)? And how about nearly a full deck devoted to a kid's world of games, entertainment, and exploration, as well as a teens-only club up top and a state-of-the-art video arcade at sea?

And then there's Mickey. Disney is always quick to admit that it all started with a mouse. Mickey and his friends are there, making cameo appearances at the childrens' clubs and an occasional visit to the pools and restaurants. Goofy will sometimes appear on the dance floor in one of the clubs, or Minnie may make a visit to the shopping district. But, in truth, the Disney characters have a very low-key presence aboard ship. They're there if you look for them, but on my eight days at sea on the two ships, the cartoon characters seemed to fade into the background, outshone by the vessels themselves.

And if you want to show off your vacation photographs to friends who might turn up their noses at all things Disney, pass around the pictures of the classic lines of the ship, her black hull knifing through the blue waters off the Bahamas. They don't have to know that on the stern of the *Disney Magic* there's a 15-foot statue of Goofy hanging upside down in a boatswain's chair, the victim of a painting accident.

The Disney Experience

Until August of 2000, the *Disney Magic* and her near-identical twin *Disney Wonder* sail out of Port Canaveral, Florida on alternating three- and four-day cruises to Nassau in the Bahamas and to Disney's private beach island, Castaway Cay. Disney promotes its cruises as part of a week-long vacation that includes a few days at Walt Disney World in Orlando, about an hour away from the cruise port; you can, though, choose to book just a cruise.

Beginning in August, the *Disney Magic* will embark on a new week-long itinerary from Port Canaveral, visiting St. Maarten and St. Thomas in the Caribbean, plus a stop at Castaway Cay.

The Disney experience begins as soon as you arrive at the pier. No ordinary shared terminal was good enough for this Mickey Mouse operation. Instead, Disney secured its own pier and built a handsome $35 million terminal. The terminal echoes the Art Deco style of the ships, from its exterior arches and curves to the interior decorations that include a terra cotta Terrazzo tile map of Florida and the Western Caribbean on the floor of the reception area.

Our stateroom, in the "deluxe" category on both ships, which lies in the middle of the range from Royal Suite to Standard Inside, was an unusually roomy and cheery accommodation, more than adequate for a close-knit family . . . at least for the duration of a four-night cruise.

The kids had a pair of beds in the main cabin area; behind a hanging curtain was another sleeping area for my wife and myself. And beyond the bed chambers was a sliding glass door that lead to our favorite private spot on the ship—a comfortable veranda. It was our choice way to begin the day and end the evening.

About three quarters of the 875 staterooms have outside views, and nearly half have verandas—a welcome modern touch. And most of the cabins offer a bath-and-a-half design in which one bathroom holds a sink and toilet, the other a sink and bathtub/shower.

Dining Disney-Style

About those four restaurants: One of the most interesting things Disney has done with its Megaship is find a way to avoid a single massive dining room for 1,000 guests at a time. Instead, there are three full-service restaurants aboard, and guests rotate from one to the next over the course of a cruise, accompanied by their assigned wait staff. Each of the restaurants has its own interesting character and décor as well as a distinct cuisine.

On the *Disney Magic*, Lumière's is a casually elegant restaurant, styled after the grand dining rooms of the old ocean liners and decorated with touches from Disney's "Beauty and the Beast" beneath sparkling chandeliers and candlelight tones. The cuisine is a light continental fare. The equivalent restaurant on the *Disney Wonder* is Triton's.

On both ships, Animator's Palette presents a tribute to Disney's cartoon heritage. You'll enter a room decorated in black and white, from the simple sketches and drawings on the walls to the stark outfits of the dining room staff. Gradually, with each new course, the room begins to take on color—on the walls, on the tables, and even the uniforms of the staff—until by dessert time the Animator's Palette is a riot of color and motion.

Parrot Cay is decidedly a laid-back Caribbean setting, with giant palms, a gingerbread-trimmed veranda roof, and a menu offering a taste of the tropics that's built around fresh fish, fruits, vegetables, and island spices. It's sort of an Enchanted Tiki Room at sea (ask a fan of the Disney theme parks if you don't catch the connection).

The fourth restaurant on both vessels is an adults-only intimate bistro known as Palo, located way up high and offering a 270-degree ocean view; the back half of the restaurant is a show kitchen. The fare is classical and Northern Italian. This restaurant is outside the regular dining rotation on the ship; if you want to escape to Palo you'll need to make a reservation for one of the nights of the cruise, and it is here the bistro's small size causes trouble: make your reservations as soon as you get on the ship.

Broadway at Sea

The Walt Disney Theatre is a 975-seat showplace that would be the envy of most Broadway producers. The stage is used for nightly performances of Disney-produced shows that are entertaining, but not to be confused with "Les Misérables" or "Chicago." Facilities include three elevators for special effects, indoor fireworks, and lasers; there's a talented cast of about 20.

There are no casinos onboard the ship, something Disney executives said would be at odds with the corporate mission. However, they point out, if you've got the itch to gamble, there are casinos in Nassau and St. Maarten where the proprietors will be happy to take your money.

Also onboard is the Buena Vista Theatre, a full-screen, 270-seat cinema that presents Disney classics and contemporary films.

Disney claims the largest dedicated area of children's space on any ship. Children ages 3–8 have Disney's Oceaneer Club, a supervised playroom. Older youngsters through age 12 can spend their time at Disney's Oceaneer Lab, which includes giant video walls and computer activities. Parents can borrow a pager so they can head off on their own while staying in touch aboard ship.

But my teenagers were thrilled to be granted admission to Common Grounds, a trendy coffee bar setting where they could dance, listen to music, play video games, and generally hang out in an environment where adults were politely encouraged not to visit.

Armed with their own key to the stateroom and a shipboard credit card, my kids would head off in the morning on their own schedule, meeting up with us for dinner and a show and trusting us to find a way to enjoy ourselves without them.

Ports of Call

On three- and four-day itineraries, the first port call is Nassau, about 50 miles off the coast of Florida, on a line with Miami. The Bahamas, an independent nation, includes nearly 700 islands of various sizes spread over 90,000 square miles reaching down to the Windward Passage between Cuba and Haiti.

Cruise ships dock at Prince George Wharf, which juts out from the heart of the town of Nassau, the largest settlement on the island of New Providence; it is the capital of the nation of The Bahamas.

The native Arawak tribe, though they were reported to be docile and cooperative, were brutally exterminated by Spanish troops in the sixteenth century. The islands of Eleuthera and New Providence were first colonized in 1647 and 1656 by British settlers from Bermuda. The inhabitants were beset with troubles from pirates, including Blackbeard and Henry Morgan, who used the islands as bases. Great Britain took a more formal hold on the islands in 1718, forcing out or killing many of the pirates.

Nassau still has vestiges of the old British empire, including a statue of Queen Victoria and some very fancy formal uniforms for the local constabulary. There are some fine snorkeling and fishing opportunities, and there's a golf course in the hills. And there is the gaudily impressive Atlantis Casino, a place that would catch your eye even in Las Vegas.

The port is one of the most active in the Caribbean. On one of our visits, there was something like $1 billion in hardware tied up alongside each other: the *Disney Magic*, Royal Caribbean's *Sovereign of the Sea* and *Empress of the Sea*, and the comparatively elderly Premier's Big Red Boat *Oceanic*.

Disney offers a decent array of shore excursions including trips to isolated beaches, fishing expeditions, and casino tours. Guests can walk from the dock into town where there are your basic souvenir markets and a few upscale clothing and jewelry stores; a few blocks away is the Straw Market where you'll find a mix of interesting native handicrafts, including carvings and straw hats as well as manufactured goods. You'll also find some less attractive come-ons, including little children who will offer to sing a song for a dollar.

Nassau, like a number of other Caribbean island towns, knows the importance of protecting the safety of tourists and the money they bring with them; there have been, though, a few violent incidents involving tourists who strayed to remote corners of the island. Consult the cruise line's shore excursion desk for advice; and use common sense, especially at night.

Beginning in August of 2000, every other four-day trip on the *Disney Wonder* will include a stop at Freeport, another island in the Bahamas.

The new seven-day itinerary for the Disney Magic begins with two days at sea and then consecutive-day stops at St. Maarten and St. Thomas. On the way back home, the ship makes a stop at Castaway Cay.

Castaway Cay: Disney's Own Country

The final stop on each of the Disney cruises is Castaway Cay, an uninhabited 1,000-acre Bahamian island, about 50 miles north of Nassau off Abaco Island.

Although the Walt Disney Company has created its own worlds in California, Florida, Tokyo, and France, this was the first opportunity for the Imagineers to design their own little country. In typical Disney style, they ended up making a place that is more real than the real thing, an idealized island paradise with perfect white sand beaches, palm trees, and a huge megaliner parked at a dock around the corner.

Ironically, local lore says an abandoned military landing strip on the island was formerly employed by drug runners. There was no local workforce, no electricity, and no running water before Disney took over. The result was an almost complete remake of the island with new vegetation, a cruiseship dock, restaurants, bicycle paths, and a set of handsome beaches and a 15-acre marked and maintained snorkeling path inside a protected lagoon.

Disney puts on an upscale barbecue for lunch; on our most recent visit the fare included grilled lobster tails along with more ordinary burgers and hot dogs.

The main beach is divided into kiddie and family areas. The north side of the island offers a mile-long "quiet" beach for adults only. You can also rent bicycles, paddle boats, sea kayaks, and other forms of transportation and entertainment. The price for renting snorkeling gear is rather steep, pretty close to the price you would pay to purchase equipment. We bought our own masks the day before in Nassau, but we were excluded from the Disney official snorkeling grounds.

Kids have their own camp on the island—with games and activities, including an excavation at the site of the remains of a (simulated) 35-foot beached whale.

Disney Days

Disney makes no apology about its family-oriented, humorously skewed view of the world. But they have done a marvelous job of creating a floating world where travelers can have an adult vacation, a family vacation, or a kid's vacation.

An Elegant Woman of a Certain Age: The *Universe Explorer* from Vancouver to Alaska

At first glance, the *Universe Explorer* sends a mixed message. There's no way to sugar coat this: She's old, a bit tired, dented and dinged-up, and smaller than the younger models all around. But she also has the classic design of an ocean liner and she carries about her the aura of a woman who has seen the world.

Now in her fifth decade (and ninth name), the *Universe Explorer* unpretentiously carries happy explorers deep into Alaska each summer and into Latin America and the Western Caribbean in the fall. For the rest of the year, she travels the four corners of the planet as a floating university; in 1999, the ship was featured in an extended series on the MTV network.

We caught up with the *Universe Explorer* in Vancouver, sailing with her on a week-long trip to Juneau and back. The passengers ranged from an Elderhostel group to a number of independent European travelers to a group of serious birders, whale-watchers, and nature lovers.

The *Universe Explorer* is not the place to look for a five-story, chrome-and-neon atrium, splashy Broadway-style shows, or fantasy suites with verandas and hot tubs. This is much more of a ship than a floating resort hotel. Prices are somewhat lower than those on newer ships from major cruise lines.

One of the last remaining steam turbine ships, she moves nicely and is relatively stable in most sea conditions. There is fairly little engine noise or vibration on most of the ship; there were several times, though, when a shower of soot issued forth from the ship's stack onto guests who were gathered on the expansive stern deck.

Cabins are clean and presentable, average-sized for cruise ships. Many of the cabins have portholes or small windows, and many are obstructed by low-hanging lifeboats.

There is nothing extraordinary about the setting for the Hamilton Dining Room, either, with low ceilings and small windows on the port side only. But again, the ship's crew did a good job with an attractively presented menu that included fresh fish picked up at Alaskan ports, including (almost) too much wonderful salmon.

The *Universe Explorer* carries a floating library of some 15,000 books with an emphasis on Alaska and other travel destinations, perhaps the largest seagoing collection anywhere. Some of the books are related to the Semester at Sea program. Even better, the library replaces the casino that had previously occupied the space. Nearby is a room full of computers—like the ship, they're a bit elderly but still hard-working; the ship conducts classes on computers and Internet use.

The Mid-Ocean Lounge is an attractive but simple lounge that extends across the width of the ship on the promenade deck, the heart of the ship that includes the pleasant but plain Harbour Grill and the ordinary but agreeable pool deck.

A curved amphitheater of couches faces the stage area, and tables flank the windows. The lounge is used as the main classroom for an interesting series of lectures by college professors. On our cruise from Vancouver to Alaska, the ship carried a geologist, a biologist, an anthropologist, and a guest artist. During the lovely trip north through the Inside Passage of British Columbia and then Alaska, these experts set the stage with fascinating discussions of the native cultures, the geology of glaciers and mountain ranges, and the marine and land-based wildlife, birds, and plants all around us.

While on some cruises the only real education may entail discussions of the operating hours for the casino or the health spa, by the end of a week on the *Universe Explorer* we could speak relatively intelligently about the differences between the Kwakautil and Tlingit cultures of Alaska, understand the origin of glaciers and the reason they assume such an other-worldly shade of blue, and discuss the feeding habits of the sperm whales that sometimes followed our ship.

Are you getting the picture here? On the *Universe Explorer*, the spectacle lies *outside*, in the narrow canyons of Tracy Arm and Glacier Bay, the untouched watery highway of the Inside Passage, and the wonders that lie outside the small towns of Alaska where she makes port calls.

That's not to say we didn't find something interesting to do within the walls of the ship. Our ship's professors gave lectures anticipating ports we were about to visit or discussed sights we would soon see from the decks.

We set sail from Vancouver on a week-long trip north through the Inside Passage with stops in the Alaskan ports of Wrangell, Sitka, Juneau, and Ketchikan. The *Universe Explorer* offers a mix of trips up to 14 days in length. (For most of the summer, the *Universe Explorer* operates extended two-week journeys that travel further north in Alaska.)

Alaska's Gold Rushes

In the 1800s, Alaska's first economic boom was "soft gold"—the export of beaver pelts to Europe and New England. The beaver was mostly used in the manufacture of hats; the business turned out to be a fad that passed by late in the century. It was the discovery of real gold in the 1890s, across the border in Canada's Yukon, that started Alaska's next boom. In more modern times, the development of "black gold" in the Alaskan oilfields has propelled the economy. And today, a fourth wave of gold in the form of tourist dollars is being distributed by cruise ships making stops along the Inside Passage to Juneau.

Wrangell is a small fishing town dating back to a Russian stockade built in 1834; the British leased the redoubt in 1840 and they held it until 1868 when the territory came under American control. Hard-hit by the closure of a pulp mill in 1994, Wrangell hopes to expand its tourism industry.

The biggest lure here is fishing and wildlife expeditions up the rugged Stikine River. On shore near the ferry terminal is a small beach that is home to a few dozen petroglyphs that are visible at low tide; these rock drawings may be several thousand years old, although some anthropologists date them as considerably younger.

On the road to the beach is "Our Collection," one of the weirder museums of eclectic stuff, and well worth a short visit. Proudly on display in an old barn are items from Barbie dolls to old mining tools, as well as a piece of plastic water pipe damaged by wolverines.

Sitka is one of the more dramatic settings in Alaska, which is saying quite a lot in this state of superlatives. The city is on the Pacific Ocean, in the shadows of Mt. Edgecumbe, a dramatic cone-shaped extinct volcano. The city retains much of its early Russian flavor; explorers from Russia landed in the area in the 1740s briefly, perhaps driven off by the Tlingits. They returned about 1799, establishing the first non-native settlement in Southeast Alaska. The fort they built just above the present location of town was the center of the Russian sea otter trade for several years before Tlingits, armed with guns obtained from British and American traders, overran the fort and killed most of the settlers. Alexander Baranof returned in 1804, this time with a Russian Navy warship, which pounded what was now a Tlingit fort. He re-established a settlement, now known as New Archangel; the town took its present name of Sitka after the American purchase of Alaska in 1867.

Today, Sitka retains a great deal of Russian flavor, centered around St. Michael's Cathedral in the city center. Originally constructed in 1848, it served for more than 100 years until it was destroyed by fire in 1966. While the fire spread, most of the cathedral's priceless icons and paintings were saved by townsfolk in a sort of bucket brigade. The building was reconstructed and today is open for visits.

The Episcopal Church in Sitka has an attractive stained glass window in front that sports a Star of David, which had been destined for a synagogue. It was six years from the time the window was ordered until the wrong glass arrived in Alaska; parishioners decided they liked the window anyhow.

At the Sitka Visitor Bureau in the Centennial Building, townsfolk daily put on Russian dance and folklore shows during cruise ship visits.

We also visited the Alaska Raptor Rehabilitation Center, a non-profit organization devoted to nursing back to health eagles, owls, hawks, and other birds of prey that are sick or injured. For many of us, this is as close as we can hope (or want) to get to a bald eagle. There's also a lovely nature trail nearby that heads into a small but entrancing rain forest.

But the unusual highlight of Sitka for us was an off-the-beaten-paths tour to the top of Harbor Mountain just west of town, the former site of a top-secret radar station constructed between 1941 and 1942 as a lookout for Japanese planes feared to be planning an attack on the Navy seaplane base on Sitka's Japonski Island. Guide Howard Ulrich of Harbor Mountain Tours [(907) 747-8294] takes guests up the rough road built by the military.

The six-and-a-half-mile road climbs 2,500 feet past stands of fireweed and salmonberries and dense forests of western hemlock and Sitka spruce, and there are spectacular views at every turn stretching across Sitka Sound toward Mt. Edgecumbe. There at the top were the crumbling remains of the radar station, an all-but-forgotten relic of World War II. The tour ends with a visit to the Starrigavan River, which includes an elevated wooden walkway through an estuary and a view from late July through September of massive shoals of spawning salmon.

The state capital of Juneau is a bit of a surprise, a state capital that shares space with honky-tonk saloons and towering hills; it's also the only seat of government I know of that has a major glacier in its backyard.

The tourist draw of downtown is the Red Dog Saloon, a place that gives "tacky tourist dive" a new meaning; here is celebrated all things kitsch. I liked best one of the signs on the wall: "If our food, drinks, and service ain't up to your standards, please lower your standards."

Much more glorious is the Mendenhall Glacier, located about 10 minutes outside town and reachable by city bus or one of several shuttle services; it is also a stop on nearly every bus tour.

Mendenhall Glacier is one of the rivers of ice formed during the Little Ice Age of nearly 3,000 years ago. The 12-mile-long glacier is fed by icefields high in the Coast Mountains, a frozen sheet of ice covering some 1,500 square miles. Annual snowfall on the icefield often exceeds 100 feet; the cold temperatures in the mountains and the tremendous pressure of the ice cause the glacier to flow forward at a pace of about two feet per day.

Scientists say the glacier was continuing to advance until about 1750 when its face was approximately two-and-a-half miles further down the valley. In the succeeding two centuries, the melt at the bottom of the glacier has exceeded the forward flow and it has slowly pulled back, revealing land that has been buried under ice for centuries. The ice that "calves" off the face of the glacier is 80 to 100 years old.

There's a small visitor's center at the glacier and a pathway that takes you down to a viewing point about half a mile from the face. Adventuresome—and well-equipped—hikers can explore several trails that lead up the mountainside.

Back in town, alongside the cruise ship dock, is an aerial tramway that rises up Mount Roberts.

A Brighter Shade of Blue

The undisputed highlight of the cruise was a slow passage up the narrow fjord of Tracy Arm to the face of the South Sawyer Glacier.

The steep-walled watery canyon is approximately 50 miles south of Juneau, branching eastward off Stephens Passage. The *Universe Explorer* steamed slowly through the fog at the entrance to the deep fjord and then followed the twists and turns of the canyon for nearly two hours, steering around some large ice floes along the way. Finally, the ship came to the end of the passageway and we came face-to-face with a massive electric blue wall of ice.

The color of a glacier is almost always a surprise to visitors. The ice at the face has been compressed and most of the air within has escaped. What remains is highly crystallized; as light strikes the surface, all colors of the spectrum are absorbed except for blue, which is reflected back.

The 600-foot-long *Universe Explorer* approached within 100 feet of the glacier and then used her bow thrusters to slowly turn 180 degrees and make a graceful exit. All the while we served as the afternoon's entertainment for a family of seals on a bobbing ice floe.

Flying into the Bush

The town of Ketchikan is a setting-off point for a wide range of Alaskan adventures, including nature expeditions by boat and plane and a large collection of native art and cultural items, including Totem Bight, a state historical park that has more than a dozen restored or recreated totems and a large community house in a lovely setting overlooking Tongass Narrows on the Inside Passage.

The most surreal experience from Ketchikan was a "flightseeing" adventure to the huge Misty Fjords National Monument. We boarded a Taquan Air floatplane from the terminal just above town and taxied out into the harbor for takeoff alongside the *Universe Explorer*.

Misty Fjords is one of the least-known treasures of America; it encompasses 2.3 million acres, almost four times the area of the state of Rhode Island. Accessible only by boat or floatplane, it's a world of cascading waterfalls, hundreds of untouched lakes, and wildlife—including brown and black bear, Sitka black-tailed deer, wolves, moose, and bald eagles.

Our plane flew low and slow through canyons that had 3,000-foot-high, sheer granite walls carved by ancient glaciers, over seal rocks and a pair of breaching whales, and in for a swooping landing on tiny Nooya Lake. Our pilot taxied to shore and then tied the plane to a tree stump; we walked on the pontoons to dry land and soaked up the wilderness—six humans in a place rarely touched by our kind.

Taquan Air [(800) 770-8800] is the largest of a number of floatplane operators, with service from Ketchikan, Sitka, and other ports. Among its other interesting offers: You can hitch a ride on one of the line's daily scheduled mail and freight runs to isolated bush communities.

From the Pacific to the Atlantic in High Style: The *Radisson Diamond* from Costa Rica Through the Panama Canal

We made a slow and deliberate passage through the Panama Canal aboard the *Radisson Diamond*, a floating island of high-tech luxury passing through what was once one of the most inhospitable places on earth.

We sat on the private veranda of our stateroom sipping cool drinks and watching the sheer rock of the Gaillard Cut and the dense jungle go by. As we passed through the locks, the walls were just inches away from the railing of our balcony, and we were able to reach out and touch the concrete, bridging the old and new worlds of technology.

A Ship Like No Other

The *Radisson Diamond* is one of a kind, the largest multihull cruise ship afloat; there are a handful of small catamaran ferries and cruise ships, but no others in her class of size or luxury. She has a capacity of 20,295 tons but carries no more than 320 passengers; other ships of her size carry as many as 800 guests.

You can think of the *Diamond* as a luxury hotel mounted atop a pair of submarines. Unlike high-speed catamarans that have more than one hull but very shallow drafts, the unusual *Diamond* floats on "tubes" that extend about 23 feet below the surface of the water; each contains a separate engine room.

The ship was intended as a great breakthrough in design, and on some counts it has been a success. The two hulls and their deep draft give the ship somewhat more stability than other cruise ships. The *Diamond* also presents an unusual profile and a startling head-on appearance; she attracts attention on the high seas and in every port. There are also some spectacular interior spaces including a two-story lounge that has a wall of windows at the bow (the appropriately named Windows Lounge) and an open observation deck at the top that hangs over the bridge.

The ship is made up of three floors of cabins (all with outside views, and two levels with private verandas) plus an elegant dining room, an intimate lounge, and a pool and sun deck. The design puts most of the public rooms and the sparkling atrium down the central spine of the ship, with cabins to the outside.

All of this sits atop a tunnel approximately 60 feet wide and 30 feet tall that runs 400 feet down the full length of the ship.

The ship is relatively short at 420 feet but is a full 103 feet wide, a barge-like shape that just barely squeezes through the Panama Canal. Her deep draft means she must anchor offshore in many ports, sometimes a bit further out than larger, more conventional craft.

The ship includes four stabilizers, one each at the bow and stern of each tube. Unlike every other cruise ship afloat, the stabilizers move inward from the tubes into the tunnel between them. You can feel the ship start to roll and then correct itself in the other direction. The short swings can take a few hours to get used to, but after a while the voyage will likely be a bit more comfortable for travelers who are concerned about seasickness. The design works well at top speed, not quite so well at slower speeds.

The design, though, proved to be a not particularly efficient one, at least in terms of fuel usage and speed. The underwater body and decidedly non-aerodynamic shape of the front of the ship (it's hard to call it a "bow" since it is more like a ski slope than a classic narrow cake wedge) result in a top cruising speed of just 14 knots and a monumental fuel bill of as much as twice that of a more conventional shape. The contour of the tubes result in a short, weak side wake—a wall of water the *Diamond* must plow through. And the squat design of the ship makes it somewhat susceptible to twisting in winds or seas that move across her amidships.

A single control room on Deck 6 oversees the operation of two separate engine rooms in the underwater pontoons of the ship. Down in the submarine tubes are four engines—two on each side; engineers must scurry down five flights of stairs to one or the other tube. Up and over is a trip of 10 flights—there is no connection between the pontoons below the water line.

One of the sustaining memories of our trip came when the tender boat returning us from a visit to shore made a transit down the length of the tunnel between the hulls. The white walls of the pontoons and the "roof" of the tunnel contrasted with a gorgeous iridescent Caribbean sea; at one end of the tunnel was the green jungle of San Andres Island and at the other end, the bright tropical sun.

Traveling in Style

Like every other cruise ship, the *Radisson Diamond* has a dining room and lots of food, there are passenger cabins with a place to sleep and a bathroom, and there are showrooms and bars and lounges.

But at every turn, the *Radisson Diamond* delivers it all in great style.

The Grand Dining Room is one of the most elegant rooms at sea . . . or on land, for that matter. The two-floor-high glass wall at the stern of the ship offers spectacular views all through the day. There are also more than enough tables for two, as well—a relative rarity on many cruise lines. Because of the stability of the ship, and also because this is a "customer is king" operation, the tables can be moved around the dining room and rearranged to create tables large or small.

And there is an open seating policy in the dining room, with guests free to arrive at any time during serving hours. The dining room staff, by the way, features female servers from Europe, not all that common on cruise ships.

That's the good news. The bad news, for some cruise veterans, is that you won't have the comfort of an assigned wait staff who will learn your favorites and become your short-term best friend aboard ship.

But the other good news is that the ratio of guests to staff is low and the dedication to service so high that the entire crew seems devoted to your needs. My wife and I found a particular section of the dining room we liked, and a pair of waitresses we enjoyed, and by three days into the trip, the maitre d' knew our preferences.

One other nice point: Tips are included in the cruise fare on Radisson ships. This means that members of the staff are paid a decent wage and are not reliant on gratuities from guests. Put another way, you do not feel that the waitresses, the maitre d', the wine steward, and the cabin attendant are calculating the size of their tip each time they greet you or offer a service.

Of course, nothing is free—the cost of higher wages is reflected in stateroom charges. But for my money, I would just as soon see all cruise lines go this route. There certainly was no lack of effort, courtesy, or attention to detail on the tipless *Diamond.* In fact, the service was as good as, or better than, any we have received on a cruise ship.

Captain Jan Blindheim and his wife were gracious hosts, mingling with guests, more accessible than most officers on cruises we have taken.

Entertainment Aboard: Less Is More

There are no lavish production shows, no parade of waiters with flaming Baked Alaska (thank goodness), and no painful guest talent shows or costume balls onboard (even more thanks).

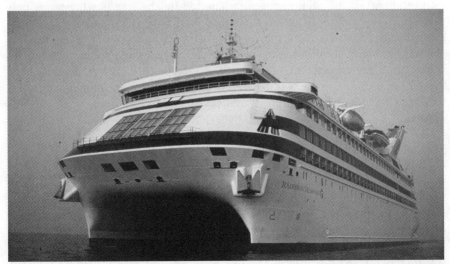

The Radisson Diamond
Radisson Seven Seas Cruises

Instead, the *Diamond* presents a very laid-back atmosphere, a less-is-more philosophy. On our cruise there was a talented piano and violin duo who gave a few recitals and performed at dinner. The cruise director, an amiable Briton who had a respectable background in theater and cabaret, sang show tunes and pop songs. Each afternoon, the staff conducted an informal trivia quiz in the lounge during tea time.

There is a short jogging and walking track on the topmost deck, and a golf driving net. At the stern, the *Diamond* includes a small marina that can be lowered into the sea to allow guests to use jet skis and sailboats; the marina is mostly used in Europe and was not available on our particular cruise.

But the real entertainment was a lovely ship with superb service and luxurious accommodations and food. This is a cruise for the self-sufficient.

And Now for Something Completely Different

However, lest you fear that everything aboard the *Diamond* is prim and proper, there is also "An Evening at Don Vito's," the alternative dining experience that is not to be missed.

Most evenings, the casual grill on the tenth deck is transformed into a small Italian bistro. Guests are offered an eclectic evening, a cross between a fine Italian restaurant—the food would win raves anywhere on land—and a rollicking burlesque.

The evening starts out with a talented singer and musician playing Italian songs. Sometime around the second appetizer, the waiters begin to join in on the songs, and by the salad course there's a full chorus of wisecracking, singing, and dancing clowns bringing you your dinner. On our visit, a talented ringer suddenly took the stage; a young Fillipino waitress who had quietly been pouring wine took the microphone and contributed a lovely song in phonetic Italian.

By the end of the night, somewhat abetted by the free-flowing wine, one matron was in a near-swoon on the dance floor with the maitre d' Guiseppe, and another took over from the singer for the final chorus.

There are only about 50 seats in the restaurant, enough room on a typical cruise for every passenger to visit once. After our first visit we immediately staked out a place on the waiting list for a second pass; we happily returned to Don Vito's for the final night of our cruise.

A Sparkling Itinerary

The *Diamond* makes a grand circuit each year from the Pacific to the Caribbean and on to Europe for the summer. The ship is also regularly chartered to major corporations for special events and "incentive" rewards.

We flew to San José, Costa Rica to meet up with the *Diamond* for a trip through the Panama Canal that would end in Fort Lauderdale, Florida. Most of the guests on our cruise began their adventure with a day trip to a Costa Rican rain forest and animal preserve; we caught up with the group on the second day for a visit to the spectacular Poás volcano. From there we traveled the mountainous countryside to a private plantation for a peasant-style lunch. Late in the day we were delivered to Puntarenas, a port on an inlet of the Pacific Ocean.

Our first full day was spent cruising south down the untouched jungle coast of Costa Rica and northern Panama. We were accompanied in the morning by several schools of dolphins who happily played in the ship's broad wake, launching themselves a few feet into the air.

Then on the second day, we arrived just before dawn at Panama City. As the sun came up we found ourselves threading our way through a few dozen freighters waiting their turn to enter the Panama Canal. At our appointed time, we passed beneath the Bridge of the Americas and entered the canal.

The construction of the Panama Canal stretched over more than 30 years, begun in 1880 with the tragic French effort and finished in 1914 under the sheer bravado of Teddy Roosevelt, George Goethals, and the not-insignificant solution to the deadly malaria-and-yellow-fever plagues by Dr. William Gorgas.

The 10-hour passage through the six locks (three up and three down) of the canal was a fascinating voyage along the border where one of mankind's greatest feats of engineering meets nature's wildest challenges. We passed through the spectacular Gaillard Cut, where thousands of men labored for decades to cut a passage; from there we moved into Gatun Lake, a body of water brought about by a huge earthen dam in the jungle.

At the end of the day, as night fell, we exited the canal and entered the Caribbean Ocean, passing through another floating waiting line of freighters heading for the Pacific.

Our first stop in the Caribbean was at San Andres island, a somewhat obscure possession of Colombia. From there we moved on to Grand Cayman Island and Cozumel, Mexico. On the last full day of the 10-day cruise, we moved along the mountainous northern coast of Cuba, en route to debarkation in Fort Lauderdale, Florida.

Cuba is a Holy Grail for cruise lines. Nearly every company has plans already on the shelf for trips to the large, culturally rich and exotic island that has been off-limits to most Americans for nearly 40 years. Lying just 90 miles south of Miami, Cuba will likely one day be a popular destination for ships sailing out of Florida and the Gulf of Mexico.

Can a Luxury Cruise Represent a Good Deal?

The published cruise fare in 1999 on the *Radisson Diamond* for a 10-day passage from Costa Rica to Fort Lauderdale through the Panama Canal ranges from $5,195 to $6,295 per person for a deluxe outside cabin with a sitting room or a private veranda.

Compare this to a 10-day Holland America cruise through the Panama Canal on the *Maasdam*; Holland America is an above-average mass-market line. The listed price for an outside mini-suite with veranda was $4,725; the lowest price outside stateroom sold for $3,425 per person.

On the face of it, this makes a trip on the *Radisson Diamond* about $350 to $400 more per person per day.

Now, of course, the savvy consumer doesn't pay full fare. At the time of my cruise in early 1999, both Radisson and Holland America offered substantial discounts to their fares. Radisson's deal was a 50 percent discount for the second person in a cabin; Holland America offered a break of 25 percent for early booking. (Both deals work out to 25 percent off the fare for a couple.)

The reduced fare prices, then, were:

Radisson	$3,896 to $4,721 per person
Holland	$2,621 to $3,606 per person

You may also be able to obtain a discount or rebate from a travel agency.

Then, when you consider a luxury cruise, be sure you compare apples to apples:

Radisson includes airfare from major U.S. cities and transfers from the airport to the pier on most of its cruises. You can accept their arrangements or make your own and deduct a substantial allowance from cabin prices.

On the *Diamond* and other ships in the luxury Radisson fleet, all staterooms are outside. About two-thirds of the cabins on the *Diamond* include a lovely, private veranda; those that don't offer a comfortable sitting room alongside a picture window.

The quality of food and its presentation on the *Diamond* is comparable to that of a top restaurant on shore. Put another way, a dinner on the *Diamond*, with appetizer, soup, salad, entrée, dessert, and wine, would probably cost $70 to $90 per person (with tip) in a major city. On a more ordinary cruise line, the value would be about half that.

For the trip through the Panama Canal, passengers also received two days in a luxury hotel in San José, Costa Rica plus two days of escorted tours to rain forests, volcanoes, and a peasant lunch in the countryside en route to the port at the start of the cruise.

When you include the value of airfare, transfers from the airport, two nights in a hotel, two days of shore excursions in the port of embarkation, the cost of a luxury cruise becomes a lot closer to the mass market. The difference may work out to only a few hundred dollars.

Once you are onboard, what else do you get for your extra dollars? The answer is dozens of little niceties.

Our cabin was decorated with an arrangement of exotic live flowers, an echo of decorations throughout the ship. The bathroom was equipped with extra-plush towels and bathrobes. A refrigerator in the room was kept filled with soda, mixers, and bottled water.

When we boarded the ship, there was a bottle of French champagne on ice set up on the table. The cabin was also stocked with a personal bar set up with more liquor than I could personally consume over the course of a 10-day voyage; if you did manage to go through the bar, additional supplies were available for purchase.

When you return from a shore excursion in a tropical port, a uniformed waitress stands just inside the reception area with a tray of chilled champagne or juice.

The cabin stewardess discreetly noted our schedule each day and made at least three visits to make the beds, remake them, and turn them down.

A small pleasure: Soda and juice flows freely and without charge at any of the bars and from wandering staff members. At dinner, the steward pours from complimentary offerings of red or white wine selected to complement the evening's fare; there is also an extensive wine cellar for those who insist on paying extra.

Rooms are equipped with a video player and the ship's library has a decent collection of classic and current movies for loan.

And then there's the food. Nearly every cruise ship does a good job of feeding guests, but the offerings sometimes emphasize quantity over quality. On the *Radisson Diamond,* however, every meal was on the level of a four-star restaurant. The plates (Villeroy & Boch china, actually) were laid out like works of art. Each afternoon, the executive chef would appear on stateroom television to describe in luscious detail the menu for dinner and demonstrate the creation of a sauce or stock.

Menus do not repeat over the course of a cruise. Guests are discreetly encouraged to make reasonable special requests. I particularly enjoyed a gazpacho soup one evening; I put in a word of praise to the maitre d', and the next night I was offered a second chance at the appetizer, freshly concocted just for me in the galley. The chef will also attempt to fulfill any reasonable requests for special dishes or preparation styles.

At dinner, if you somehow find the strength to resist dessert and order "nothing," your waitress may appear with a dinner plate decorated in chocolate icing and glaze spelling out "Nothing." More than a few guests end up licking the plate in utter defeat.

Every cruise ship offers a lunchtime buffet on the upper deck, but on the *Radisson Diamond* it was more of a catered picnic than a casino smorgasbord. The silver serving dishes held rich goulash or lamb chops; an outside barbecue offered grilled fish, chicken, or beef; a cheese cart held hundreds of dollars worth of sinful international offerings. And waiters and waitresses stood by to carry your plate from station to station.

Our favorite lunch included shrimp, crab legs, cold lobster, and an assortment of seafood salads. On a more ordinary cruise ship, a "gala" buffet might have featured just one of these premium dishes.

Although on most ships I spend little time in the cabin, preferring to watch the sea from the deck or from a library or lounge, when your cabin has its own balcony all things are different. The *Radisson Diamond's* verandas are completely private from one another and sheltered from the wind. When we were out to sea, the large sliding door to the outside stood open all day.

We happily began every morning of our trip with breakfast on the veranda, delivered with clockwork precision and served on a linen tablecloth. Each night before retiring, we toasted a day of adventure or a day of blissful indolence.

Though we preferred the elegance of the Grand Dining Room, guests can also ask room service to deliver a meal ordered from the evening menu; dishes are brought course by course to your veranda or sitting room.

We toured behind the scenes with Executive Chef Peter Spörndli, who met us in the galley with a chilled bottle of wine. The bright and open workspace is blessed with an unusual feature for cruise ships—a picture window. The dining room on the *Diamond* sits high on the eighth deck; most cruise ships set their dining rooms down low. Of course, on the *Diamond*, there is no space below the seventh deck for a wide open room.

The ship's larders were like an international gourmet shop: asparagus from Guatemala, tomatoes from Costa Rica, beef from the United States, and seafood from around the world. Shelves held fresh spices, including a case of horseradish roots. We watched as a sous-chef decorated the plates for one of the night's appetizers—exquisite cold mussels from New Zealand, served with a seasoned mayonnaise concocted fresh onboard.

Another nicety—for experienced cruise travelers—is the low-key shipboard commerce. On many cruises, there is a drumbeat of sales pitches for shore excursions, bingo games, "sales" at the boutique, come-ons from the ship's photographers, auctions of "fine art," and sprawling, beeping, and flashing casinos. For many cruise companies, a large portion of their profits come from onboard marketing and bar tabs.

Each day the ship's golf pro offered lessons in the net on the small sports deck above the bridge; husband-and-wife bridge experts delivered talks on arcane strategies and conducted tournaments, and a visiting professor offered several lectures on history and economics.

But, we found it quite possible to enjoy our cruise in peaceful obliviousness to all of the shipboard sideshows. They are still there, but we didn't have to go out of our way to avoid them.

In fact, that was the way we looked at our entire cruise: We let the *Diamond* transport us on the path between the seas while we laid back in the lap of luxury.

E.T. Phone Home: From Hawaii to an Almost Untouched South Pacific Island

We caught up with the *Norwegian Dynasty* in Honolulu in the late fall of 1998; she was sailing a series of 10-day cruises from Hawaii after a summer in Alaska and before repositioning through the Panama Canal to the Caribbean. The unusual itinerary included stops at four Hawaiian Islands—Oahu, Hawaii, Maui, and Kauai—interrupted by a five-day journey down to near the equator, to Fanning Island in the tiny Republic of Kiribati.

The *Dynasty* has since left the NCL fleet, moving over to become the flagship of the new Crown Cruise Line, an offshoot of Commodore; she now sails in the Caribbean and to Bermuda, as the *Crown Dynasty*.

NCL has given over the Hawaiian itinerary to the *Norwegian Wind*.

Cruising Back in Time

We left Honolulu and sailed to Kailua on the Kona Coast on the big island of

Hawaii. Kona, which means "leeward" or sheltered side, lives up to its name. This is the calm, sunny side and home to some relatively isolated luxury resorts, golf courses, and tons of gift shops.

Then we headed south from Kona toward the Republic of Kiribati, a two-and-a-half-day, full-steam cruise toward the equator and back in time.

We approached Fanning Island (Tabueran to the locals) just after breakfast, greeted by a native in a wooden sailboat who paralleled us the last few miles to the entrance to the inner harbor.

Fanning is a broken Cheerio of an atoll, the land only a few hundred feet wide around an inner lagoon that is actually the collapsed cone of an ancient volcano. Beaches on the ocean are somewhere between tricky and dangerous. English Harbor, the interior of the atoll, is deep enough for a major ship but not wide enough for a cruise ship to comfortably enter and turn around, and the ocean currents and soft sand bottom made it impossible to set an anchor; there are also believed to be wrecks of World War II ships and planes on the bottom. The *Norwegian Dynasty* was forced to cruise slowly back and forth while passengers visited the island on tenders that surfed through the waves into the harbor.

Kiribati (pronounced *Kiribass*) is made up of the Gilbert, Line, and Phoenix islands. The island nation of 75,000 population is made up of 33 islands and just 268 square miles of land spread over 5 million square miles of ocean. Kiribati won its independence from Great Britain in 1979. The capital is Tarawa, site of some of the bloodiest battles at the end of World War II.

Fanning is located 3 degrees, or 273 miles, north of the equator. A sister island, 50 miles away, is Christmas Island, which from 1954–65 served as a base for American, British, and French atomic testing on more distant atolls. The island was discovered in 1798 by Edmund Fanning, the American captain of the ship *Betsy*. A number of whaling ships visited the uninhabited island in succeeding years. Beginning in 1848, 500 natives of other islands in the chain were moved to Fanning to operate a coconut oil plantation for a British company. A bit later in the century, the island was extensively mined for guano, and some 20,000 tons of the natural phosphate fertilizer were shipped to Honolulu.

In 1902, one of the first transoceanic telephone cables was brought ashore at Fanning. The cable stretched from near Vancouver, British Columbia to New Zealand. During World War II, a small Japanese landing party damaged the cable station on Fanning. In another footnote to history, Fanning Island was one of Amelia Earhart's waypoints on her final voyage.

Modest plantation operations continued until midway through the twentieth century. Most of the approximately 1,600 residents of Fanning are descendants of the plantation workers, abandoned when the company closed operations and pulled out.

First Contact

At the time of our visit in late 1998, the *Norwegian Dynasty* was making her third trip to the atoll, the only three times a cruise ship had ever come to

Fanning Island. Before then, only a handful of modern-day outsiders had visited here.

Still, the residents of Fanning were at the time of our visit not at all used to outsiders. Many of the residents, and especially the young children, were at least as interested in us as we were in them.

NCL paid for the construction of a small pier, built like most everything else on the island, from coconut trees.

Our arriving tenders were met by the town council and a band of about 50 dancers in grass skirts and musicians who performed continuously for the seven hours we were ashore.

We found a nearly untouched tropical paradise, where residents, the I-Kiribati, live a subsistence life grabbing bonefish and the occasional lobster from the lagoon and harvesting taro, coconuts, and a few other crops. The local livestock includes foot-wide land crabs that make their homes in large holes in and among the coconut trees.

The island is almost untouched by modern influences, without electricity, plumbing, telephone service, and little in the way of permanent changes to the coconut jungle. Most of the homes consist of open platforms a few feet above the ground with thatched coconut frond roofs. There are no doors, windows, or privacy except for the blackness of the night.

While most of the ship's passengers stayed near the pier and the pretty sand beach on the lagoon, my wife and I headed out on the packed sand road that led from the pier. We passed some of the ruins of the old plantation and phosphate mining operations, including a few dozen feet of rusted narrow-gauge rails and found a small overgrown cemetery that held the remains of some of the family members of the plantation people. Every few hundred feet we came to another little cluster of huts, each with its own name.

Children, and there were hundreds of them, peeked out at us from behind trees or came to the road to say hello. One group of little boys came forth to shake our hands.

We walked past the atoll's primary school, listening for a while to the children reciting their numbers in math class. Once we were spotted, though, class came to a halt and dozens of heads crowded the doorway to catch a glimpse of the unusual visitors.

The management of Norwegian Cruise Line was appropriately sensitive to the effects of the ship's visit to the unspoiled atoll. Guests were asked not to give money to the children to avoid creating professional beggars. The cruise line brought picnic tables and water ashore, and removed all of the garbage left behind by passengers. As a parting gift, the ship's crew brought sacks of flour and rice for distribution by the town council.

There were a small number of merchants selling a few local products, including mats, eel traps, and hats—all made from coconut products. Another table offered a few postcards and stamps of the Republic of Kiribati . . . although there was no way to reliably send mail from the atoll.

We were told a tragicomedy story of the ship's first visit to Fanning. It seems an intrepid American sailor had chosen Fanning Island as his destination for a solo journey from the West Coast of the United States. His research had told him he would be a modern-day Captain Cook, visiting a place that time had bypassed. After several weeks at sea, he arrived at the isolated speck of sand near the Equator . . . to find the *Norwegian Dynasty* pulling up with a load of 600 passengers.

Can Fanning Island remain virtually untouched? I'm afraid I have my doubts. Other cruise lines are considering calling at Fanning to meet the requirements of the Jones Act, and the more visits by outsiders the more likely the contamination of their culture.

The kids will learn to stick out their hands for a dollar when they are photographed and the native dancers will pass the hat instead of performing in welcome. And, alas, Fanning will become just another tourist island.

Back to the Future

After our return from Fanning Island, we made port at Hilo on the other side of the big island. Hilo is the takeoff point for numerous helicopter tours of the Mauna Loa volcano.

We chose instead to explore the island by car, renting a vehicle and driving to the extraordinary Volcano National Park. I have been to many strange places on this planet, but few exceed the peculiarity of a stroll across the miles of black lava left behind by dozens of recent flows; it's as close to a moonscape as most of us will ever experience and a scene that will stick with you forever. The lava is frozen in twisting ropes, undulating waves, and crunchy beaches of pumice.

The volcanoes of Hawaii are still very much alive, although eruptions are rarely violent explosions. Instead there are near-continuous slow flows of thick super-heated lava that bubbles out of cracks in the mountains and heads down the hillside and into the sea where it gives off clouds of steam that rise several miles into the sky.

Also in the park is the Thurston Lava Tube, a natural tunnel caused by a cooling lava flow; midway through a walk in the long tunnel it's like a journey to the center of the earth.

Lahaina, on the island of Maui, was once the royal capital of the Hawaiian kingdom and the seat of the power for the Kamehameha dynasty. In the early nineteenth century, Lahaina became the lusty port away from home for the American whaling fleet that had sailed all the way around the Horn of South America in search of "greasy luck"—whale oil. In a way, it became an extension of Nantucket, a whaling capital thousands of miles away in Massachusetts and the home of many of the ship owners and captains.

At the heyday of the whaling era, as many as 400 ships at a time were berthed in the harbor; whalemen said there was no God west of the Horn and conducted themselves accordingly, at least until a band of puritanical missionaries arrived from New England to attempt to clean things up. Among the sailors was Herman Melville, who wrote about the whole scene in "Moby Dick" and other works.

The weathered wooden buildings on Front Street now house boutiques, art galleries, and restaurants, but the sense of history in Lahaina is more intense than most anywhere else in the islands.

Lahaina also offered the most diverse collection of activities for visitors, from golf expeditions to helicopter and biplane routes to whale watching. We chose to make a visit to the floor of the harbor onboard one of the ships in the Atlantis Submarine fleet; the 65-foot craft descended to a depth of 125 feet and allowed us to intrude on fish and other creatures of the sea and coral beds not often seen outside an aquarium. Atlantis operates similar subs at a number of ports in the Hawaiian islands and in the Caribbean; it's a voyage worth the trip.

The last stop on the *Norwegian Dynasty*'s tour around the fiftieth state was Nawiliwili on the lush island of Kauai, the most isolated of the major islands. Here, we rented a car and drove west—there's really only one major road and it does not quite circle the island because of the severe geography of the Na Pali Coast—and went for a visit to Waimea Canyon State Park. Waimea is called the Grand Canyon of Hawaii, and with just a little bit of exaggeration involved. The steep, multicolored walls of the canyon are hidden from view until you complete a long, slow drive up the mountainside.

Kauai's scenery is unusual enough to have attracted a long line of Hollywood filmmakers who have over the years used settings on the island for scenes in films "King Kong," "South Pacific," "Raiders of the Lost Ark," and "Jurassic Park."

Enchantment, Economy Style: From New Orleans to Mexico on the *Enchanted Capri*

By Joan Manring Hull

While the author of this book and his wife were sitting on their private veranda and eating fresh-baked croissants and scones from fine china on a linen table cloth on their luxury cruise ship, my son and I were standing in a line waiting to enter a noisy and decidedly modest dining room. Behind us were the odor of smoke and the beeping and ringing of the slot machines in the nearby casino.

The *Enchanted Capri* is without doubt a budget-level cruise ship, one of two vessels operated by Commodore Cruise Lines out of New Orleans to destinations in the Gulf of Mexico.

But what the *Enchanted Capri* lacked in brass, marble and crystal was compensated by friendliness, easy atmosphere, and sincerity.

Public areas and cabins were clean but very simply decorated. Our outside cabin on the Dolphin Deck was paneled in faux wood without any decoration on the walls; the twin beds, which doubled as couches by day, were narrow. The cabin was clean, and the steward was very attentive; we received service at least twice a day.

There was no television in the room, but there was a nice double window and in port we could see barges and a small paddlewheeler moving on the brown Mississippi River.

The low-ceiling dining room, with outside windows running down one side of the room, was very simply decorated and very noisy when full. There was no health club or spa, although Commodore promises to add some exercise equipment to the ship.

The saltwater pool was small and the pool deck was too noisy for my tastes; my feet turned black with soot as I walked on the deck below the ship's funnel. The crew was busy painting and scraping, a continuous effort on a ship now in her third decade.

The *Enchanted Capri* delivers good value for cruisers who have simple tastes or limited pocketbooks; the company's *Enchanted Isle,* an older and larger vessel, offers a similar class of service. Commodore also owns the *Universe Explorer,* operated by World Explorer Cruises on Alaskan itineraries; it's also a good quality budget cruise.

The *Enchanted Capri* was built in Finland in 1975 and operated as a Russian cruise ship under the names *Arkadya* and *Azerbajian.* (Some of the signs posted around the ship were in both Russian and English, and a few of the ship's officers were from parts of the former Soviet Union.)

The 15,000-ton ship has a passenger capacity of as many as 637 if all the cabins were fully populated, which would make for a rather crowded vessel. On our trip in early February, the *Enchanted Capri* was only half full and comfortable; the dining room went to a single seating, though, which filled the space to the walls.

Onboard the *Enchanted Capri*

The food was generally acceptable, and sometimes very good—about the level of a decent neighborhood restaurant—and served attractively; but it was nothing to write home about. I did like the attitude of the staff; our waiter and busboy were charming—teasing, attentive, always smiling, and energetic.

And of course, the wait staff knew all the steps to the Macarena. They swayed their way through the dining room carrying—or balancing on their heads—the final evening's traditional special dessert, Baked Alaska. You'd expect nothing less on a basic cruise like this.

On several nights of the cruise, the dining room offered a midnight buffet, which was decorated with fanciful sculptures of vegetables, fruits, and ice—and included shrimp, crab, and fresh fruit.

There's a large-screen television in the non-smoking Sand Dollar Lounge located on the highest deck, which offers nearly a 360-degree view of the water. The ship could have used more hideaways from smokers.

Like many cruise lines, Commodore hopes to boost its earnings from onboard sales, and the loudspeakers were busy through the day with promotions for the casino—an outpost of the Isle of Capri Casino—and for bingo games and the bars.

The show lounge was home to a floor show that included four young singers who were enthusiastic and talented. However, the show itself was not very memorable. The stage and the pivoting seats were on the same level, and it was sometimes smoky. My son made a few appearances at the disco and took the microphone in a karaoke session, and we visited the ship's movie theater a few times for films.

Cruising the Gulf of Mexico

Our five-day cruise included two stops in Mexico, at Cozumel and the developing port of Progreso. On our first day at sea, we found a quiet spot for two, shaded by the lifeboats above, which had an expansive view of the sea. While others were spending time in the casino or playing scheduled games, we enjoyed our unscheduled solitude.

In Progreso, we pulled up to the four-mile-long concrete pier, which extends out from shore to service large ships. We docked next to Celebrity's *Mercury,* a behemoth compared to the *Enchanted Capri.* It's a lovely vessel, but I wondered how well we could spot flying fish from her lofty decks.

From the pier at Progreso we took an air-conditioned bus to the Mayan ruins of the royal city of Uxmal. Our distinguished and well-spoken Mexican guide fascinated us with details about Mayan architecture and society structure. Our next stop on the bus was Mérida, a colonial city established in the mid-1500s, with beautiful murals, mansions, and a lively market.

The next day we headed out on our own at Cozumel, intent on snorkeling. Commodore did offer an excursion for beginner snorkelers, but I wanted to plunge in on my own. We took a short taxi ride to Chanakanaab National Park and spent a sun-drenched afternoon of snorkeling and dozing beneath the shade of a palm tree. The large park was clean and beautifully landscaped, with walking paths of crushed shell throughout the botanical garden.

We headed across the fine, white sand to wooden stairs and slippery rocks that led us into the clear waters of the Caribbean, filled with colorful fish and coral formations.

On our return to New Orleans, we enjoyed a gourmet dinner at Arnaud's in the French Quarter. The restaurant, established in 1918 by "Count" Arnaud Cazenave, is a combination of twelve originally separate buildings, ranging from intimate to spacious in size, and furnished with dark woods, chandeliers, mosaic floors and soft colors. Upstairs, guests may visit the Mardi Gras Museum. We were fascinated by the collection of ornate gowns worn by the queen, and the costumes and photos also on display.

We enjoyed a lengthy, relaxed dinner at Arnaud's, happy only to observe the giddiness of Mardi Gras through the dining room windows, and dreamily recalling the vast, shimmering blue water that surrounded us during our Commodore cruise.

If money were no object, I would probably prefer a more luxurious ship. But in the real world, an outside cabin or one of the handful of suites on the *Enchanted Capri* is a pretty good deal for a short and simple cruise. And once you're on shore, the sights you see and the shore excursions are the same as if you came in on a luxury cruise ship.

Chapter 12
An Econoguide to Cruise Ships

So many lovely cruise ships, so little time!

In the next section of the book, I'll give you a guided tour to more than 140 cruise ships under construction from 36 cruise lines, plus previews of 25 ships under construction. This book concentrates on ships that regularly include calls at U.S. ports, the Caribbean, the Mexican Riviera, and coastal Canada.

Each section begins with information about the cruise line. You'll find telephone numbers and web pages for information. Note that only a few companies accept direct reservations from travelers; in most cases you'll be referred to travel agencies or cruise specialists. If you do call directly, though, be sure to ask about special offers and last-minute booking.

The listings of each company's fleet is organized by the size of each ship. Sister ships are grouped together; sisters may have identical specifications, but in most cases there are slight differences in public rooms and facilities.

You'll also find a preview of new ships under construction for many major cruise lines. The names, sizes, and expected dates of maiden voyages are all subject to change.

Be aware, too, that each year you can expect a few ships to be taken out of service or sold to another line. Most of the major lines tend to retire their ships somewhere around their teenage years; this trend has accelerated because many of these older ships are smaller and have fewer special features such as verandas and large showrooms than their younger cousins. The older ships are usually sold to one of the second tier of cruise lines that can happily operate a well-tended cruise ship for many decades.

Econoguide Cruise Classifications

Each of the ships in this book is judged in four categories of size, quality, and price range, plus an Econoguide Rating that separates the superb from the merely wonderful and the very good from the good enough.

Here's an explanation of the ratings:

Econoguide Rating

★★★★★★	Best luxury cruise ships
★★★★★	Best cruise ships
★★★★	Above-average
★★★	Middle of the fleet
★★	Budget
★	Below-average

Ship Size

Colossus	100,000+ gross registered tons
Megaship	70,000–100,000 GRT
Grand	40,000–70,000 GRT
Medium	10,000–40,000 GRT
Small	Less than 10,000 GRT

Category

Ultra-Luxury	A semi-private yacht
Top of the Line	Best of the large cruisers
Golden Oldie	A classic older ship
Vintage	A less-than-classic older ship
Adventure	Transport to far-flung places

Price Range

Budget $	Less than $185
Moderate $$	$186 to $250
Premium $$$	$251 to $325
Opulent $$$$	$326 to $400
Beyond Opulent $$$$$	More than $401

Prices are based on per-person, per-day brochure prices for mid-range cabins in regular season. Nearly all cruise lines offer discounts for advance booking, off-season, and special promotions. Use the price range here for comparison purposes only.

Who Owns Whom?

You're not a Carnival sort of cruiser, you say. Seabourn, or maybe Cunard sounds more like your level of luxury. That's just fine, although you might be interested to know that all three cruise lines are part of the same company.

One of the effects of the tremendous success of Carnival has been a consolidation among cruise lines into a family of brands that meet various price and luxury classes. Here's a guide to who owns whom among the major cruise lines:

Carnival Corp., the parent company for Carnival Cruise Lines, has its headquarters in Miami and has mostly American executives. The publicly held corporation, though, is registered in Panama. Controlling interest in the company is held by the family of founder Ted Arison; his son Micky is chairman.

Carnival Corp. owns Carnival Cruise Lines, Holland America Line, and Windstar Cruises. The company also has major interests in Seabourn Cruise Line, Cunard Line, and Costa Cruise Line.

Norwegian Cruise Lines fought a hostile takeover bid by Carnival in 1999, only to find more than half its shares bought by Malaysia-based Star Cruises. After another round of boardroom battles, NCL finally succumbed in early 2000 to a takeover by a new company jointly owned by Star and Carnival. Star, the largest cruise line in Asia, owns 60 percent of the new company, and Carnival 40 percent.

In 1998, Carnival completed the acquisition of Cunard Line and simultaneously completed the merger of Cunard with Seabourn Cruise Line, which was 50 percent owned by Carnival Corporation and 50 percent owned by Atle Brynestad, a Norwegian entrepreneur. Thus, Carnival owns a 68 percent stake in the newly merged company, named Cunard Line Limited, with Brynestad and a group of Norwegian investors holding 32 percent.

Royal Caribbean Cruises Ltd., which also has its headquarters in Miami, is registered as a Liberian corporation. Controlling interests are held by a

What's a knot? One knot is equal to one nautical mile per hour; a nautical mile is about 1.15 land-based miles. Here's a conversion chart:

15 knots = 17.25 mph
16 knots = 18.4 mph
17 knots = 19.55 mph
18 knots = 20.7 mph
19 knots = 21.85 mph
20 knots = 23 mph
21 knots = 24.15 mph
22 knots = 25.3 mph
23 knots = 26.45 mph
24 knots = 27.6 mph
25 knots = 28.75 mph

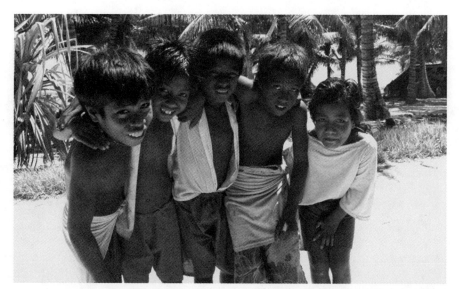

A welcoming committee on Fanning Island, Republic of Kiribati
Photo by Corey Sandler

Bahamian partnership associated with the Pritzker family of Chicago and by a shipping company owned by the Wilhelmsen family in Norway.

Royal Caribbean Cruises Ltd. owns Royal Caribbean International and Celebrity Cruises.

Crystal Cruises is owned by the huge Japanese freighter company Nippon Yupen Kaiska (NYK).

American Classic Voyages owns Delta Queen, American Hawaii, and United States Lines.

Peninsular & Oriental Steam Navigation Company of London owns Princess Cruises.

Radisson Seven Seas Cruises is part of Carlson Hospitality Worldwide; its ships are owned by a variety of international companies and marketed by Radisson Hospitality Worldwide in joint ventures.

Silversea is owned by the Lefebvre family of Rome.

Crown Cruise Line is a new premium brand, part of Commodore Cruises.

Chapter 13
Major Cruise Lines

Carnival Cruise Lines
Celebrity Cruises
Costa Cruise Lines
Crystal Cruises
Cunard Line
Disney Cruise Line
Holland America Line
Norwegian Cruise Line
Princess Cruises
Radisson Seven Seas Cruises
Royal Caribbean International
Seabourn Cruise Line
Silversea Cruises

)Carnival.

Carnival Cruise Lines
3655 N.W. 87th Ave.
Miami, FL 33178-2428
Information: (800) 227-6482, (305) 599-2600
www.carnival.com

The Carnival Fleet

Carnival Victory. (Summer 2000) 2,758 passengers, 102,000 tons

Carnival Triumph. (1999) 2,758 passengers, 102,000 tons

Carnival Destiny. (1999) 2,642 passengers, 101,353 tons

Elation. (1998) 2,040 passengers. 70,367 tons

Paradise. (1998) 2,040 passengers. 70,367 tons

Inspiration. (1996) 2,040 passengers. 70,367 tons

Imagination. (1995) 2,040 passengers. 70,367 tons

Fascination. (1994) 2,040 passengers. 70,367 tons

Sensation. (1993) 2,040 passengers. 70,367 tons

Ecstasy. (1991) 2,040 passengers. 70,367 tons

Fantasy. (1990) 2,044 passengers. 70,367 tons

Celebration. (1987) 1,486 passengers. 47,262 tons

Jubilee. (1986) 1,486 passengers. 47,262 tons

Holiday. (1985) 1,452 passengers. 46,052 tons

Tropicale. (1982) 1,022 passengers. 36,674 tons

Future Ships

Carnival Spirit. (Early 2001) 2,112 passengers, 84,000 tons

Carnival Pride. (Late 2001) 2,112 passengers, 84,000 tons

Carnival Legend. (2002) 2,112 passengers, 84,000 tons

Carnival Conquest. (Fall of 2002) 2,758 passengers, 102,000 tons

Carnival Glory. (Summer 2003) 2,758 passengers, 102,000 tons

It all began with a small cruise charter company run by Ted Arison, an Israeli who had an air freight company in New York. In 1966, when financial difficulties by a shipowner forced the removal of a leased vessel, Arison was left with several loads of passengers but no ship. Arison contacted Knut Kloster, a Norwegian shipping company operator whose vessel the *Sunward* was laid up, and the two put the passengers together with a cruise ship. Thus was born Norwegian Caribbean Lines, the predecessor of today's Norwegian Cruise Lines. That partnership came to an end in 1972.

The flagship line of what became the world's largest cruise company began in 1972 with just one ship, the aging classic *Empress of Canada,* renamed as the *Mardi Gras.* (And in a much-reported example of an inauspicious start, the *Mardi Gras* ran aground off Miami Beach on her maiden voyage.)

But Carnival got past its beginning with a well-crafted marketing plan that turned 180-degrees away from the formal and stuffy image of the great ocean liners. Instead, Carnival's fleet was made up of the "Fun Ships" and featured a near-continuous party atmosphere.

During the next 25 years, the line grew rapidly to become the largest cruise company in the world. In the mid-1980s, Carnival launched an insistent series of television commercials that brought the cruise line into middle-class America with great success.

Carnival operates sailings ranging from three to 16 days to the Bahamas, Caribbean, Mexican Riviera, Alaska, Hawaii, and the Panama Canal.

Carnival purchased Holland America Line and Windstar Cruises in 1989, and holds major interests in Seabourn Cruise Line, Cunard Line (including the *QE2*), and Costa Cruise Line. And in early 2000, Carnival entered into an agreement as a 40 percent partner with Star Cruises of Malaysia to take over Norwegian Cruise Lines.

Carnival began its rise in 1975 with the purchase of the *Empress of Britain,* which entered service as the *Carnivale.* That was followed by the refurbished *S.A. Vaal,* which entered service as the *Festivale* in 1978. The company's first brand-new cruise ship, the *Tropicale,* joined the fleet in 1982.

Three new SuperLiners followed—the *Holiday* in 1985, the *Jubilee* in 1986, and the *Celebration* in 1987. The first in a series of 2,040-passenger Megaships, the *Fantasy,* debuted in 1990, followed by the *Ecstasy, Sensation, Fascination, Imagination,* and *Inspiration* in following years. The *Mardi Gras, Carnivale,* and *Festivale* have since been retired.

And in 1996, Carnival introduced the 2,642-passenger, 101,353-ton *Carnival Destiny,* which was the largest passenger vessel afloat for several years. Four more Destiny-class ships, slightly enlarged to 102,000 tons, are due to join the fleet in coming years. The *Carnival Triumph* arrived in 1999, and the *Carnival Victory* was due in the summer of 2000. *Carnival Conquest* was due to leave the shipyards in the fall of 2002, and the *Carnival Glory* in the summer of 2003.

In 1998, Carnival debuted a pair of Fantasy-class vessels, the *Elation* and *Paradise.* The *Elation* was the first major new cruise ship to be homeported on the West Coast, sailing year-round from Los Angeles to the Mexican Riviera.

The *Paradise* is billed as the world's first smoke-free cruise ship, sailing on alternating eastern and western Caribbean itineraries.

In 2001 and 2002, Carnival will introduce the first ships in the new Spirit-Class. The 960-foot long, 2,112-passenger ships will include two decks of bars, lounges, and nightspots, one with an outdoor wrap-around promenade. Some 80 percent of the staterooms will offer ocean views, with 87 percent of those cabins including private balconies. In addition to a two-level main restaurant, a topside alternative restaurant extends out over the uppermost section of the vessel's atrium. *Carnival Spirit* is due early in 2001, and *Carnival Pride* later in the year. A third sister, *Carnival Legend,* is due in 2002.

Responding to what it says is a growing trend among North Americans for taking short, convenient getaways versus more traditional longer-length vacations, Carnival Cruise Lines was operating about half its fleet on itineraries of five or less days by mid-1999.

And in early 2001, the company expects to open a new cruise terminal in Long Beach, California, adjacent to the *Queen Mary* attraction and hotel. The terminal will include a single berth large enough to accommodate vessels of the size of Carnival's 102,000-ton Destiny-class ships. The terminal will be used as homeport for Carnival's West Coast-based ships, which currently include *Elation* and *Holiday.*

Embarking and debarking passengers can explore the *Queen Mary* and dining and shopping at the pier as well as stay the night in one of the 365 restored staterooms on the *Queen Mary*. Debarkation will take place within a section of the huge geodesic dome at the site, former home of Howard Hughes' Spruce Goose flying boat.

In early 2000, the company announced it was working with Finnish diesel engine manufacturer Wartsila to develop a smokeless diesel-electric propulsion system for future new vessels.

The Carnival Experience

Carnival lives up to its name pretty well, offering a Mardi Gras of glitz, pizazz, and hoopla. These are theme parks on water, with flashing lights, polished wood and chrome, and nearly non-stop parties, contests, and shows.

The ships feature lavish Las Vegas-style shows, magic, singers, and bands.

In other words, Carnival is not your father's Cunard Line . . . although Carnival now owns the separately operated Cunard Line. These are not ships where you will find hushed rosewood libraries and secluded deck chair hideaways; instead you'll find discos and seaborne beach blanket bingo.

Carnival attracts a slightly younger crowd, with more singles and families than many other cruise lines.

In recent years, Carnival has offered a Vacation Guarantee: If guests are dissatisfied with their cruise experience, they may disembark in the first non-U.S. port of call and receive a refund for the unused portion of their cruise fare and reimbursement for air transportation back to the ship's home port.

According to Carnival, more than 70 percent of its customers take advantage of alternative dining areas. The Seaview Bistros, available across the fleet, offer casual dinners in more intimate settings with an array of pastas, steaks, seafood, chicken, and salads. The bistros are created each evening in a section of each ship's indoor/outdoor Lido Deck restaurant.

Camp Carnival has programs for four age groups: Toddlers (2–4) on all ships except *Tropicale,* Intermediate (5–8), Juniors (9–12), and Teens (13–17).

All Carnival vessels feature at least three swimming pools, including a children's wading pool and water slide. Most staterooms can be adapted for use by families with additional berths, rollaway beds, and cribs. There are children's playrooms on all vessels; and two rooms on the six Fantasy-class vessels have toys, games, and activities for kids ages 5 to 12. The *Carnival Destiny* includes a two-level, 1,300-square-foot play area.

The *Elation* also features a high-tech Virtual World gaming center. And the *Holiday* includes a $1 million high-tech Blue Lagoon entertainment center with virtual reality games and 60 state-of-the-art video and arcade games.

Kids can dine out under the stars on the Lido Deck with members of the youth staff. All Carnival vessels have children's wading pools and twisting, turning water slides.

Paradise Echoes the *Queen Mary*

Carnival's *Paradise*—the world's first smoke-free cruise ship—joined the fleet at the end of 1998, sailing from the Port of Miami every Sunday on seven-day alternating eastern and western Caribbean itineraries.

Elements of the ship's design are intended to echo the legendary *Queen Mary,* one of the most famous trans-Atlantic ocean liners of all time. Located aft on the Promenade Deck, the Queen Mary Lounge is used for dancing, late-night comedy shows and other live entertainment. Funnel shapes are used throughout the room, along the walls, framing the sofas, lining the bar front and serving as table bases. Their lower portions are veneered in Nigerian satinwood, stained bright red to match the *Queen Mary*'s celebrated smokestacks; the upper sections are finished in black gloss lacquer. Where red meets black is a strip of lacquered ebony wood inlaid with a clear polycarbonate tube of twinkling Tivoli lights. Even the distinctive ribs that segment the funnels are recreated in ebony inlays. Set atop the large wall-mounted funnels are stylized brass-ringed "portholes," which house video monitors broadcasting vintage motion films of the celebrated *Queen Mary,* other classic liners, and life aboard the great ships of the former heyday of cruising.

Many of the vessel's interior designs are inspired by legendary ships of the past. In the case of the Rex Dance Club, the lounge takes its name from the *Rex,* a famed Italian liner of the 1930s.

Carnival plays off the name Rex, the Latin word for "king," with images of the king of the jungle and safari scenes. Floor-to-ceiling columns surrounding the lounge are stepped like the stones of ancient temples and covered with imitation animal hides which extend upward to the ceiling, creating a mosaic of zebra, leopard and tiger skin patterns.

Between the columns, lion heads in polished black lacquer with gleaming white fangs have fiber-optic eyes that glow and change color. Four of the molded lion heads are equipped with spotlights, which radiate laserlike beams throughout the room.

The dance floor accents the club's jungle motif with yellow-orange stone against black granite, like a tiger's stripes; where the two colors meet, lines of color-changing fiber optics make the floor glimmer.

The *Paradise* is to be the final vessel of the "Fantasy class" series, named for the *Fantasy.* The eight 70,000-ton, 2,040-passenger ships comprise the most cruise ships ever built of a single design.

Fantasy, delivered in 1990, was the first newly built cruise liner that had a diesel-electric AC propulsion and power system; a joystick-controlled navigation system; and it was the first to have a seven-deck central atrium. Sister ships include *Ecstasy, Sensation, Fascination, Imagination, Inspiration,* and *Elation.*

Elation also introduced a new propulsion system known as Azipod, which pulls instead of pushes the vessel through the water, and eliminates the need for drive shafts, rudders and stern thrusters. Carnival claims a savings of 40 tons of fuel per week, improved maneuverability, and higher operating speed with this vessel.

Special Programs

Carnival has added golf packages on all its ships, giving passengers a chance to play courses in the Bahamas, Mexico and the Caribbean. More than a dozen golf courses are featured, including The Links at Safe Haven on Grand Cayman. Greens fees, lessons, cart rental and transportation are included in the port-of-call packages. Equipment rental is also available.

Shipboard lessons from PGA instructors will be offered in a netted driving range, where golfers' swings are videotaped and analyzed by computer.

Carnival has extended its special discount program for members of the American Association of Retired Persons (AARP), with savings of up to $200 per stateroom on specific ships, itineraries and departures through the end of the year 2000.

Carnival Destiny

Econoguide rating:	★★★★★
Ship size:	**Colossus**
Category:	**Top of the Line**
Price range:	**Premium $$$**
Registry:	Panama
Year built:	1996
Sister ships:	*Triumph, Victory, Conquest,* and *Glory*
Itinerary:	Eastern and Western Caribbean
Information:	(305) 599-2600, (800) 227-6482
Website:	www.carnival.com
Passenger capacity:	2,642 (double occupancy)
Crew:	1,070 International
Passenger-to-Crew Ratio:	2.5:1
Tonnage:	101,353
Passenger Space Ratio:	38.6
Length:	893 feet
Beam:	116 feet
Draft:	27 feet
Cruising speed:	22.5 knots
Guest decks:	12
Total cabins:	1,321
Outside:	758
Inside:	515
Suites:	48
Wheelchair cabins:	25
Cuisine:	Contemporary and low-fat, low-calorie Nautica spa fare
Style:	Casual, with one or two semi-formal nights
Price notes:	Single occupancy premium 150 percent to 200 percent
Tipping suggestions:	$9 pp/pd

The first ship to zoom past the 100,000-ton barrier and the holder, for a while, of the largest passenger load afloat. The *Destiny* is the namesake of Carnival's Destiny class of ships, now joined by the *Triumph,* which is ever-so-slightly larger; the *Victory* is due in the summer of the year 2000.

In recent years, *Destiny* sailed from Miami on alternating Eastern (San Juan, St. Croix, St. Thomas) and Western (Cozumel, Grand Cayman, Ocho Rios) Caribbean cruises.

In September of 2000, *Destiny* will be the first mega-liner to operate cruises from San Juan, Puerto Rico, which will become its new home port. The ship will depart every Sunday on alternating, week-long cruises to the southern Caribbean. The first itinerary includes St. Thomas, St. Lucia, Curaçao, and Aruba. The second route features calls at St. Thomas, Antigua, Guadeloupe, and Aruba.

Destiny replaced the *Inspiration* which will move from San Juan to New Orleans.

Prior to repositioning to San Juan, the Carnival Destiny will offer a variety of one- to five-day cruises from Charleston and Newport News in May 2000 including itineraries to the Bahamas; three- and four-day cruises from Boston to Canada, also in May; and a series of four- and five-day cruises to the Canadian Maritime Provinces from New York from June through August 2000.

The *Destiny* replaces the older and smaller *Fascination* on spring sailings from Charleston and Newport News.

From New York, four-day cruises will call at Halifax, Nova Scotia; five-day voyages include an additional stop at St. John, New Brunswick.

Like its near-twin the *Triumph,* the *Destiny* has only a handful of obstructed-view staterooms—the forward-facing cabins on the Upper and Empress Deck. The lifeboats and most other machinery are limited to decks 3, 4, and 5, which are used for public rooms including restaurants, lounges, and bars.

One other unusual feature, if you can call it that: there are a handful of "Night Owl Staterooms" offered at deep discounts of 50 percent or more off the least-expensive rates. But, of course, you'll have to be a Night Owl yourself because these rooms are intended for guests who "love to party late into the night." In other words, these rooms—all inside twin/king cabins—are very close to the noisy late-night action.

At the other end of the spectrum are a set of "family staterooms" that give mom and dad a bit of privacy from the kids. Camp Destiny offers programs for children from ages 5 through 12.

Carnival Triumph

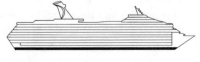

Econoguide rating:	★★★★★
Ship size:	**Colossus**
Category:	**Top of the Line**
Price range:	**Premium $$$**
Registry:	Panama
Year built:	1999
Sister ships:	*Destiny, Victory, Conquest,* and *Glory*
Itinerary:	Eastern and Western Caribbean
Information:	(305) 599-2600, (800) 227-6482
Website:	www.carnival.com

Passenger capacity:	2,758 (double occupancy)
Crew:	1,150 International
Passenger-to-Crew Ratio:	2.4:1
Tonnage:	102,353
Passenger Space Ratio:	37.0
Length:	893 feet
Beam:	116 feet
Draft:	27 feet
Cruising speed:	22.5 knots
Guest decks:	13
Total cabins:	1,379 (estimated)
Outside:	458
Inside:	526
Suites:	64
Wheelchair cabins:	20 (estimated)
Cuisine:	Contemporary and low-fat, low-calorie Nautica spa fare
Style:	Casual, including one or two semi-formal nights
Price notes:	Single occupancy premium 150 percent to 200 percent
Tipping suggestions:	$9 pp/pd

The second ship in the *Destiny* series, a slightly larger version of Carnival's first post-100,000-ton ship.

There are 13 decks, numbered from 1 to 14 (with an eye toward the superstitious, there's a numerical skip between the Sun and Sky decks). The Sky deck is a small observation platform and the entrance to the water slide down to the pool.

The nine-story main atrium is The Capitol, with a spectacular sky dome showing the sky above a lobby bar way down below. Public rooms take their theme from the great cities of the world. There is a pair of bi-level dining rooms, London and Paris; you can also dine bistro-style in the laid-back South Beach Club Restaurant.

Las Vegas-style revues are presented in the three-level Rome Lounge. Drinks and cigars can follow at a cigar bar, or cappuccino and pastry at the Vienna Café. Underground Tokyo is a cavern-like video arcade. Youngsters can join Camp Carnival for daily activities.

The design of the tall ship puts the lifeboats and other obstructions in front of decks 3, 4, and 5 where there are no staterooms. This means there are hardly any outside cabins with obstructed views—the only exceptions are a scant 19 cabins at the bow of the ship with forward facing windows partially blocked by equipment there.

More than 60 percent of the staterooms have ocean views, and of those 70 percent have private balconies.

Balconies are on Upper, Empress, Verandah, Lido, and Panorama decks. Way up top on the Spa deck are 14 cabins that have floor-to-ceiling windows.

After an inaugural series of cruises from New York to Canada, the ship was due to be positioned in Miami for Eastern (San Juan, St. Thomas, St. Croix) and Western (Cozumel, Grand Cayman, Ocho Rios) Caribbean cruises.

Public rooms are inspired by the world's great cities, with decorations commissioned from a crew of international artists.

Among the most spectacular is a series of three-dimensional, map-like murals in glass created by renowned Venetian artist Luciano Vistosi. Depicting the planet's continents, the murals are positioned along the 525-foot-long World's Way promenade. Vistosi also created "Moebius," an expansive, tricolor glass sculpture that dominates the *Triumph's* three-deck-high aft atrium. The eight-foot-high by eight-foot-long abstract sculpture, which took nearly a year to complete, is composed of intertwining blue, green and white glass prisms woven together in a unique free-flowing pattern.

Adorning the *Triumph's* elevator lobbies and passenger stair landings are a series of 35 original murals by Israeli artist Calman Shemi, whose works can also be seen aboard Carnival's *Sensation, Elation* and *Paradise.* Citing influences ranging from Jules Vernes' *Around the World in Eighty Days* to twentieth century French impressionist Raoul Dufy, Shemi's vibrant, multi-hued murals depict such landmarks as Paris' Eiffel Tower, New York's towering skyscrapers, and India's ancient temples.

British artist Susanna Holt's four stone sculptures are located adjacent to the Universe pool on Lido Deck; the vase-like sculptures feature a variety of unique and exquisite materials from around the world including small horn-shaped Bullia Vittata shells from India, sea urchin spines from the Gulf of Mexico, and several varieties of star-shaped Terebra Turritella shells from Taiwan and the Phillipines.

Carnival Victory

Econoguide rating:	★★★★★
Ship size:	**Colossus**
Category:	**Top of the Line**
Price range:	**Premium $$$**
Registry:	Panama
Year built:	2000
Sister ships:	*Destiny, Triumph, Conquest,* and *Glory*
Itinerary:	Eastern and Western Caribbean
Information:	(305) 599-2600, (800) 227-6482
Website:	www.carnival.com
Passenger capacity:	2,758 (double occupancy)
Crew:	1,150 International
Passenger-to-Crew Ratio:	2.4:1
Tonnage:	102,000
Passenger Space Ratio:	37.0
Length:	893 feet
Beam:	116 feet
Draft:	27 feet
Cruising speed:	22.5 knots
Guest decks:	13
Total cabins:	1,379 (estimated)
Outside:	853
Inside:	526
Suites:	64
Wheelchair cabins:	27
Cuisine:	Contemporary and low-fat, low-calorie Nautica spa fare
Style:	Casual, including one or two semi-formal nights
Price notes:	Single occupancy premium 150 percent to 200 percent
Tipping suggestions:	$9 pp/pd

The centerpiece is Oceanic Hall, a nine-deck atrium decorated in watery hues of turquoise, green, gold, and blue. Handmade glass-tile mosaics of mermaids, the sea god Neptune, and other aqueous themes are displayed; overhead, an illuminated dome is decorated in Tiffany-style glass.

The oceanic theme is continued in the names and decor of public rooms including the Coral Sea Café, laid out with displaus of coral.

After she is delivered to Carnival from the Fincantieri shipyards in Monfalcone, Italy, the *Carnival Victory* will set sail to introduce herself to the American East Coast, beginning in August of 2000 with a series of four- and five-day voyages from New York to the Canadian Maritime Provinces. The program starts with a four-day Labor Day weekend cruise to St. John, New Brunswick, departing Aug. 31, 2000. Next, she'll work her way south, operating a series of voyages from several mid-Atlantic ports, including Newport News, Virginia, and Charleston, South Carolina en route to her home port in Miami.

Beginning in mid-October of 2000, the *Carnival Victory* will operate a year-round schedule of seven-day cruises from Miami, alternating weekly to the eastern and western Caribbean, taking over the program that had been offered on the *Carnival Destiny*. Eastern Caribbean cruises visit San Juan, St. Croix and St. Thomas, while western Caribbean sailings feature Playa del Carmen/Cozumel, Grand Cayman and Ocho Rios.

Fantasy

Econoguide rating:	★★★★
Ship size:	**Megaship**
Category:	**Top of the Line**
Price range:	**Moderate $$**
Registry:	Liberia
Year built:	1990
Sister ships:	*Ecstasy, Imagination, Elation, Paradise, Sensation, Fascination,* and *Inspiration*
Itinerary:	Bahamas from Port Canaveral
Information:	(305) 599-2600, (800) 227-6482
Website:	www.carnival.com
Passenger capacity:	2,056 (double occupancy)
Crew:	920 International
Passenger-to-Crew Ratio:	2.2:1
Tonnage:	70,367 tons
Passenger Space Ratio:	34.4
Length:	855 feet
Beam:	103 feet
Draft:	25.9 feet
Cruising speed:	21 knots
Guest decks:	10 decks
Total cabins:	1,022
Outside:	566
Inside:	402
Suites:	54
Wheelchair cabins:	22
Cuisine:	Contemporary and low-fat, low-calorie Nautica spa fare
Style:	Casual during the day. For one or 2 nights, formal dress or dark suit suggested
Price notes:	Single occupancy premium 150 percent to 200 percent
Tipping suggestions:	$9 pp/pd

The namesake ship of Carnival's Fantasy class of ships, which also includes *Ecstasy, Imagination, Elation, Paradise, Sensation, Fascination,* and *Inspiration.*

Fantasy, delivered in 1990, was the first newly built cruise liner with a diesel-electric AC propulsion and power system, and joystick-controlled navigation. Of more interest to most cruisegoers, the *Fantasy* also was the first cruise ship to have a seven-deck central atrium, the Grand Spectrum.

Among her more unusual features is Cleopatra's Bar, a great place to get mummified; the appointments are right out of Egypt by way of Las Vegas.

Sailing out of Port Canaveral, the ship's three-day itinerary visits Nassau while the four-day itinerary adds Freeport.

Ecstasy

Econoguide rating:	★★★★
Ship size:	**Megaship**
Category:	**Top of the Line**
Price range:	**Moderate $$**
Registry:	Liberia
Year built:	1991 (Refurbished in 1998)
Sister ships:	*Fantasy, Imagination, Elation, Paradise, Sensation, Fascination,* and *Inspiration*
Itinerary:	Bahamas, Key West, Cozumel
Information:	(305) 599-2600, (800) 227-6482
Website:	www.carnival.com
Passenger capacity:	2,052 (double occupancy)
Crew:	920 International
Passenger-to-Crew Ratio:	2.2:1
Tonnage:	70,367 tons
Passenger Space Ratio:	34.5
Length:	855 feet
Beam:	103 feet
Draft:	25.9 feet
Cruising speed:	21 knots
Guest decks:	10
Total cabins:	1,022
Outside:	566
Inside:	402
Suites:	54
Wheelchair cabins:	22
Cuisine:	Contemporary and low-fat, low-calorie Nautica spa fare
Style:	Casual with one or two semi-formal evenings
Price notes:	Single occupancy premium 150 percent to 200 percent
Tipping suggestions:	$9 pp/pd

Carnivals' *Ecstasy* sails out of Miami on alternating three- and four-day cruises. The shorter trip makes a 24-hour stop in Nassau; the longer voyage makes port calls at Key West and Cozumel.

A member of the *Fantasy* class of Carnival ships, *Ecstasy* includes three dining areas, 10 bars and lounges, a spa and health club, casino, three swimming pools, jogging tracks, and two children's playrooms.

In July of 1998, *Ecstasy* suffered a minor fire soon after she left the Port of Miami and was forced to return. The ship was refurbished and returned to service.

Elation

Econoguide rating:	★★★★
Ship size:	**Megaship**
Category:	**Top of the Line**
Price range:	**Moderate $$**
Registry:	Panama
Year built:	1998
Sister ships:	*Fantasy, Ecstasy, Imagination, Paradise, Sensation, Fascination,* and *Inspiration*
Itinerary:	From Los Angeles to Mexican Riviera
Information:	(305) 599-2600, (800) 227-6482
Website:	www.carnival.com
Passenger capacity:	2,052 (double occupancy)
Crew:	920 International
Passenger-to-Crew Ratio:	2.2:1
Tonnage:	70,367 tons
Passenger Space Ratio:	34.5
Length:	855 feet
Beam:	103 feet
Draft:	25.9 feet
Cruising speed:	21 knots
Guest decks:	10
Total cabins:	1,020
Outside:	564
Inside:	402
Suites:	54
Wheelchair cabins:	22
Cuisine:	Contemporary and low-fat, low-calorie Nautica spa fare
Style:	Casual, with one or two semi-formal nights
Price notes:	Single occupancy premium 150 to 200 percent
Tipping suggestions:	$9 pp/pd

The first new cruise ship homeported on the West Coast in decades, the *Elation* sails a year-round program of seven-day Mexican Riviera voyages departing from Los Angeles to Puerto Vallarta, Mazatlan, and Cabo San Lucas. She replaced the smaller *Jubilee*, which was shifted to Alaska and Hawaii.

Elation is a member of the *Fantasy* class of Carnival ships. She was the first company ship to include the innovative Azipod propulsion system, which pulls instead of pushes the vessel through the water, and eliminates the need for drive shafts, rudders and stern thrusters. The system dramatically improves maneuverability and delivers higher operating speed, all at a significant savings in fuel.

Fascination

Econoguide rating:	★★★★
Ship size:	**Megaship**
Category:	**Top of the Line**
Price range:	**Moderate $$**
Registry:	Panama
Year built:	1994
Sister ships:	*Fantasy, Ecstasy, Imagination, Elation, Paradise, Sensation,* and *Inspiration*

Itinerary:	Southern Caribbean
Information:	(305) 599-2600, (800) 227-6482
Website:	www.carnival.com
Passenger capacity:	2,052 (double occupancy)
Crew:	920 International
Passenger-to-Crew Ratio:	1:2.22
Tonnage:	70,367 tons
Passenger Space Ratio:	34.4
Length:	855 feet
Beam:	103 feet
Draft:	25.9 feet
Cruising speed:	21 knots
Guest decks:	10
Total cabins:	1,022
Outside:	566
Inside:	402
Suites:	54
Wheelchair cabins:	22
Cuisine:	Contemporary and low-fat, low-calorie Nautica spa fare
Style:	Casual, with one or two semi-formal nights
Price notes:	Single occupancy premium 150 percent to 200 percent
Tipping suggestions:	$9 pp/pd

Fascination brought Hollywood, or at least life-sized likenesses of the stars, to the cruising world. The ship's main drag is Hollywood Boulevard on the Promenade Deck.

The ship sails from San Juan on one-week itineraries to St. Thomas, St. Maarten, Dominica, Martinique, and Barbados, making more port calls than many other Carnival ships in the Caribbean.

Imagination

Econoguide rating:	★★★★
Ship size:	**Megaship**
Category:	**Top of the Line**
Price range:	**Moderate $$**
Registry:	Panama
Year built:	1995
Sister ships:	*Fantasy, Ecstasy, Elation, Paradise, Sensation, Fascination,* and *Inspiration*
Itinerary:	Western Caribbean; Key West
Information:	(305) 599-2600, (800) 227-6482
Website:	www.carnival.com
Passenger capacity:	2,052 (double occupancy)
Crew:	920 International
Passenger-to-Crew Ratio:	2.2:1
Tonnage:	70,367 tons
Passenger Space Ratio:	34.5
Length:	855 feet
Beam:	103 feet
Draft:	25.9 feet
Cruising speed:	21 knots
Guest decks:	10
Total cabins:	1,022
Outside:	566
Inside:	402

Suites:	54
Wheelchair cabins:	22
Cuisine:	Contemporary and low-fat, low-calorie Nautica spa fare
Style:	Casual with one or two semi-formal nights
Price notes:	Single occupancy premium 150 percent to 200 percent
Tipping suggestions:	$9 pp/pd

Imagination is a member of Carnival's *Fantasy* class. Her décor emphasizes some unusual corners of human fancy, from the Curiosity Library to the Shangri-La and Xanadu lounges and the El Dorado Casino.

Imagination sails a year-round schedule of four- and five-day western Caribbean cruises from Miami. Four-day cruises departing Thursdays visit Key West and Cozumel. Five-day cruises departing Mondays call at Grand Cayman and Calica/Cancun. Five-day cruises departing Saturdays stop at Grand Cayman and Ocho Rios.

Inspiration

Econoguide rating:	★★★★
Ship size:	**Megaship**
Category:	**Top of the Line**
Price range:	**Moderate $$**
Registry:	Panama
Year built:	1996
Sister ships:	*Fantasy, Ecstasy, Imagination, Elation, Paradise, Sensation,* and *Fascination*
Itinerary:	West Caribbean from New Orleans
Information:	(305) 599-2600, (800) 227-6482
Website:	www.carnival.com
Passenger capacity:	2,052 (double occupancy)
Crew:	920 International
Passenger-to-Crew Ratio:	2.22:1
Tonnage:	70,367 tons
Passenger Space Ratio:	34.5
Length:	855 feet
Beam:	103 feet
Draft:	25.9 feet
Cruising speed:	21 knots
Guest decks:	10
Total cabins:	1,022
Outside:	566
Inside:	402
Suites:	54
Wheelchair cabins:	22
Cuisine:	Contemporary and low-fat, low-calorie Nautica spa fare
Style:	Casual, including one or two semi-formal nights
Price notes:	Single occupancy premium 150 percent to 200 percent
Tipping suggestions:	$9 pp/pd

A member of Carnival's Fantasy class of ships, *Inspiration* will sail from San Juan with a pair of alternating routes to the southern Caribbean, offering stops at four islands in seven days. One route featured St. Thomas, Antigua, Guadeloupe, and Aruba; the other itinerary offered stops at St. Thomas; St. Lucia, Curaçao, and Aruba.

In September of 2000, *Inspiration* will become the largest cruise ship ever to be based in New Orleans. The ship will sail week-long cruises every Sunday with stops at Montego Bay, Jamaica; George Town, Grand Cayman; and Playa del Carmen/Cozumel, Mexico.

The Inspiration's interior design pays tribute to the popular and fine arts, with rooms such as the Avant-Garde Lounge, featuring statues and wall designs reminiscent of the cubist art form, and the Shakespeare Library, whose ceiling is lined with some of the playwright's most famous quotations.

Paradise

Econoguide rating:	★★★★
Ship size:	**Megaship**
Category:	**Top of the Line**
Price range:	**Moderate $$**
Registry:	Panama
Year built:	1998
Sister ships:	*Fantasy, Ecstasy, Imagination, Elation, Sensation, Fascination,* and *Inspiration*
Itinerary:	Eastern and Western Caribbean from Miami
Information:	(305) 599-2600, (800) 227-6482
Website:	www.carnival.com
Passenger capacity:	2,040 (double occupancy)
Crew:	920 International
Passenger-to-Crew Ratio:	2.2:1
Tonnage:	70,367 tons
Passenger Space Ratio:	34.5
Length:	855 feet
Beam:	103 feet
Draft:	25.9 feet
Cruising speed:	21 knots
Guest decks:	10
Total cabins:	1,020
Outside:	564
Inside:	402
Suites:	54
Wheelchair cabins:	22
Cuisine:	Contemporary and low-fat, low-calorie Nautica spa fare
Style:	Casual, including one or two semi-formal nights
Price notes:	Single occupancy premium 150 percent to 200 percent
Tipping suggestions:	$9 pp/pd

The world's first smoke-free cruise ship, from cabins to dining rooms to the open decks. Carnival is pretty serious about its commitment to healthy air; according to press reports, a pair of travel agents was discovered sneaking a smoke during the ship's christening ceremonies and were made to walk the plank. Luckily, the ship was tied up in New York at the time.

Vacationers who light up onboard the ship may find it's the most expensive cigarette they've ever smoked. Guests who violate the no-smoking policy will be required to disembark at the next port of call and return home at their own expense without any refund of their cruise fare, and $250 in "liquidated damages" will be charged to the passenger's onboard charge account. And the company sent out a press release in December of 1998 when the first passenger was put off the ship because of a transgression of the rules.

Paradise sails from Miami on alternating week-long tours to the Eastern

Caribbean (San Juan, Virgin Gorda, Tortola, and St. Thomas) and the Western Caribbean (Playa del Carmen, Cozumel, Grand Cayman, and Ocho Rios). Among her special places is the Blue Riband Library, which has models of record-breaking ships and a ceiling featuring the route of the transatlantic race for which the room and trophy was named.

Like *Elation* before her, *Paradise* uses the innovative Azipod propulsion system, which pulls instead of pushes the vessel through the water.

Sensation

Econoguide rating:	★★★★
Ship size:	**Megaship**
Category:	**Top of the Line**
Price range:	**Moderate $$**
Registry:	Panama
Year built:	1993
Sister ships:	*Fantasy, Ecstasy, Imagination, Elation, Paradise, Fascination,* and *Inspiration*
Itinerary:	Western Caribbean
Information:	(305) 599-2600, (800) 227-6482
Website:	www.carnival.com
Passenger capacity:	2,040 (double occupancy)
Crew:	920 International
Passenger-to-Crew Ratio:	2.2:1
Tonnage:	70,367 tons
Passenger Space Ratio:	34.5
Length:	855 feet
Beam:	103 feet
Draft:	25.9 feet
Cruising speed:	21 knots
Guest decks:	10
Total cabins:	1,022
Outside:	566
Inside:	402
Suites:	54
Wheelchair cabins:	22
Cuisine:	Contemporary and low-fat, low-calorie Nautica spa fare
Style:	Casual, with one or two semi-formal nights
Price notes:	Single occupancy premium 150 percent to 200 percent
Tipping suggestions:	$9 pp/pd

Sensation, a member of Carnival's *Fantasy* class of ships, sails from Tampa, with week-long tours to the Western Caribbean including calls in Grand Cayman, Playa del Carmen/Cozumel, and New Orleans.

Holiday

Econoguide rating:	★★★
Ship size:	**Grand**
Category:	**Top of the Line**
Price range:	**Budget to Moderate $–$$**
Registry:	Panama
Year built:	1985
Sister ships:	*Celebration* and *Jubilee*
Itinerary:	Los Angeles to Baja Mexico
Information:	(305) 599-2600, (800) 227-6482

Website:	www.carnival.com
Passenger capacity:	1,452 (double occupancy)
Crew:	660 International
Passenger-to-Crew Ratio:	2.2:1
Tonnage:	46,052 tons
Passenger Space Ratio:	31.7
Length:	727 feet
Beam:	92 feet
Draft:	24.7 feet
Cruising speed:	21 knots
Guest decks:	9 decks
Total cabins:	726
Outside:	437
Inside:	279
Suites:	10
Wheelchair cabins:	15
Cuisine:	Contemporary and low-fat, low-calorie Nautica spa fare
Style:	Casual during the day. For one or two nights, formal dress or dark suit suggested
Price notes:	Single occupancy premium 150 percent to 200 percent
Tipping suggestions:	$9 pp/pd

Along with the *Celebration* and the *Jubilee*, the *Holiday* is one of the older sisters of Carnival, but still pretty flashy for an older woman.

In typical Carnival fashion, the *Holiday*'s deck-long Broadway on the Promenade Deck features a bus parked outside the Casino. The nightclub is the western-themed Doc Holiday's.

On this class of ship, lifeboats sit way up high, resulting in very few obstructed views, affecting just four suites on the Veranda Deck.

The ship's three-day cruise to Ensenada departs Friday night and returns to Los Angeles Monday morning; not a bad way to stretch a weekend. Four-day cruises add a stop at Catalina Island.

Celebration

Econoguide rating:	★★★
Ship size:	**Grand**
Category:	**Top of the Line**
Price range:	**Moderate $$**
Registry:	Liberia
Year built:	1987
Sister ships:	*Holiday* and *Jubilee*
Itinerary:	Caribbean from New Orleans
Information:	(305) 599-2600, (800) 227-6482
Website:	www.carnival.com
Passenger capacity:	1,486 (double occupancy)
Crew:	670 International
Passenger-to-Crew Ratio:	2.2:1
Tonnage:	47,262 tons
Passenger Space Ratio:	31.8
Length:	733 feet
Beam:	92 feet
Draft:	24.7 feet
Cruising speed:	21 knots
Guest decks:	9 decks
Total cabins:	743

Outside:	443
Inside:	290
Suites:	10 with balconies
Wheelchair cabins:	14
Cuisine:	A casual café-like setting at least once during week-long cruise. Contemporary and low-fat, low-calorie Nautica spa fare
Style:	Casual with one or two semi-formal nights
Price notes:	Single occupancy premium 150 percent to 200 percent
Tipping suggestions:	$9 pp/pd

Celebration, and her sister ships the *Holiday* and *Jubilee*, are (in relative terms) the old ladies of the Carnival fleet. Only the *Tropicale* has been in service longer.

But these ships have held up pretty well; they were early examples of the Carnival flash, introducing the broad internal "boulevard" on the Promenade Deck. Bourbon Street runs down the length of the starboard side of the ship from the Islands in the Sky Lounge to the Astoria Lounge, passing by the Galaxz Dance Club, the Rainbow Club Casino, and the drydocked trolley parked nearby.

On this class of ship, lifeboats sit way up high, resulting in very few obstructed views, affecting just four suites on the Veranda Deck.

Celebration sails week-long Western Caribbean tours from New Orleans until September of 2000, when it is due to move to Galveston to begin year-round four- and five-day Western Caribbean cruises. Four-day cruises call at Playa del Carmen/Cozumel, Mexico, operating Thursday to Monday for long weekend getaways. Five-day sailings, departing alternate Mondays and Saturdays, feature Cozumel and Calica/Cancun, Mexico.

Jubilee

Econoguide rating:	★★★
Ship size:	**Grand**
Category:	**Top of the Line**
Price range:	**Moderate to Premium $–$$$**
Registry:	Panama
Year built:	1986
Sister ships:	*Holiday* and *Celebration*
Itinerary:	Alaska from Vancouver and Seward, Hawaii, Panama Canal Caribbean
Information:	(305) 599-2600, (800) 227-6482
Website:	www.carnival.com
Passenger capacity:	1,486 (double occupancy)
Crew:	670 International
Passenger-to-Crew Ratio:	2.2:1
Tonnage:	47,262 tons
Passenger Space Ratio:	31.8
Length:	733 feet
Beam:	92 feet
Draft:	24.7 feet
Cruising speed:	21 knots
Guest decks:	9 decks
Total cabins:	743
Outside:	443
Inside:	290
Suites:	10
Wheelchair cabins:	14

Cuisine:	Contemporary and low-fat, low-calorie Nautica spa fare
Style:	Casual, with one or two semi-formal nights
Price notes:	Single occupancy premium 150 percent to 200 percent
Tipping suggestions:	$9 pp/pd

Jubilee moves with the seasons: sailing in Alaska in the summer, heading south from Vancouver to Hawaii in the fall, then on to Ensenada, and from there to transit the Panama Canal to the Caribbean for the winter.

Sister ship to the *Celebration* and *Holiday*, and therefore among the oldest vessels in the fleet, the *Jubilee* still knows how to party.

On this class of ship, lifeboats sit way up high, resulting in very few obstructed views, affecting just four suites on the Veranda Deck.

The *Jubilee's* 10- and 11-day southern Caribbean cruises visit Aruba, Trinidad/Tobago, and St. Kitts. 11-day cruises include a full day cruising through the San Blas Islands as well as a partial transit of the Panama Canal.

In Alaska, the ship sails seven-day Alaska Glacier Route cruises, northbound from Vancouver and southbound from Seward/Anchorage. In the spring, the ship embarks on a 12-day voyage up the coast from Ensenada, Mexico, to four stops in the Hawaiian Islands. Then a new load of passengers begins in Hawaii and moves on to Alaska; the process is reversed in the fall.

Tropicale

Econoguide rating:	★★
Ship size:	**Medium**
Category:	**Middle Age**
Price range:	**Budget to Moderate $$**
Registry:	Liberia
Year built:	1982
Itinerary:	Western Caribbean from Tampa
Information:	(305) 599-2600, (800) 227-6482
Website:	www.carnival.com
Passenger capacity:	1,022 (double occupancy)
Crew:	550 International
Passenger-to-Crew Ratio:	1.9:1
Tonnage:	36,674 tons
Passenger Space Ratio:	35.9
Length:	660 feet
Beam:	85 feet
Draft:	23 feet
Cruising speed:	20 knots
Guest decks:	10 decks
Total cabins:	511
Outside:	312
Inside:	187
Suites:	12
Wheelchair cabins:	11
Cuisine:	Contemporary and low-fat, low-calorie Nautica spa fare
Style:	Casual, with one or two semi-formal nights
Price notes:	Single occupancy supplement 150 percent to 200 percent
Tipping suggestions:	$9 pp/pd

The oldest and smallest ship in the Carnival fleet, in recent years the *Tropicale* has sailed a schedule of four-day and five-day cruises from Tampa to Key

West and Playa del Carmen/Cozumel on shorter trips, adding Grand Cayman to longer journeys.

When the ship was commissioned in 1978, industry experts declared that she was too big and too expensive to ever make a profit; instead, the *Tropicale* blazed a path for the birth of the cruising industry and helped make Carnival a major success.

In September of 1999, *Tropicale* suffered a fire that disabled its engines in the Gulf of Mexico as a tropical storm approached; after drifting for nearly a day, the crew was able to restart one engine and the ship limped out of the way of the storm. After a few weeks of repairs, the ship returned to service, but passengers complained of problems with toilets and other amenities.

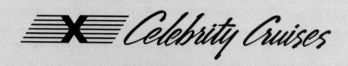

Celebrity Cruises
1050 Caribbean Way
Miami, FL 33132-2096
Information: (800) 437-3111, (305) 262-6677
www.celebrity-cruises.com

Celebrity Cruises Fleet

Millennium. (2000) 1,950 passengers. 91,000 tons

Galaxy. (1996) 1,870 passengers. 77,713 tons

Mercury. (1997) 1,870 passengers. 77,713 tons

Century. (1995) 1,750 passengers. 70,606 tons

Zenith. (1992) 1,375 passengers. 47,255 tons

Horizon. (1990) 1,354 passengers. 46,811 tons

Future Ships
Infinity. (February 2001) 1,950 passengers. 91,000 tons

Unnamed Millennium-class. (August 2001) 1,950 passengers. 91,000 tons

Unnamed Millennium-class. (April 2002) 1,950 passengers. 91,000 tons

X marks the spot for this upscale cruise line that sits somewhere between middle-of-the-market lines such as Royal Caribbean International and the small super-luxury ships of companies such as Crystal and Seabourn.

The Celebrity logo "X" refers to the Greek character used to spell Chandris Group, the original founder of the company; Celebrity will also have you believe the symbol recalls the "X" ancient mariners would use to mark their destinations.

In June of 2000, the first of four Millennium-class ships arrived, becoming the new flagships of the line. The 91,000-ton, 1,950-passenger ships, built at Chantiers de l'Atlantique in St. Lazaire, France, feature balconies for about 70 percent of staterooms as well as some of the largest luxury suites afloat. Along with cousins at Royal Caribbean, they are the first cruise ships to use clean-burning gas turbines for propulsion.

The first ship, *Millennium,* features a unique maritime treasure: the specialty dining room is decorated with the actual interior paneling of the R.M.S. *Olympic,* sister ship to the R.M.S. *Titanic.* The wood paneling in the 134-seat Olympic restaurant once graced the a la carte dining room onboard the glamorous R.M.S *Olympic,* launched in 1911. The paneling was discovered in a private English residence and purchased at auction at Sotheby's.

The restaurant also offers the industry's first demonstration galley, along with a dine-in wine cellar. And speaking of wine, Celebrity also was the winner of an auction at Christie's in New York for three rare bottles of 1907 Heidsieck Monopole champagne; the bottles of bubbly are displayed in the wine cellar. The champagne was salvaged in 1998 from the wreck of the *Jonkoping,* a Swedish merchant ship, which was sunk in the Baltic Sea in 1916 by German sailors who believed the ship was carrying contraband: 5,000 bottles of top-quality French champagne destined for the czar of Russia.

Wine experts say the champagne survived, with corks intact, in 35-degree water and total darkness. The same champagne was believed to be onboard the R.M.S. *Titanic* when it sank in 1912.

The second ship in the class is the *Infinity,* due in February of 2001. She will sail from Fort Lauderdale to Costa Rica and back before heading to Hawaii and on to Alaska for the summer of 2001.

The Millennium ships will head up a fleet that includes the elegant *Galaxy* and *Mercury* sisters and the close cousin *Century,* each with dramatic two-story dining rooms and a great deal of pizazz in public areas. Two older sisters are the smaller *Horizon* and *Zenith.*

Celebrity Cruises was founded in 1989 by the Athens-based Chandris Group as an upscale cruise line. The company's first vessel was the *Meridian,* formerly known as the *Galileo,* completely rebuilt and launched in 1990. That same year Celebrity brought onto the line a new ship, *Horizon.*

One of Celebrity's claims to fame is the quality of its food; among the company's first steps was the hiring of three-star "Guide Michelin" chef and restaurateur Michel Roux to design the food service and train the executive restaurant staff. Roux continues as a consultant, sailing unannounced on the vessels and revising and updating menus every six months.

Roux also supervises an elegant formal tea served weekly aboard all ships, elaborate midnight buffets featuring exquisite ice carvings and theme meals.

The *Meridian* was sold to a Singapore company in 1997 when the *Galaxy* and *Mercury* sisters came on line. That same year, the Chandris family sold Celebrity to Royal Caribbean International.

Long-term plans for Celebrity call for the line to be positioned as a premium brand, with its ships and itineraries marketed separately from Royal Caribbean.

New Celebrity itineraries featuring Europe and South America are planned. Beginning in the year 2000, the Zenith will introduce a new South American itinerary with a pair of sailings in the winter and spring from San Juan and points in the Caribbean.

Overall, Celebrity represents good value for money, a reasonable step up in quality and price from the middle of the pack.

The Celebrity Experience

In the main dining room, the dress code is just a bit more formal than on other lines; jackets and ties are requested for men on formal and informal nights, with time off for good behavior on casual nights only.

At the same time, Celebrity has introduced more casual dining options most nights on every cruise, served in the Palm Springs Grill and pool area on *Mercury*, at the Oasis Grill and pool area on *Galaxy*, the Coral Seas Cafe on *Horizon*, the Windsurf Café on *Zenith*, and in the Sky Bar on *Century*. A typical casual menu would offer lasagna, broiled salmon steak, spit-roasted chicken and grilled sirloin steak—simpler fare than offered in the main dining rooms.

Indulgences onboard include the AquaSpa program offering treatments and facilities from Middle Eastern, Asian, and European sources, including a 115,000-gallon Thalassotherapy pool on the *Century*, hydrotherapy spa baths of seaweed, minerals, or aromatherapy oils, and aqua meditation. There's also the Rasul treatment that includes a seaweed soap shower, medicinal mudpack, herbal steam bath, and massage. Treatments can be booked individually or as part of packages extending over the course of a voyage.

The line's Family Cruising Program serves Ship Mates (3–6), Celebrity Cadets (7–10), Ensigns (11–13), and Teens (14–17) with events that include pool Olympics, scavenger hunts, video games, arts and crafts, ship tours, pizza and ice cream parties.

During summer and seasonal sailing periods, the youth program includes a "Summer Stock Theater." A play is performed by Ship Mates and Celebrity Cadets, produced and directed by the Ensigns.

The Young Mariners Club offers a behind-the-scenes look at cruising, allowing youngsters to interact with departments of the cruise ship, including navigation, food and beverage departments, and the entertainment staff.

Millennium

Econoguide rating:	★★★★★
Ship size:	**Megaship**
Category:	**Top of the Line**
Price range:	**Premium $$$**
Registry:	Liberia
Year built:	2000
Sister ships:	*Infinity* and two other *Millennium*-class ships under construction

Itinerary:	Europe, Caribbean from Fort Lauderdale
Information:	(305) 262-6677
Website:	www.celebrity-cruises.com
Passenger capacity:	1,950 (double occupancy)
Crew:	999 International
Passenger-to-Crew Ratio:	2:1
Tonnage:	91,000
Passenger Space Ratio:	46.7
Length:	965 feet
Beam:	105.6 feet
Draft:	26.3 feet
Cruising speed:	24 knots
Guest decks:	11
Total cabins:	975 staterooms
Outside:	780
Inside:	195
Suites:	50
Wheelchair cabins:	9
Cuisine:	Continental and International
Style:	Informal with two or three formal evenings
Price notes:	Single occupancy available for about 125 percent premium
Tipping suggestions:	$9 pp/pd

The first of Celebrity's Millennium-class ships took to the seas in the summer of 2000, sailing in Europe until November when she was to cross the pond to Fort Lauderdale to begin a season of alternating eastern and western Caribbean tours.

The handsome ships employ environmentally friendly gas turbines and high-tech engine pods for maneuverability.

Infinity (Preview)

Econoguide rating:	★★★★★
Ship size:	**Megaship**
Category:	**Top of the Line**
Price range:	**Premium $$$**
Registry:	Liberia
Year built:	February, 2001
Sister ships:	*Millennium* and two other *Millennium*-class ships under construction
Itinerary:	Caribbean, Hawaii, Alaska
Information:	(305) 262-6677
Website:	www.celebrity-cruises.com
Passenger capacity:	1,950 (double occupancy)
Crew:	999 International
Passenger-to-Crew Ratio:	2:1
Tonnage:	91,000
Passenger Space Ratio:	46.7
Length:	965 feet
Beam:	105.6 feet
Draft:	26.3 feet
Cruising speed:	24 knots
Guest decks:	11
Total cabins:	975 staterooms
Outside:	780
Inside:	195
Suites:	50
Wheelchair cabins:	9
Cuisine:	Continental and International

Style:	Informal with two or three formal evenings
Price notes:	Single occupancy available for about 125 percent premium
Tipping suggestions:	$9 pp/pd

The second of four ships in Celebrity's Millennium class is due to begin service in early 2001. The ship's two penthouse suites feature marble floors, separate living and dining rooms, a baby grand piano, a high-tech flat screen entertainment system, fax machine, and a private veranda with a whirlpool for times when you absolutely need to get away from it all.

Century

Econoguide rating:	★★★★★
Ship size:	**Megaship**
Category:	**Top of the Line**
Price range:	**Premium $$$**
Registry:	Liberia
Year built:	Entered service 1995
Sister ships:	*Galaxy* and *Mercury*
Itinerary:	Eastern and Western Caribbean from San Juan in winter, Europe in summer
Information:	(305) 262-6677
Website:	www.celebrity-cruises.com
Passenger capacity:	1,750 (double occupancy)
Crew:	858 International
Passenger-to-Crew Ratio:	2:1
Tonnage:	70,606 tons
Passenger Space Ratio:	40.3
Length:	815 feet
Beam:	105 feet
Draft:	25 feet
Cruising speed:	21.5 knots
Guest decks:	10
Total cabins:	875
Outside:	517
Inside:	306
Suites:	52
Wheelchair cabins:	8
Cuisine:	Continental and International
Style:	Informal with two or three formal evenings
Price notes:	Single occupancy available for about 125 percent premium
Tipping suggestions:	$9 pp/pd

Celebrity's *Century* is a close sister to handsome *Galaxy* and *Mercury* twins. *Century* will enter the growing European market in 1999, moving across the Atlantic from Fort Lauderdale in April and returning from Genoa, Italy in November to resume her schedule of trips to the Eastern and Western Caribbean.

The spectacular 1,080-seat two-level Grand Restaurant surrounds diners with the blue of the sea in a setting of old world elegance.

Lifeboats on the handsome ship hang recessed into the Entertainment and Promenade decks, leaving very few obstructed views from passenger cabins above and below.

Galaxy

Econoguide rating:	★★★★★
Ship size:	**Megaship**
Category:	**Top of the Line**
Price range:	**Premium $$$**
Registry:	Liberia
Year built:	1996
Sister ships:	*Century* and *Mercury*
Itinerary:	Pacific Coast to Vancouver; Alaska, Panama Canal, Southern Caribbean
Information:	(305) 262-6677
Website:	www.celebrity-cruises.com
Passenger capacity:	1,870 (double occupancy)
Crew:	909 International
Passenger-to-Crew Ratio:	2.1:1
Tonnage:	77,713
Passenger Space Ratio:	41.6
Length:	866 feet
Beam:	105.6 feet
Draft:	25.5 feet
Cruising speed:	21.5 knots
Guest decks:	10
Total cabins:	935
Outside:	419
Inside:	296
Suites:	220 with private balconies
Wheelchair cabins:	5
Cuisine:	Pacific Northwest cuisine for Alaska cruises
Style:	Informal with two or three formal evenings
Price notes:	Single occupancy available for about 125 percent premium
Tipping suggestions:	$9 pp/pd

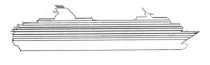

Along with *Century* and *Mercury,* one of the flagships of the Celebrity fleet.
The lifeboats are recessed into Entertainment and Promenade decks, all but eliminating obstructed views from passenger cabins that are all located above or below the boats. The Promenade deck, though, does not allow a full circuit of the deck, blocked at the bow and stern by the Celebrity Theater and the Orion Restaurant respectively.

In recent years, *Galaxy* cruised Alaska in the spring and summer, moving to the Caribbean through the Panama Canal in October; she reverses her migration in late April of each year.

Mercury

Econoguide rating:	★★★★★
Ship size:	**Megaship**
Category:	**Top of the Line**
Price range:	**Premium $$$**
Registry:	Panama
Year built:	1997
Sister ships:	*Century* and *Galaxy*
Itinerary:	Alaska, Pacific Coastal to Vancouver, Panama Canal, Western Caribbean
Information:	(305) 262-6677
Website:	www.celebrity-cruises.com
Passenger capacity:	1,870 (double occupancy)
Crew:	909 International

Passenger-to-Crew Ratio:	2.1:1
Tonnage:	77,713
Passenger Space Ratio:	41.6
Length:	866 feet
Beam:	105.6 feet
Draft:	25.5 feet
Cruising speed:	21.5 knots
Guest decks:	10
Total cabins:	935
Outside:	419
Inside:	296
Suites:	220 with private balconies
Wheelchair cabins:	8
Cuisine:	Gourmet pizza delivery. Pacific Northwest, Continental
Style:	Informal with two or three formal nights per cruise
Price notes:	Single cabins available at about 125 percent premium
Tipping suggestions:	$9 pp/pd

Near-twin to the handsome *Galaxy*, the *Mercury* summers in Alaska, sailing from Vancouver and Seward, moving south to San Diego and through the Panama Canal in October and November. At the end of 2000, she will sail a new set of itineraries in South America from La Guaira to Rio de Janerio, and around Cape Horn, returning to Fort Lauderdale in March of 2001 for Caribbean cruises.

The ship's shopping space resembles a European piazza.

Recreation facilities include an indoor Palm Springs pool area, two outdoor La Playa pools and four outdoor whirlpools. A sports deck offers basketball, a golf simulator and volleyball; there's also trap shooting off the ship.

Horizon

Econoguide rating:	★★★★
Ship size:	**Grand**
Category:	**Top of the Line**
Price range:	**Premium $$$**
Registry:	Liberia
Year built:	1990 (Refurbished 1998)
Sister ships:	*Zenith*
Itinerary:	Bermuda from New York, Caribbean and Panama Canal from Aruba
Information:	(305) 262-6677
Website:	www.celebrity-cruises.com
Passenger capacity:	1,354 (double occupancy)
Crew:	642 Greek officers, international crew
Passenger-to-Crew Ratio:	2.1:1
Tonnage:	46,811
Passenger Space Ratio:	34.6
Length:	682 feet
Beam:	95 feet
Draft:	24 feet
Cruising speed:	21.4 knots
Guest decks:	9
Total cabins:	677
Outside:	513
Inside:	144
Suites:	20
Wheelchair cabins:	4 ocean-view staterooms
Cuisine:	Continental and International

Style:	Informal with two or three formal evenings
Price notes:	Single occupancy available for about 125 percent premium
Tipping suggestions:	$9 pp/pd

In relative terms, one of the more "intimate" ships in the Celebrity fleet, albeit still a rather large vessel with more than 2,000 passengers and crew onboard most voyages. The *Horizon* is a near-twin to the *Zenith*.

The *Horizon* will sail from New York to Bermuda from May through October of 2000, moving to Aruba to sail in the Southern Caribbean and through the Panama Canal through April of 2001.

Most of the cabins on the Bermuda Deck have views obstructed by the lifeboats that hang outside the windows there.

In 1998, *Horizon* underwent a $4.5 million refurbishment that brought it up to the comfort and elegance specs of Celebrity's *Century*-class vessels. The Gemini Disco was gutted and redesigned to form a grand entrance area, with the intimate Michael's Club, a cigar and cognac club (complete with a high-tech fireplace). Also in the entrance area is a card room and library, complete with personal computers and printers; the former card room and library on Galaxy Deck was redesigned as a Martini Bar, art gallery, and boutique.

Horizon's COVA Café, in the former Plaza Bar, is based on the famed Milan coffeehouse Pasticceria Confetteria COVA. The intimate café features cappuccino, espresso, macchiato, a variety of teas, liqueurs, and chocolates.

The Fantasia bar on the Sun Deck was remade as *Horizon*'s AquaSpa, including a beauty salon, five treatment rooms, and a fitness and aerobics area.

A similar redesign was undertaken in late 1999 for Celebrity's *Zenith*, sister ship to the *Horizon*.

Zenith

Econoguide rating:	★★★★
Ship size:	**Grand**
Category:	**Top of the Line**
Price range:	**Premium $$$**
Registry:	Liberia
Year built:	1992
Sister ships:	*Horizon*
Itinerary:	Bermuda, Panama Canal, Mexico
Information:	(305) 262-6677
Website:	www.celebrity-cruises.com
Passenger capacity:	1,375 (double occupancy)
Crew:	670 International
Passenger-to-Crew Ratio:	2:1
Tonnage:	47,255
Passenger Space Ratio:	34.4
Length:	682 feet
Beam:	95 feet
Draft:	24 feet
Cruising speed:	21.4 knots
Guest decks:	9
Total cabins:	687
Outside:	519
Inside:	146
Suites:	22

Wheelchair cabins:	4
Cuisine:	Continental and International
Style:	Informal with two or three formal evenings
Price notes:	Single occupancy available for about 125 percent premium
Tipping suggestions:	$9 pp/pd

Near-twin to the *Horizon,* the *Zenith* received a major refurbishment in late 1999 along the lines of the remake of *Horizon.*

She will sail from New York to Bermuda from April to October of 2000, moving south to Fort Lauderdale for Caribbean cruises until April of 2001.

The ship's observation lounge includes telescopes; the pool lies beneath a retractable sliding glass sunroof.

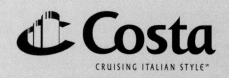

Costa Cruise Lines
80 Southwest 8th St.
Miami, FL 33130-3097
Information: (800) 332-6782, (305) 358-7325
www.costacruises.com

Costa Cruise Line Fleet

CostaAtlantica. (2000) 2,112 passengers, 84,000 tons

CostaVictoria. (1996) 1,950 passengers, 76,000 tons

CostaRomantica. (1993) 1,350 passengers, 54,000 tons

CostaClassica. (1991) 1,308 passengers, 53,000 tons. Sails in Europe.

CostaAllegra. (1992) 820 passengers. 28,500 tons. Sails in Europe.

CostaMarina. (1990) 776 passengers. 25,500 tons. Sails in Europe.

Costa puts the emphasis on its Italian roots, even though today it travels mostly to the Caribbean and is operated out of Miami by a corporation registered in Panama that was founded by an Israeli.

Nevertheless, its ships do have a distinctive Italian flavor in their design, cuisine and activities. And its distinctive appearance is enhanced with bright yellow smokestacks that bear the company's "C."

In the summer of 2000, all five of Costa's vessels were due to be deployed in Europe, from May to October, sailing from the ports of Genoa, Venice, Barcelona, Amsterdam, and Copenhagen on trips to the eastern and western Mediterranean, Canary Islands, Black Sea, the Baltic, and the fjords of Scandinavia. In November of 2000, the new *CostaAtlantica* and the *CostaVictoria* were due to sail from Fort Lauderdale to the Caribbean for the winter.

Costa's history can be traced back to 1860 when Giacomo Costa began an olive oil business in Genoa, Italy. In 1916, his three sons inherited the family business; in 1924, they purchased the *Ravenna*, a 1,100-ton freighter, to reduce the transportation costs for their oil empire.

By 1935, seven more freighters had joined the fleet, with two more by 1942. World War II reduced the fleet back to a single ship, but by 1948 the company had rebounded to a 12-ship fleet.

Passenger service began in 1948 with the 12,000-ton, 850-passenger *Anna C*, carrying passengers between Genoa and South America. The service was an immediate success, and within four years Costa added three more vessels. In the late 1950s, the company constructed its first brand-new ships.

Costa's year-round North American cruise operation began in 1959 with seven-day cruises into the Caribbean from Miami on the *Franca C*. The company continued to grow in North America and Europe, introducing in 1985 its North American flagship, the 984-passenger *CostaRiviera*, which remains in service today in Europe and the Middle East after a recent refurbishment. After more than 100 years under the ownership of the Costa family, in 1989 the company opened to outside investors, ushering in a new era of expansion.

In 1997, Costa Crociere (Costa Cruises) was purchased by Carnival Corporation and Airtours plc.

The *CostaAtlantica*, a handsome 84,000-ton, 2,112-passenger ship, joined the fleet in the spring of 2000. It is similar to Carnival's Spirit-class vessels.

After an inaugural season in Europe, the *CostaAtlantica* will cross her namesake ocean to Fort Lauderdale and sail the Caribbean from there.

The company offers cruises of seven days and longer in the Caribbean, Mediterranean, Northern Europe, South America, and Transatlantic.

The Costa Experience

Costa promotes "cruising Italian Style" with Italian theme nights, Italian language lessons, cooking lessons, and its famously quirky entertainments, including the Festa Italiana, which is billed as an Italian Street Festival at Sea with bocce ball tournaments, Tarantella dance lessons, pizza dough tossing contests, Italian Karaoke, and the like.

Another theme night is Notte Tropical, when the evening's activities take place out on deck, including ice carving demonstrations and a sumptuous midnight alfresco buffet.

But Costa is most famous for the "Roman Bacchanal" toga party on the last night of its Caribbean cruises; for the evening, passengers don togas and enjoy a Bacchanal parade and other such preplanned debauchery. (By the way, passengers no longer have to create their own togas from bedsheets—ready-made off-the-shoulder models are available from the cruise staff.)

In 1999, Costa added Ristorante Magnifico by Zeffirino to the *CostaVictoria* as an alternative dining experience; the same offering will be available on *CostaAtlantica*. Zeffirinos has been a favorite restaurant in Genoa since 1939. Seating is by reservation, and a service charge of $18.75 per person is applied.

The *CostaRomantica* and *CostaVictoria* offer the Golf Academy at Sea, with onboard golf clinics and seminars conducted by a PGA Member Golf Instructor. Guests can also be accompanied by a PGA Instructor as they play on some of the Caribbean's best golf courses, such as Mahogany Run in St. Thomas, the Links at Safe Haven in Grand Cayman, Runaway Bay and Sandals Golf Resorts in Ocho Rios, Cable Beach Golf Course in Nassau, Key West Golf Course in Key West, and Teeth of the Dog or The Links at the Casa de Campo Resort in the Dominican Republic.

Costa's private beach is Catalina Island just off the coast of the Dominican Republic. Entertainment includes a beach barbecue, chaise lounges, water floats, and land and water sports.

The Costa Kids Club and the Costa Teens Club offer special activities, including Nintendo competitions, tours of the bridge and galley, arts and crafts, scavenger hunts, and more. Two full-time youth counselors are available on each Caribbean sailing, with additional staff members available when there are more than 12 children on a cruise.

Depending on demand, the program may offer activities while the ship is in port. And Costa also offers the Parents Night Out; on two different nights, parents can enjoy an evening alone while the children enjoy a supervised buffet or pizza party, as well as fun activities.

Group baby sitting for ages 3 and up is available on request in the evening while the ship is at sea, and during the day when the ship is in port. There is an extra charge for sitting services.

Special Deals

Passengers who book at least 120 days in advance can take advantage of Costa's "Andiamo Rates" of about $500, which can work out to as much as one-third off per person on the less-expensive cabins and still a decent break on more-expensive accommodations.

Costa Cruise Savers offers additional savings for senior citizens, children, and single parents on selected ships and sailing dates. Savings are also available for passengers who combine two 7-night cruises.

CostaAtlantica

Econoguide rating:	★★★★★
Ship size:	**Megaship**
Category:	**Top of the Line**
Price range:	**Moderate to Premium $$–$$$**
Registry:	Liberia
Year built:	Summer of 2000
Itinerary:	Alternating eastern and western Caribbean in fall and winter from Fort Lauderdale; Greece and Turkey in spring and summer
Information:	(800) 332-6782
Website:	www.costacruises.com
Passenger capacity:	2,112 (double occupancy)
Crew:	900 (estimated)
Passenger-to-Crew Ratio:	2.4:1
Tonnage:	84,000

Passenger Space Ratio:	39.8
Length:	960 feet
Beam:	106 feet
Draft:	25 feet
Cruising speed:	22 knots
Guest decks:	12
Total cabins:	1,057
Outside:	787
Inside:	212
Suites:	58
Cuisine:	Italian/Continental
Style:	Informal with two formal nights per cruise. One casual night is a Roman Bacchanal, with guests invited to wear togas
Price notes:	Single occupancy premium 150 percent to 200 percent
Tipping suggestions:	$8.50 pp/pd

The largest, fastest, and splashiest Costa ship joins the fleet in the summer of 2000.

Nearly three-quarters of the cabins on the $400 million ship feature verandas. The ship has three pools, including one featuring a retractable magrodome, which allows swimming in all weather.

The 12 passenger decks of the ship are all named after motion pictures by famed Italian director Federico Fellini; among them, *La Dolce Vita, Amarcord, I Clowns,* and *La Strada.*

The *CostaAtlantica* features a replica of the famed Caffé Florian, the landmark café located under the arcades of the Procuratie Nuove in St. Mark's Square in Venice. The original café opened in 1720 and became the most famous botega da caffé of its time. Along the years, the Caffé Florian has entertained notables who include Casanova, who hung out there in search of beautiful women; composers Antonio Vivaldi and Igor Stravinsky; and author Charles Dickens.

In addition to the two-level Tiziano main restaurant, the Botticelli Buffet, and the Napoli Pizzeria, guests can also opt for an alternative dining experience at the Ristorante Magnifico by Zeffirino.

CostaRomantica

Econoguide rating:	★★★★★
Ship size:	**Grand**
Category:	**Top of the Line**
Price range:	**Moderate $$**
Registry:	Liberia
Year built:	1993 (entered service)
Itinerary:	Spring and summer Northern Europe and Mediterranean; fall and winter in South America
Information:	(800) 332-6782
Website:	www.costacruises.com
Passenger capacity:	1,356 (double occupancy)
Crew:	610
Passenger-to-Crew Ratio:	2.2:1
Tonnage:	53,000
Passenger Space Ratio:	39
Length:	722 feet

Beam:	102 feet
Draft:	25 feet
Cruising speed:	18.5 knots
Guest decks:	10
Total cabins:	678
Outside:	428
Inside:	216
Suites:	34
Wheelchair cabins:	6
Cuisine:	Italian/Continental
Style:	Informal with two formal nights per cruise.
Price notes:	Single occupancy premium from 150 percent to 200 percent; single cabins available
Tipping suggestions:	$4.50 pp/pd

A bit of European sophistication at sea, including almost $20 million invested in original works of art, including sculptures, paintings, murals, and wall hangings. There's a primarily Italian and international hotel and dining staff, and within is the Via Condotti elegant European shopping promenade. The ship's decks are named after great cities of Europe: Monte Carlo, Madrid, Vienna, Verona, Paris, London, Copenhagen, and Amsterdam.

The Piazza Italia Grand Bar on the Verona Deck is one of the largest lounges afloat with a capacity of 300; it has a teak dance floor and offers live entertainment. L'Opera Theatre is a 630-seat Renaissance-style amphitheater setting, extending to the Vienna Deck above. A disco atop the ship offers 360-degree views

Oversized staterooms average 200 square feet, with 34 luxurious suites with as much as 580 square feet; there are only 10 verandas, though. An inside Standard room is a still-spacious 175 square feet.

In 2000, the ship sailed away from the Caribbean, switching over to a schedule that puts her in Europe in the spring and summer and South America in the fall and winter.

The Costa Kids Program features morning, afternoon and evening events for children ages 3 to 17.23

CostaVictoria

Econoguide rating:	★★★★★
Ship size:	**Megaship**
Category:	**Top of the Line**
Price range:	**Moderate $$**
Registry:	Liberia
Year built:	1996 (entered service)
Information:	(800) 332-6782
Itinerary:	Alternating eastern and western Caribbean from Fort Lauderdale in fall and winter, Europe in spring and summer
Website:	www.costacruises.com
Passenger capacity:	1,928 (double occupancy)
Crew:	800
Passenger-to-Crew Ratio:	2.4:1
Tonnage:	76,000
Passenger Space Ratio:	39
Length:	828 feet

Beam:	105.5 feet
Draft:	26 feet
Cruising speed:	23 knots
Guest decks:	10
Total cabins:	964
Outside:	555
Inside:	389
Suites:	20
Wheelchair cabins:	6
Cuisine:	Italian/Continental
Style:	Informal with two formal nights per cruise. One casual night is a Roman Bacchanal, with guests invited to wear togas
Price notes:	Single occupancy premium 150 percent to 200 percent
Tipping suggestions:	$8.50 pp/pd

An unusual design in this day of Megaships; the *CostaVictoria* is almost squared off at the stern and pinched like a pumpkin seed at the bow with a very steep forward slope. From the side it looks like a horizontal skyscraper. Inside is the central Planetarium Atrium, seven decks high and covered by a large glass dome. Four panoramic elevators take passengers to the upper deck. Decks are named after classic operas, including "Madame Butterfly," "Rigoletto," "Norma," "Tosca," "Othello," "Carmen," "Traviata," and "Boheme."

In recent years, the *CostaVictoria* cruised the Eastern and Western Caribbean on alternating 7-night journeys out of Ft. Lauderdale in the fall and winter. The Eastern circuit included San Juan, St. Thomas/St. John, Serena Cay/Casa de Campo, and Nassau. Heading west, the ship stopped at Key West, Cozumel, Ocho Rios, and Grand Cayman. In the summer and fall, the ship sailed to Greece and Turkey.

The Costa Kids program features events for children ages 3 to 17.

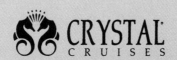

Crystal Cruises
2049 Century Park East, Suite 1400
Los Angeles, CA 90067
Information: (800) 820-6663, (310) 785-9300
www.crystalcruises.com

Crystal Cruises Fleet

Crystal Symphony. (1995) 940 passengers, 51,044 tons

Crystal Harmony. (1990) 940 passengers, 49,400 tons

Crystal Cruises is a luxury cruise line that has a most unusual pedigree. Founded in 1988, Crystal offers a world of attendants in white gloves, leaded crystal wine glasses filled with the contents of a world-class wine cellar at sea,

Wedgwood bone china, teak deck furniture, goose down pillows and mohair lap blankets.

At about 50,000 tons each, these are large ships by any measure. But they are half the size of the current heavyweight champions and they carry only about one-third the number of passengers. On each of the ships, 545 crew members serve about 940 passengers, resulting in a very large amount of space per passenger.

All this from a company that is much more used to hauling around grain and auto parts. Crystal Cruises is owned by the Japanese company Nippon Yupen Kaiska (NYK), the largest freighter shipping company in the world with more than 500 vessels in its fleet.

The Crystal Experience

Crystal's two ships are very similar, although they were built oceans apart: the *Crystal Harmony* in Nagasaki, Japan in 1990 and the *Crystal Symphony* in Turku, Finland in 1995. They shared the same lead designer. The newer *Crystal Symphony* includes a larger atrium and restaurants.

Most of the cabins have private verandas, and the most spectacular suites are, well, spectacular. The penthouse suites are nearly 1,000 square feet in size, including a private Jacuzzi with an ocean view. The *Crystal Harmony* has a small number of inside cabins while the Crystal Symphony offers outside accommodations for all. The lobby of each ship showcases a "crystal" piano (made of lucite, actually, but still an impressive objet d'art).

Shipboard dining is a high priority. The elegant Crystal Dining Room never repeats a menu, even on three-month World Cruises, although guests can order past favorites. The *Crystal Harmony* offers Japanese cuisine in the Kyoto dining room, and *Crystal Symphony* offers Asian specialties at Jade Garden. A third choice, the Italian bistro Prego, is offered on both ships. The small alternative restaurants can only accommodate a portion of the total number of guests, though.

In early 2000, the line announced plans to build a third ship similar in size and configuration to the *Crystal Harmony* and *Crystal Symphony*.

Onboard entertainment ranges from "Some Enchanted Evening," the first licensed shipboard production show of Rodgers and Hammerstein music, to a performance by a concert pianist, or a nightclub comedian.

And if you haven't spent enough money already, you can go to a Caesars Palace casino at sea.

The Crystal Visions Enrichment Program features authors, journalists, historians, and famed chefs. In 1998, the line presented a lecture program in cooperation with *The New Yorker* magazine, presenting authors, cartoonists, and editors.

Crystal was also among the first cruise lines to allow guests to send and receive e-mail messages to anywhere in the world from onboard the ship at a price much less than the cost of a satellite phone call.

In the spring of 2000, Crystal Cruises' European season began in London with trips to Western Europe and the Mediterranean, with summer visits throughout Europe, Scandinavia, and the Baltic.

Crystal's 2000 Theme Cruise schedule includes a voyage to the Summer Games in Sydney in the company of ten Olympic greats. Other theme cruises include Classical Music, Opera, Art & Architecture; Wine & Food Festival; Big Band and Jazz, and Golf.

Membership in the Crystal Society (for previous customers) brings with it a 5 percent discount on future sailings.

Crystal Harmony

Econoguide rating:	★★★★★★
Ship size:	**Grand**
Category:	**Ultra-Luxury**
Price range:	**Beyond Opulent $$$$$**
Registry:	Bahamas
Year built:	1988
Sister ships:	*Crystal Symphony*
Itinerary:	Panama Canal, Mexican Riviera, Alaska, Canada, New England, Caribbean, South America, South Pacific
Information:	(800) 820-6663
Website:	www.crystalcruises.com
Passenger capacity:	940 (double occupancy)
Crew:	545 (Norwegian and Japanese officers)
Passenger-to-Crew Ratio:	1.7:1
Tonnage:	49,400
Passenger Space Ratio:	52.6
Length:	790 feet
Beam:	105 feet
Draft:	24.6 feet
Cruising speed:	22 knots
Guest decks:	8
Total cabins:	480
Outside:	461 (260 with verandas)
Inside:	19
Suites:	62
Wheelchair cabins:	4
Cuisine:	Continental and American. Two specialty restaurants: Japanese, Italian cuisine
Style:	Casual with at least three formal evenings per cruise
Price notes:	Single occupancy supplement 125 percent to 200 percent of advance booking fares. Discounts available for bookings made six months or more in advance, and cruises booked onboard a previous cruise. An adult or child 12 or older in a third berth pays minimum fare. Children 11 and younger pay 50 percent of the minimum fare when accompanied by two full-fare paying adults
Tipping suggestions:	$10.50 pp/pd

High-tone elegance and service on one of the largest of the luxury ships. The *Crystal Harmony* has eight guest decks, including four 948-square-foot Crystal Penthouses that have verandas, 58 other suites that have verandas, and 198 outside deluxe staterooms that have verandas. The smallest cabins are 19 Inside Staterooms, a not-too-tiny 183 square feet in size.

Entertainment includes the Caesars Palace at Sea Casino with 115 slot machines, seven tables and a roulette wheel. The domed Vista Observation Lounge up forward offers three levels of seating and a 270-degree view.

The Crystal Dining Room offers international cuisine and a world-class wine list; Crystal also offers a pair of alternative restaurants. The Kyoto restaurant features a Japanese menu, not surprising for a ship line owned by a Japanese freight line. Typical menu items include tempura; Pacific salmon with shiitake mushrooms, and traditional sukiyaki dinner with filet mignon. The Prego restaurant offers intimate Italian dining.

Recreation facilities include a full-length lap pool and an indoor/outdoor pool, a paddle tennis court, golf driving ranges and putting greens, and a sumptuous spa.

Crystal Symphony

Econoguide rating:	★★★★★★
Ship size:	**Grand**
Category:	**Ultra-Luxury**
Price range:	**Beyond Opulent $$$$$**
Registry:	Bahamas
Year built:	1992
Sister ships:	*Crystal Harmony*
Itinerary:	Panama Canal, South America, Mexican Riviera, Caribbean, South Pacific, World Cruise, Mediterranean, Baltic Sea, Africa, Asia
Information:	(800) 820-6663
Website:	www.crystalcruises.com
Passenger capacity:	940 (double occupancy)
Crew:	545 (Norwegian and Japanese officers)
Passenger-to-Crew Ratio:	1.7:1
Tonnage:	51,044
Passenger Space Ratio:	54.3
Length:	781 feet
Beam:	99 feet
Draft:	24.9 feet
Cruising speed:	22 knots
Guest decks:	8
Total cabins:	480
Outside:	416 (278 with verandas)
Inside:	0
Suites:	64
Wheelchair cabins:	7
Cuisine:	International; specialty restaurants: Italian, Asian
Style:	Casual with three formal nights per cruise
Price notes:	Single occupancy supplement 125 percent to 200 percent of advance booking fares. Reduced rates for third in cabin.
Tipping suggestions:	$10.50 pp/pd

The younger and near-identical sister to the *Crystal Harmony* includes a larger Caesars Palace at Sea casino and a different alternative restaurant in addition to the Crystal Dining Room.

The Jade Garden restaurant features a broad Asian menu and offers items such as Peking duck with plum sauce; spicy coconut chicken with eggplant, lemongrass and basil; and orange-glazed beef with red chilies and basil.

There's also the Prego restaurant for classic Italian cuisine served in a Venetian atmosphere.

CUNARD

**Cunard Line
6100 Blue Lagoon Drive, Suite 400
Miami, FL 33126
Information: (800) 528-6273, (305) 463-3000
www.cunard.com**

The Cunard Fleet

Queen Elizabeth 2. (1969) 1,715 passengers. 70,326 tons

*Caronia. (*Formerly *Vistafjord.)* (1973) 677 passengers. 24,492 tons

Cunard is one of the most storied of passenger lines, dating back to 1839 when Samuel Cunard of Halifax, Nova Scotia won the contract to deliver the mail across the Atlantic from Great Britain to North America. Today she operates one of the best-known ships afloat, the *Queen Elizabeth 2*, as well as another fine old ship renamed in 1999 to carry on the name of another classic vessel, *Caronia.*

And in late 2003, Cunard Line will reintroduce another great name with a fabulous vessel, the *Queen Mary 2.* Plans call for a massive vessel of more than 150,000 tons, 1,130 feet in length, to be built at the famed Chantiers de L'Atlantique shipyards in France. The huge ship will carry a relatively small passenger load of 2,800. Constructed as a liner with a deep draft and more speed than most other cruise ships, plans call for a dramatic raked prow, with the hull painted matte black, a Cunard tradition dating back nearly 160 years. Among unusual features planned for the ship are a pub with its own onboard microbrewery and a museum of ocean liner history.

"We believe there is an eager and growing audience for the drama, elegance and shipboard ambience exemplified by sailing aboard a true Atlantic ocean liner," said a company spokesman. "No one has built a true ocean liner in more than 30 years. It is nearly a lost art. We are recreating history."

The original *Queen Mary* of Cunard White Star Line entered transatlantic service in May 1936, winning the Blue Riband for the fastest crossing for the first time in August of that year; in 1938, the ship won the Blue Riband again, and held the award until 1952.

After service as a troop transport during World War II, the *Queen Mary* was refitted and re-entered the transatlantic liner service. But as air travel increased, that trade declined, and in 1967 the ship was sold to the city of Long Beach, California, where she serves today as a floating hotel and conference center.

The company, originally known as the British and North American Royal

Mail Steam Packet Company, began service in 1840 with the 1,154-ton paddlewheel steamer *Britannia* and three near-sister ships *Arcadia, Caledonia,* and *Columbia.*

Cunard's ships could cross the Atlantic voyage in 14 days, and the four ships permitted weekly departures from Liverpool. Novelist Charles Dickens was an early passenger on the *Brittania*; his description of the sleeping and eating facilities was not of the sort that would be reprinted in a sales brochure. From that beginning, Cunard went on to become one of the most successful transatlantic lines. Among its most famous liners were the *Lusitania* and the *Mauretania*, launched in 1906 and 1907; the *Mauretania* held the "Blue Riband" for 22 years.

Cunard carried more than 1 million troops and 10 million tons of cargo during the First World War; 20 vessels, including the *Lusitania,* were lost.

The *Queen Mary* and the *Queen Elizabeth*, launched in 1938, were requisitioned for use in World War II, carrying more than 1.5 million troops.

By the 1950s, Cunard had 12 liners in service, carrying one-third of all trans-Atlantic passengers. But after the first jet plane crossed the pond in 1959, the liners went into decline. When Cunard launched the *Queen Elizabeth 2* in 1969, it was the first major liner designed for both transatlantic and cruise service. The *QE2* held the title as the largest passenger ship ever built from 1940 until 1996.

Today, Cunard is the only cruise line to sail a regular schedule of transatlantic service, with 17 crossings in 1999; at other times, the *QE2* makes a spectacular world cruise and makes special cruises in Europe, the Americas, and the Caribbean.

During recent years, Cunard has gone through a number of incarnations; in 1998, the company was acquired by Carnival Corporation and a group of Norwegian investors. Carnival then merged Cunard into its Seabourn Cruise Line division.

Cunard Line Limited operates two cruise vacation brands, Cunard and Seabourn. According to Seabourn, the combined eight-vessel fleet commands almost 50 percent of the luxury cruise market worldwide.

For 2000, the fleet was reshuffled. Cunard's *Vistafjord* was renamed as *Caronia*, harkening back to one of the classic old liners of the heyday of the transatlantic ferry. At the same time, the *Royal Viking Sun, Sea Goddess I,* and *Sea Goddess II* were transferred to Seabourn, to sail under new names of *Seabourn Sun, Seabourn Goddess I,* and *Seabourn Goddess II.*

The Cunard Experience

Travelers will find Cunard a bit more formal than other cruise lines. On most transatlantic crossings, every night except the first and last calls for formal dress, and the guests like it that way very much, thank you.

In January of 2000, the *QE2* embarked on its 104-day Millennium World Cruise, sailing from New York through the Americas to Polynesia, Australia,

Indonesia, and the Orient, and then on to South Africa and Europe, with calls at 37 ports. The cruise was available as one journey, or as segments. Later in the year, she began her series of themed transatlantic crossings, including Food & Wine, British Theatre, Big Bands at Sea, *QE2* Goes to the Movies, British Comedy, the Floating Jazz Festival, and the Blues Cruise.

Caronia was to sail a collection of Caribbean and European voyages.

Queen Elizabeth 2

Econoguide rating:	★★★★
Ship size:	**Megaship**
Category:	**Vintage/Luxury**
Price range:	**Premium $$$**
Registry:	Great Britain
Year built:	1969 (In 1987, the *QE2* was re-engined from steam to diesel electric. Major refurbishments in 1994, 1996, and 1999.)
Itinerary:	18 transatlantic crossings in 2000, cruises to the Caribbean, New England, the Mediterranean, Northern Europe, British Isles, South Africa, Canary Islands, World Tour
Information:	(305) 463-3000
Website:	www.cunard.com
Passenger capacity:	1,778 (double occupancy)
Crew:	921
Passenger-to-Crew Ratio:	1.9:1
Tonnage:	70,327 tons
Passenger Space Ratio:	39.5
Length:	963 feet
Beam:	105 feet
Draft:	32 feet
Cruising speed:	28.5 knots cruising speed, 32.5 knots maximum
Guest decks:	12
Total cabins:	950
Outside:	671
Inside:	279
Suites:	187
Wheelchair cabins:	4
Cuisine:	International
Style:	Informal with several formal nights per cruise
Price notes:	Single cabins available
Tipping suggestions:	$10-$13 pp/pd

With apologies to Her Majesty, the *QE2* is one of the grand old ladies of the sea. As she moves into her fourth decade, she's still an elegant, luxurious way to travel.

She also offers one of the best glimpses back to the days of the great trans-Atlantic liners; the *QE2* was one of the last of the breed, launched after jets began flying over the route of the Atlantic Ferry.

The ship was designed as a replacement for the *Queen Mary* and *Queen Elizabeth*. In the face of competition from the jets, the designers chose to build a slightly smaller liner that could pass through the Panama and Suez canals and combine service as a liner and as a cruise ship. She was originally intended to spend half the year on the Atlantic Ferry route between Southampton and

New York and the other half in cruising; today the *QE2* still sails a dozen or more crossings, cruises in the Caribbean, and conducts one major around-the-world voyage each year.

The ship's impressive offerings include a 13-car garage, a florist, kennels, seven restaurants, a foreign exchange bank, 20-channel television, e-mail and financial fax service. The engines can reach a top speed of 32.5 knots.

The *QE2* was requisitioned for service in the Falklands War in 1982; helicopter flight decks and a modern communications system were hurriedly added. And in May of that year, the ship left Southampton for the Falklands with an infantry brigade of Scots and Welsh Guards and the Gurkhas aboard. Arriving two weeks later, the ship took onboard the survivors of a Royal Navy ship and quickly steamed out of harm's way.

The ship was out of service for approximately six months in 1986 and 1987 for the installation of modern diesel electric engines and propellers. Passenger accommodations were also upgraded at that time.

A major interior redesign was accomplished in 1994. Among changes at the time was a reduction in passenger cabins from 1,750 to 1,500, and a changeover of all restaurants to permit single seatings.

In late 1999, the ship emerged from a month-long $18 million refurbishment program at Lloyd Werft Shipyard in Bremerhaven, Germany.

From the Grand Lounge and the Queens Room to the renowned restaurants and the Golden Lion Pub, there are new furnishings, draperies, carpeting, and woodworking throughout. In addition, *QE2* added Harrods, the London-based luxury department store, to the shops of its Royal Promenade.

The Queens Grill received new furniture and new carpeting, upholstery, and lighting, as well as etched glass doors and a completely new galley. Following a complete makeover, the Caronia Restaurant displays the elegance and luster of an English country house, with rich mahogany paneling, new table lighting, crystal chandeliers, carpeting, curtains, and chairs, as well as a new stereo system. New etched-glass doors and a "rainfall" pattern air-conditioning system eliminates drafts.

The Queens Room received major treatment, including all new furniture and new royal blue carpeting interwoven with gold Tudor roses. The walls were repaneled in mahogany, and the famed bust of Her Majesty the Queen was relocated to the most prominent position within the room.

Two new Grand Suites, category QS, were added. The 575-square-foot Caledonia Suite on the port side of Boat Deck directly adjacent to and forward of the Queens Grill features marble master and guest bathrooms, separate dining area, and large picture windows. The 777-square-foot Aquitania Suite forward of the Midships Lobby on the starboard side of Two Deck offers similar luxury appointments.

All suites and cabins have been refurbished with elegant decor including new carpeting, bedspreads, valances, and draperies.

Caronia

Econoguide rating:	★★★★
Ship size:	**Medium**
Category:	**Vintage/Luxury**
Price range:	**Premium $$$**
Registry:	Great Britain
Year built:	1973, for Norwegian America Line. Refurbished 1997. Renamed from *Vistafjord* in 1999. (Refurbished 1999)
Itinerary:	South Africa, Transatlantic, Caribbean, Scandinavia, Russia, Mediterranean, Canary Islands
Information:	(305) 463-3000
Website:	www.cunard.com
Passenger capacity:	677
Crew:	379 (British)
Passenger-to-Crew Ratio:	1.8:1
Tonnage:	24,492 tons
Passenger Space Ratio:	36.2
Length:	627 feet
Beam:	82 feet
Draft:	27 feet
Cruising speed:	20 knots
Guest decks:	9
Total cabins:	379
Outside:	325
Inside:	54
Suites:	13
Wheelchair cabins:	6
Cuisine:	International
Style:	Semi-formal with several formal nights per cruise.
Price notes:	Single cabins available
Tipping suggestions:	$10–$13 pp/pd

The *Vistafjord* was renamed and reflagged as *Caronia* under the Union Jack in a ceremony in Liverpool in December of 1999. In keeping with Cunard tradition, the ceremony was carried out not with champagne but with wine. Unlike the *Queen Mary*, *Queen Elizabeth*, and *QE2*, though, the *Caronia* was ceremonially doused not with Australian wine but with a bottle from the British Isle of Wight.

Prior to the cermony, the ship underwent a multimillion dollar refurbishing. Today, she's a well-kept middle-aged lady with some touches of Scandinavian elegance. The enlarged and redesigned Dining Room can accommodate all passengers in a single seating. Unusually large windows offer views of the sea from nearly all tables. There's also Tivoli, a 40-seat alternative Italian restaurant.

In an earlier update, a pair of lavish penthouses were added forward; the bi-level suites include a large private veranda and a seaside whirlpool.

In 2000, Caronia will sail 13 theme cruises, including an African Wildlife tour from Southampton, England to Cape Town, South Africa, the Classical Strings transatlantic positioning cruise from Southampton to Fort Lauderdale, and Theater at Sea, a Greek Isles cruise with a cast of stars of stage and screen.

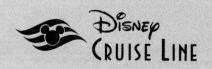

Disney Cruise Line
210 Celebration Place, Suite 400
Celebration, FL 34747-4600
Information: (800) 326-0620
www.disneycruise.com

Disney Cruise Line Fleet

Disney Wonder. (1999) 1,750 passengers, 85,000 tons

Disney Magic. (1998) 1,750 passengers, 85,000 tons

OK, let's get this out of the way right now: The Disney Cruise Line is a Mickey Mouse operation.

But this is the Mickey Mouse of *Fantasia*, the cultured gentleman in tuxedo and tails.

The *Disney Magic* and her nearly identical sister ship *Disney Wonder* are two of the most stunning, beautifully realized cruise ships on the water today. From the moment they welcomed their first paying passengers in mid-1998 and the summer of 1999 respectively, the ships were instant classics.

Until August of 2000, both ships sail from Port Canaveral on three- or four-day cruises to Nassau and Castaway Cay, Disney's private Bahamas beach.

Beginning in August of 2000, the *Disney Magic* will sail the line's first week-long itinerary, departing each Saturday from Port Canaveral for St. Maarten, St. Thomas, and Castaway Cay; the trip includes three days at sea. At the same time, the *Disney Wonder* will alter its schedule on every-other four-day cruise to include a second stop in the Bahamas, at Freeport.

The two Disney Megaships pay homage to oceanliners of the past, adding elements of creativity and whimsy in the celebrated manner of the Walt Disney Company. The black hull and white superstructure with its knife-edge bow and decorative golden filigree, topped off by a pair of nicely proportioned red smokestacks bring to mind the *Queen Mary* and other classic ships of our collective memory.

But . . . on the *Disney Magic*, there's also a large cartoon drawing of Goofy hanging onto the stern of the ship for dear life, his painter's scaffold dangling toward the sea.

About those handsome smokestacks: Only one of them is required for the modern power plant. The second structure is there because the ships look more like the perfect cruise ship of our imagination with two stacks. But as long as you're going to build another stack, why not make use of it: Put a hideaway sports club way up high and a pair of kid's clubs at its base. And as long as you're going to have a ship's whistle in that smokestack, why not have it play a note different from a mournful C-flat? Disney's whistle plays the first seven notes of "When You Wish Upon a Star."

Within the massive ship are no less than four separate and distinct dining rooms, a huge theater for live productions, and an entire entertainment district for adults.

Disney says its marketing target is the vast majority of Americans who have never taken a cruise. But experienced cruisers are also likely to enjoy the many lovely touches onboard this elegant ship. A good deal of its marketing is also aimed at tying a cruise into a visit to the Walt Disney World theme park; you can purchase a four-night cruise and a three-night stay at the park, or a three-night cruise and a four-night stay. Or you can book a three-, four-, or seven-day cruise by itself.

Although Mickey, Minnie, Goofy and others can be found onboard the ship, and the entertainment package features Disney characters in most productions, it is also possible to avoid most things Disney. The company has created a lovely adults-only restaurant and also endeavors to place most families who have children in the early dining seating for the other restaurants. And then there is Beat Street, the nightclub area down below on Deck 3 onboard the *Disney Magic* where there are lively jazz, comedy, and country-western clubs . . . and neither kids nor cartoon characters are expected. The equivalent on the *Disney Wonder* is Route 66.

Only on a ship of this size owned by a company like Walt Disney would you reasonably expect to find most of an entire deck devoted to supervised children's activities—Disney's Oceaneer Lab and Disney's Oceaneer Club. There's even a kids-only buffet. And up top on the pool deck is a coffee bar just for teenagers; adults are carded at the door and asked to step outside.

In an interesting nod toward the needs and expectations of youngsters and the overburdened wallets of adults, in 2000 Disney added an all-you-can-drink soda pass for youngsters ages 12 and younger; the package costs $4 per day.

The seven-day cruises depart on Saturday from Port Canaveral, spending two days at sea before arriving at St. Maarten on Tuesday, moving on to St. Thomas on Wednesday. After another day at sea, the ship arrives at Castaway Cay, returning to Port Canaveral on Saturday.

Disney's plans for the seven-day cruises includes some special Disney magic as well as some more traditional cruising fare. For the first time, cruisers can attend a black tie formal dinner with the captain. The tony Palo restaurant will be open during the day for a champagne brunch and high tea, and Disney will offer its first midnight buffet—in the galley.

New programs will include backstage peeks at the extensive theater facilities on the ship as well as tours of the bridge, galley, and other places not ordinarily open to guests. Another program will focus on sea lore, from the days of the pirates to modern cruise ships. The nightly shows will expand to include an hour-long magic extravanganza starring a nineteenth-century prestidigitator who magically arrives on ship.

The Disney Experience

Disney is a young cruise line without a grand history on the seas. And some purists will find fault with Goofy hanging on the stern, or Mickey and Minnie lounging by the pool.

But in some ways, Disney has come up with a ship that is more true to our memories or dreams of grand ocean liners than are many of the Colossuses now being launched, ships that are more like floating vacation resorts or shopping malls.

Blessed with the deep pockets of Walt Disney Company, the Disney Cruise Line purchased a pair of stunning ships from one of the most advanced shipyards, and has brought in a staff of cruise line veterans to run its operations.

The only serious glitch—and it has a positive spin—was the fact that the maiden voyage of the *Disney Magic* was postponed twice because of construction delays at the Italian shipyard where it was being built. Disney took the position that it wanted its ships to be near-perfect and refused delivery before they were.

About those restaurants: Onboard the *Disney Magic* there's an elegant Continental restaurant known as Lumiere's that mixes a grand dining room of a classic ocean liner with chandeliers and candlesticks whimsically derived from Disney's *Beauty & the Beast*. The equivalent dining room on the *Wonder* is Triton's, based on *The Little Mermaid*.

Parrot Cay, on both ships, is an informal eatery bedecked with palms and flowers and gingerbread-trimmed verandas, a Disney magnification of the mind's-eye of the Bahamas and the Caribbean.

And then on both ships there is Animator's Palette, one of the most unusual settings for a restaurant at sea or on land. The very room itself is an actor in the evening's entertainment. The meal begins in a room that is entirely outlined in black and white—from the linens on the table and the uniforms on the serving staff to the line art sketches on the wall. As the meal progresses, though, dabs of color work their way into the drawings, onto the table, and onto the uniforms. By the end of meal, the room is a riot of color, including a rainbow dessert you paint on your plate.

And the fourth restaurant is Palo, an adults-only sophisticated Italian bistro perched way up high in the second smokestack. You'll need a reservation.

Among Disney's innovations is "rotation dining." Guests are assigned to one of the three main restaurants each day; their servers and tablemates move with them from dining room to dining room. As this book goes to press, it is unclear how the rotation will be adjusted for the week-long Magic cruises that were to begin in August of 2000.

Disney's attention to detail begins at the $27 million Art Deco-style terminal it constructed in Port Canaveral; it's all part of the company's packaging of its ships as a return to the golden era of cruising. Many guests will arrive at the terminal by bus from Disney World, about one hour away; even the buses have been molded and painted in an artist's vision of a streamlined conveyance of the 1930s and 1940s.

All of this does not come cheap. Disney's list prices for cruises are approximately 15 percent to 30 percent higher than other similar operations, placing the cruise line somewhere between Moderate- and Premium-priced classes. However, like most cruise lines, cruises with Disney are often available at deep discounts from travel agencies; Disney also books its cruises directly.

Disney's Bahamian Theme Park

Imagine yourself a castaway on an idyllic remote island . . . with pristine beaches, an outdoor barbecue shack, a marina, and a spectacular 1,750-passenger cruise ship pulled up to a pier nearby.

In typical Disney fashion, the company created a lovely private island experience for its guests, fashioning a story of pirates and whales and a bit of Sybaritic indulgence for the adults.

Castaway Cay, a 1,000-acre island north of Nassau, was reworked by Disney Imagineers in a massive $25 million effort that included the construction of a dock for the ships and the moving of some 50,000 truckloads of sand dredged from the floor of the Atlantic during creation of a channel.

In an interesting irony, the island formerly known as Gorda Cay had been used in recent years as a hideaway for drug smugglers; a short World War II-era runway on the island was believed to have been used by the smugglers.

Only about 55 acres of the island have been developed, with the remainder mostly open for hiking and biking paths. Salt water desalination and sewage treatment plants, as well as a small village of housing for staff members, are well hidden from view.

The main beach is the Snorkeling and Swimming Lagoon, which features a snorkeling "track" with underwater objects and marine objects to explore; you'll need to rent snorkels and a flotation vest to swim the track. Nearby are Scuttle's Cove, a supervised children's water area, and the Teen Beach. Again in keeping with Disney's promise to offer grown-ups an escape, the north side of the island has a somewhat isolated "quiet" beach for adults only.

Disney Magic

Econoguide rating:	**★★★★★**
Ship size:	**Megaship**
Category:	**Top of the Line**
Price range:	**Premium $$$**
Registry:	Bahamas
Year built:	1998
Sister ship:	*Disney Wonder*
Itinerary:	3 or 4 days from Port Canaveral to Bahamas. Beginning August 2000, seven-day cruises to St. Maarten and St. Thomas.
Information:	(800) 326-0620
Website:	www.disneycruise.com
Passenger capacity:	1,750 (double occupancy)
Crew:	915 European and American staff
Passenger-to-Crew Ratio:	1.9:1
Tonnage:	85,000
Passenger Space Ratio:	48.6

Length:	964 feet
Beam:	106 feet
Draft:	25.3 feet
Cruising speed:	21.5 knots
Guest decks:	11
Total cabins:	875
Outside:	547
Inside:	246
Suites:	82
Wheelchair cabins:	14
Cuisine:	Continental, American. Three restaurants in rotation
Style:	Casual, informal resort atmosphere
Price notes:	Single occupancy premium 175 percent to 200 percent. Reduced rates for third through seventh occupant of cabins or suites
Tipping suggestions:	$11 pp/pd

A spectacular ship that looks back fondly on the grand old liners of the past. Disney's Imagineers worked with Italian designers to create a thoroughly modern Megaship that comes very close to our mind's eye view of what a cruise ship should look like.

Disney's attention to detail include wondrous parallel worlds for children and adults. There's an adults-only restaurant and adults-only swimming pool and a kids-only buffet and pool. There's most of an entire deck of the huge ship devoted to kids' programs, and an adult entertainment district that has a set of swinging nightspots.

The Walt Disney Theatre is a tribute to grand theatrical palaces, with a different live musical stage show each night of the cruise.

Disney Wonder

Econoguide rating:	★★★★★
Ship size:	**Megaship**
Category:	**Top of the Line**
Price range:	**Premium $$$**
Registry:	Bahamas
Year built:	1999
Sister ship:	*Disney Magic*
Itinerary:	3 or 4 days from Port Canaveral to Bahamas, Disney's Castaway Cay
Information:	(800) 326-0620
Website:	www.disneycruise.com
Passenger capacity:	1,750 (double occupancy)
Crew:	915 European officers and crew
Passenger-to-Crew Ratio:	1.9:1
Tonnage:	85,000
Passenger Space Ratio:	48.6
Length:	964 feet
Beam:	106 feet
Draft:	25.3 feet
Cruising speed:	21.5 knots
Guest decks:	11
Total cabins:	875
Outside:	547
Inside:	246
Suites:	82
Wheelchair cabins:	14
Cuisine:	Continental, American. Three restaurants in rotation

Style:	Casual, informal resort atmosphere
Price notes:	Single occupancy premium 175 percent to 200 percent. Reduced rates for third through seventh person in cabin or suite
Tipping suggestions:	$11 pp/pd

The art theme for *Disney Wonder* is Art Nouveau, differing from the *Disney Magic*'s Art Deco concept. New designers have applied their marks to the lobby and staterooms.

The showplace dining room on the *Wonder* is Triton's, derived from the Little Mermaid story. The menu, of course, emphasizes seafood. Animator's Palette and Parrot Cay are the same as the eateries on the *Magic*.

The adult entertainment district on the *Wonder* is Route 66, and includes a dance club known as Cadillac's, the Brew Ha Ha (themed like a brew pub) comedy club, and the Wave Bands jazz club. The upper deck buffet is the Beach Blanket Buffet.

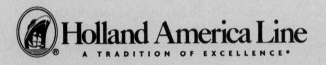

Holland America Line—Westours Inc.
300 Elliott Avenue West
Seattle, WA 98119
Information: (800) 227-6482, (800) 426-0327
www.hollandamerica.com

Holland America Fleet

Zaandam. (2000) 1,440 passengers. 63,000 tons

Volendam. (1999) 1,440 passengers. 63,000 tons

Amsterdam. (Fall 2000) 1,380 passengers. 61,000 tons

Rotterdam. (1997) 1,316 passengers. 60,000 tons

Veendam. (1996) 1,266 passengers. 55,451 tons

Ryndam. (1994) 1,266 passengers. 55,451 tons

Maasdam. (1993) 1,266 passengers. 55,451 tons

Statendam. (1993) 1,266 passengers. 55,451 tons

Westerdam. (1988) 1,494 passengers. 53,872 tons

Noordam. (1984) 1,214 passengers. 33,930 tons

Nieuw Amsterdam. (1983) 1,214 passengers. 33,930 tons. Will leave Holland America fleet in the Fall of 2000 to join United States Line, reflagged as the *Patriot*.

Future Ships
Unnamed. (Fall 2002) 1,800 passengers. 84,000 tons

Unnamed. (Summer 2003) 1,800 passengers. 84,000 tons

Holland America was the floating highway for nearly 1 million European immigrants who traveled to the New World at the end of the nineteenth and the beginning of the twentieth centuries.

Today, it continues as one of the premier cruise lines, carrying Americans and others to holidays in the Caribbean, Alaska, and through the Panama Canal. Holland America is the largest cruise tour operator in Alaska and Canada's Yukon and the ninth largest private motorcoach company in North America.

The company was founded in 1873 as the Netherlands-America Steamship Company for shipping and passenger service. Because it provided service to the Americas, it became known as Holland America Line.

The company's first ocean liner was the original *Rotterdam*, which made its maiden voyage from the Netherlands to New York on Oct. 15, 1872. Within 25 years, the company owned a fleet of six cargo and passenger ships and also provided service between Holland and the Dutch East Indies via the newly constructed Suez Canal.

Today, the company's Holland America–Westours is the largest cruise tour operator in Alaska and Canada's Yukon, with a fleet of 176 buses, and several dozen tourism railroad cars. Westours owns Gray Line of Alaska, Gray Line of Seattle, and the Westmark Hotels and Inns group with 14 hotels in Alaska and the Yukon Territory. And the company also owns the *Ptarmigan,* a small ship that operates tours to the face of Portage Glacier, and the *Yukon Queen* on the Yukon River between Dawson City in the Yukon Territory to Eagle, Alaska.

In January of 1989, Holland America Line–Westours, Inc. became a wholly owned subsidiary of The Carnival Corporation.

Holland America also owns Windstar Cruises, which operates four computer-directed luxury sailing cruise ships in the Mediterranean, Caribbean, and Costa Rica.

Many Caribbean cruises include a stop at Half Moon Cay, a 2,500-acre private Bahamian island purchased in 1997 and lightly developed by Holland America Line. The crescent-shaped isle, just two miles long and a third of a mile across, was an unihabited cay known as Little San Salvador. The nation of the Bahamas honored the tourist dollars of HAL guests with a special postage stamp that has an image of the *Ryndam* and a small Holland America Line logo.

The Holland America Experience

Holland America cultivates an air of refinement aboard its ships, and its clientele has historically been slightly older and more experienced than those on other cruise lines. Fresh flowers, in some cases flown in from Holland, decorate the ship. An art and history tour is scheduled on each cruise to inform guests about the $2 million of art and artifacts aboard each ship.

On most cruises introductory Dutch language classes are offered; Spanish instruction is available on all Caribbean cruises. All Alaska cruises feature an onboard naturalist who presents slide lectures on the wildlife and natural history of the area.

In 1999, Holland America featured its University at Sea program on four Panama Canal cruises, offering courses on various subjects including history and finance; for a program fee, guests can earn college credits for the courses.

Each ship has a priest onboard for all sailings; cruises of 10 days or longer also have a Protestant minister. A rabbi is onboard for all sailings during Jewish holidays; cruises during Passover feature a Seder dinner.

For families traveling with children, Holland America's Club HAL youth program provides activities for youngsters ages 5–17. Additional youth counselors are onboard for Christmas/New Year's and Easter cruises.

The ships also offer more traditional cruise activities—dance lessons, bingo, "horse" racing, trap shooting, a mileage pool, passenger talent show, and karaoke. The show lounge features a Broadway or Las Vegas–style revue or variety entertainment.

Harking back to its Dutch roots, HAL employs mostly Indonesian and Filipino crew members, training them in its own school in Jakarta.

Holland America promotes a "No Tipping Required" policy, which means just what it says; however, most guests do leave a gratuity for members of the staff.

Guests aboard all eight Holland America Line cruise ships are now offered a casual Lido dining option for dinner on several nights of their cruise. Serenaded by a pianist, diners order from a set menu with choices including Caesar salad, shrimp cocktail, and entrees including fillet of salmon, sirloin steak, roast chicken, and lasagna.

New Year's Eve will never end on Holland America ships in 2000. That's because every cruise over the course of the year will include "Dick Clark's New Year's Rockin' Eve," an hour-long theme show with a video introduction by Clark, live production numbers, historical footage from New York's Times Square, and a countdown that ends with champagne toasts and confetti salutes.

The sister ships *Volendam* and *Zaandam* are the first of a new generation of luxury cruise ships. The interior décor of the *Volendam* features a flower theme, while the *Zaandam* is based around musical themes.

The two new ships have the same length and width as the *Rotterdam* but their gross tonnage is larger, about 63,000 tons versus 59,652 tons, because they have more passenger staterooms.

In the fall of 2000, Holland America will add a new ship with an old name. The *Amsterdam*, will have the same length and beam as the *Rotterdam* but have a slightly larger gross tonnage (61,000 gross tons) because of an increase in the number of staterooms to 660. The new ship's all-suite deck will be extended and the number of suites that have verandas will be increased. The new ship also will feature 120 deluxe mini-suites with verandas, 385 large outside staterooms and 133 large inside staterooms, for a total of 690 staterooms.

The *Statendam, Maasdam, Ryndam,* and *Veendam* are close sisters. The *Ryndam* and *Maasdam* were redeployed to the Caribbean in the fall of 1998; the new *Volendam* will also sail a schedule of trips from there.

And beginning in 2000, Holland America will offer a range of shorter cruises of five days or less along the Pacific Coast in the spring and fall. Ports of call will include Acapulco, Puerto Vallarta, Mazatlan, and Cabo San Lucas in Mexico, and Victoria and Vancouver in Canada. Ships will depart from or arrive in San Diego, Los Angeles, San Francisco, Portland, and Seattle.

Holland America offers Early Booking Fares with a 25 percent discount for a limited number of staterooms.

Future Plans

New ships under constuction include four 84,000-ton behemoths; the 951-foot-long, 1,800-passenger ships are due to join the line in the Fall of 2002, the Summer of 2003, late in 2003, and 2004. The ships mark the beginning of a new class of vessels for Holland America, and will introduce a number of new features including the first "exterior elevators" on a cruise ship. The lifts, located on the port and starboard sides, will connect 10 decks of the ship, offering panoramic sea views from glass walls. About 85 percent of the cabins on the new ships will be outside, with about 80 percent of those offering private verandas.

Other features include two interior promenade decks, an exterior covered promenade deck encircling the entire ship, and HAL's trademark Lido area pool with a retractable dome.

The third and fourth vessels will include a unique propulsion system that is based on a diesel-electric power plant backed up by a gas turbine as an additional power source. Holland America also has an option with Italian shipbuilder Fincantieri to build a fifth ship of the same design.

Volendam

Econoguide rating:	★★★★★
Ship size:	**Grand**
Category:	**Top of the Line**
Price range:	**Premium $$$**
Registry:	Netherlands
Year built:	1999
Sister ship:	Zaandam
Itinerary:	Caribbean, Central America, Mexico, South America
Information:	(206) 283-2687, (800) 426-0327
Website:	www.hollandamerica.com
Passenger capacity:	1,440 (double occupancy)
Crew:	N/A
Passenger-to-Crew Ratio:	N/A
Tonnage:	63,000
Passenger Space Ratio:	43.8
Length:	781 feet

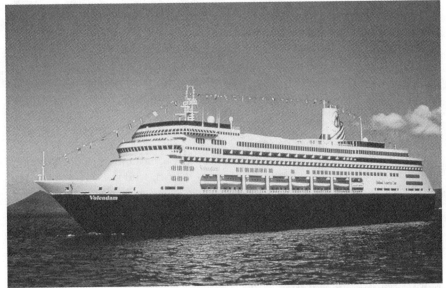

Holland America's Volendam

Holland America Line

Beam:	105.8 feet
Draft:	N/A
Cruising speed:	23 knots
Guest decks:	10
Total cabins:	720
Outside:	552
Inside:	139
Suites:	29
Wheelchair cabins:	23
Cuisine:	International
Style:	Elegantly casual to formal in evening
Price notes:	Single occupancy premium 150 percent to 190 percent. Single Partners Program: agree to share a stateroom with another nonsmoking guest of the same sex, and you pay only the per-person, double-occupancy rate
Tipping suggestions:	No tipping required

This spectacular Holland America Line ship is the third in the company's 125-year history to bear the *Volendam* name. In her inaugural season, she was due to spend the winter in the Caribbean, sailing out of Fort Lauderdale.

After then, she was due to reposition in April of 2000 to Vancouver, British Columbia, via the Panama Canal, with a 10- to 17-day cruise featuring Half Moon Cay; Cartagena, Colombia; the Panama Canal transit; Puntarenas, Costa Rica; Santa Cruz Huatulco, Acapulco, and Cabo San Lucas, Mexico; and San Diego.

From May through early September, the *Volendam* will sail week-long Glacier Bay Inside Passage cruises from Vancouver with visits to Juneau, Skagway, Glacier Bay National Park, and Ketchikan. Then In October of 2000, she will return to Fort Lauderdale through the Panama Canal and resume sailings in the Caribbean.

Slightly larger than the *Rotterdam*, the new design moves the oudoor swimming pool one deck higher to Lido Deck and extends Navigation Deck aft to accommodate 48 additional mini-suites with verandas.

A sister ship, the *Zaandam*, is due to join the fleet in 2000. The basic layout of the public rooms of both of the new ships is the same as that of the *Rotterdam*, including the alternative dining restaurant.

The predominant theme of *Volendam's* interior décor is flowers, from the seventeenth to the twenty-first centuries. Flowers are featured in the ship's artwork, doors, and other design elements.

The three-deck-high central atrium features a monumental crystal sculpture titled "Caleido" by Italian artist Lucian Vistosi, who also created the towering glass sculptures onboard the *Maasdam* and *Veendam*.

The *Volendam's* Marco Polo Restaurant, an alternative to the dining room, is a recreation of a classic European "artist's bistro," a place where the walls are lined with works of art traded for plates of spaghetti.

The walls are a pastiche across time, with works by unknown contemporary artists as well as etchings by Rubens and Rembrandt and works by Henry Moore, Matisse, and Picasso.

Diners at the 88-seat restaurant are offered "California-style" Italian cuisine for lunch or dinner; there is no extra charge, but advance reservations are required. Typical pasta menu items include Fettucine con Gamberetti, fettucine pasta with rock shrimp, chopped tomato, spinach, garlic and toasted pine nuts, and Linguine ala Friulana, linguine pasta with Italian sausage, peppers, onions, tomato and sangiovese wine sauce.

Entrees include Pollo ala Aglio e Rosmarino, marinated chicken breast in garlic puree and rosemary; Lombata de Vitello al Carbone, a large veal chop grilled with sage and rosemary, and Agnello Arosto alla Chiretto, pan-roasted lamb loin with red wine sauce.

Luncheon offerings include Pizza Rustica with goat cheese, salami, coppa, mushrooms, calamata olives, crisp pancetta, tomato sauce, fontina cheese, and oregano, and Nissarda con Salmon, a poached salmon nicoise salad with potatoes, eggs, green beans, tomato, red onions, cucumber, capers and a light mustard dressing.

The Casino Bar, in addition to being the ship's sport bar, features cinematic memorabilia, including costumes, props, photos, and posters of movies and the stars who made them.

The ship's main show lounge features colorful colonnades against satiny dark wood walls, harkening back to the Art Deco era, with a design inspired by the famed Tuschinski Theater in Amsterdam.

On both the *Volendam* and *Zaandam*, the Navigation Deck was extended aft to accommodate the additional staterooms, moving the outdoor swimming pool to the lido deck, one level above its location on the Rotterdam and Statendam-class ships. This design change permits direct access between the indoor and outdoor swimming pools and the Lido Restaurant.

Zaandam

Econoguide rating:	★★★★★
Ship size:	**Grand**
Category:	**Top of the Line**
Price range:	**Premium $$$**
Registry:	Netherlands
Year built:	2000
Sister ships:	*Volendam, Rotterdam*
Itinerary:	Caribbean, U.S. Virgin Islands, Bahamas, Southern Caribbean
Information:	(206) 283-2687, (800) 426-0327
Website:	www.hollandamerica.com
Passenger capacity:	1,440 (double occupancy)
Crew:	N/A
Passenger-to-Crew Ratio:	N/A
Tonnage:	63,000
Passenger Space Ratio:	43.8
Length:	780 feet
Beam:	105.8 feet
Draft:	N/A
Cruising speed:	23 knots
Guest decks:	10
Total cabins:	720
Outside:	552
Inside:	139
Suites:	29
Wheelchair cabins:	23
Cuisine:	International
Style:	Elegantly casual to formal in evening
Price notes:	Single occupancy premium 150 percent to 190 percent. Single Partners Program: agree to share a stateroom with another nonsmoking guest of the same sex, and you pay only the per-person, double-occupancy rate
Tipping suggestions:	No tipping required

Near-twin to the *Volendam* and sister to the *Rotterdam,* the *Zaandam* is due to join the Holland America fleet in the spring of 2000.

The interior theme is music, featured throughout public rooms but most prominently in the Casino Bar, which will showcase music memorabilia from jazz and blues to rock 'n' roll and the classics.

The centerpiece of the *Zaandam*'s grand atrium is a towering pipe organ that has mechanical figures of dancing musicians.

Maasdam

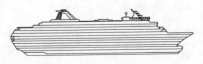

Econoguide rating:	★★★★
Ship size:	**Grand**
Category:	**Top of the Line**
Price range:	**Premium $$$**
Registry:	Netherlands
Year built:	1993
Sister ships:	*Ryndam, Statendam* and *Veendam*
Itinerary:	Caribbean, Central America, Mexico, South America, Panama Canal
Information:	(206) 283-2687, (800) 426-0327
Website:	www.hollandamerica.com
Passenger capacity:	1,266 (double occupancy)
Crew:	588

Passenger-to-Crew Ratio:	2.2:1
Tonnage:	55,451
Passenger Space Ratio:	43.8
Length:	720 feet
Beam:	101 feet
Draft:	24.6 feet
Cruising speed:	22 knots
Guest decks:	10
Total cabins:	633
Outside:	336
Inside:	148
Suites:	149
Wheelchair cabins:	6
Cuisine:	International
Style:	Elegantly casual to formal in evening
Price notes:	Single occupancy premium 150 percent to 190 percent. Single Partners Program: Agree to share a stateroom with another nonsmoking guest of the same sex, and you pay only the per-person, double-occupancy rate
Tipping suggestions:	No tipping required

The fifth Holland America Line ship to carry the name, the *Maasdam* features a $2 million collection of art and artifacts, a company trademark.

A three-deck grand atrium, featuring a monumental glass sculpture by Italian artist Luciano Vistosi, extends from Lower Promenade Deck to Upper Promenade. An escalator provides access upward from the Main Deck to staterooms on Lower Promenade Deck.

Located on Promenade and Upper Promenade Decks, the Rotterdam Dining Room seats 657 on two levels connected by a pair of grand curved staircases. An antique marble fountain from Argentina is the centerpiece of the lower level. Windows on two sides and the stern offer panoramic views of the sea, accented by murals by Danish ceramic artist Bjorn Wiinblad.

At the opposite end of the ship, the two-deck, 600-seat Rembrandt Show Lounge features Broadway-style entertainment. The room is decorated with Delft ceramic tiles from Holland as well as plush, brocaded fabrics, gold-tinted mirrors and mahogany panels to recall the era of seventeenth Century Dutch master Rembrandt van Rijn, whose portrait is etched into the glass doors.

Ryndam

Econoguide rating:	★★★★
Ship size:	**Grand**
Category:	**Top of the Line**
Price range:	**Premium $$$**
Registry:	Netherlands
Year built:	1994
Sister ships:	*Maasdam, Statendam* and *Veendam*
Itinerary:	Alaska, Caribbean, Central America, Mexico, South America, Panama Canal
Information:	(206) 283-2687, (800) 426-0327
Website:	www.hollandamerica.com
Passenger capacity:	1,266 (double occupancy)

Crew:	588
Passenger-to-Crew Ratio:	2.2:1
Tonnage:	55,451
Passenger Space Ratio:	43.8
Length:	720 feet
Beam:	101 feet
Draft:	24.6 feet
Cruising speed:	22 knots
Guest decks:	10
Total cabins:	633
Outside:	336
Inside:	148
Suites:	149
Wheelchair cabins:	6
Cuisine:	International
Style:	Elegantly casual in evening to formal in evening
Price notes:	Single occupancy premium 150 percent to 190 percent. Single Partners Program: agree to share a stateroom with another nonsmoking guest of the same sex, and you pay only the per-person double-occupancy rate
Tipping suggestions:	No tipping required

The *Ryndam,* third in the company's history to carry the name, is a sister ship to the *Maasdam, Statendam,* and *Veendam* with most of the same interior features.

The Rotterdam Dining Room, with side and stern windows, is decorated with four large murals by a Dutch artist depicting elaborately costumed seventeenth century Dutch noblemen against a backdrop of period sailing ships. The Vermeer Show Lounge has a tulip motif throughout, in light fixtures, wall panels, lamps, and carpeting.

Statendam

Econoguide rating:	★★★★
Ship size:	**Grand**
Category:	**Top of the Line**
Price range:	**Premium $$$**
Registry:	Netherlands
Year built:	1993
Sister ships:	*Maasdam, Ryndam,* and *Veendam*
Itinerary:	Alaska, Hawaii, Caribbean, Central America, Mexico, South America, Panama Canal
Information:	(206) 283-2687, (800) 426-0327
Website:	www.hollandamerica.com
Passenger capacity:	1,266 (double occupancy)
Crew:	588
Passenger-to-Crew Ratio:	2.2:1
Tonnage:	55,451
Passenger Space Ratio:	43.8
Length:	720 feet
Beam:	101 feet
Draft:	24.6 feet
Cruising speed:	22 knots
Guest decks:	10
Total cabins:	633
Outside:	336

Inside:	148
Suites:	149
Wheelchair cabins:	6
Cuisine:	International
Style:	Elegantly casual to formal in evening
Price notes:	Single occupancy premium 150 percent to 190 percent. Single Partners Program: agree to share a stateroom with another nonsmoking guest of the same sex, and you pay only the per-person, double-occupancy rate
Tipping suggestions:	No tipping required

A three-deck atrium features the ornate, 26-foot-high "Fountain of the Sirens," extending from the Lower Promenade Deck to Upper Promenade.

The dramatic Rotterdam Dining Room seats 700, spread across two levels connected by a pair of grand curved staircases, with windows on both sides and the stern.

At the opposite end of the ship, the two-deck, 600-seat Van Gogh Show Lounge features Broadway-style entertainment. The show room is themed to Dutch artist Vincent van Gogh's paintings, "The Starry Night" and "Irises."

The *Statendam* is sister ship to the *Maasdam, Veendam* and *Ryndam*.

Veendam

Econoguide rating:	★★★★
Ship size:	**Grand**
Category:	**Top of the Line**
Price range:	**Premium $$$**
Registry:	Bahamas
Year built:	1996
Sister ships:	*Maasdam, Ryndam,* and *Statendam*
Itinerary:	Alaska, Caribbean, Central America, Mexico, South America, Panama Canal
Information:	(206) 283-2687, (800) 426-0327
Website:	www.hollandamerica.com
Passenger capacity:	1,266 (double occupancy)
Crew:	588
Passenger-to-Crew Ratio:	2.2:1
Tonnage:	55,451
Passenger Space Ratio:	43.8
Length:	720 feet
Beam:	101 feet
Draft:	24.6 feet
Cruising speed:	22 knots
Guest decks:	10
Total cabins:	633
Outside:	456
Inside:	148
Suites:	29
Wheelchair cabins:	6
Cuisine:	International
Style:	Elegantly casual to formal in evening
Price notes:	Single occupancy premium 150 percent to 190 percent. Single Partners Program: agree to share a stateroom with another nonsmoking guest of the same sex, and you pay only the per-person, double-occupancy rate
Tipping suggestions:	No tipping required

The Rotterdam Dining Room, seating 657 on two levels connected by a pair of grand curved staircases, is decorated by enormous paintings of flowers based on details from seventeenth century Dutch still lifes.

The Rubens Show Lounge, named for 16th Century Flemish master painter Pieter Paul Rubens, is done in copper brown and gray tones with accents of gold leaf and brass. Glass cutouts of dancers' forms radiate from large columns. The three-deck grand atrium features "Jacob's Staircase," a glass sculpture by Luciano Vistosi of Italy.

The *Veendam* is sister ship to the *Statendam, Ryndam,* and *Maasdam.*

Rotterdam

Econoguide rating:	★★★★★
Ship size:	**Grand**
Category:	**Top of the Line**
Price range:	**Premium $$$**
Registry:	Netherlands
Year built:	1997
Itinerary:	World Tour, Caribbean, Bermuda, Central America, Hawaii, Mexico, Panama Canal
Information:	(206) 283-2687, (800) 426-0327
Website:	www.hollandamerica.com
Passenger capacity:	1,316 (double occupancy)
Crew:	644
Passenger-to-Crew Ratio:	2:1
Tonnage:	62,000
Passenger Space Ratio:	47.1
Length:	778 feet
Beam:	105.8 feet
Draft:	25.5 feet
Cruising speed:	25 knots
Guest decks:	10
Total cabins:	658
Outside:	381
Inside:	117
Suites:	160
Wheelchair cabins:	20
Cuisine:	International
Style:	Elegantly casual to formal in evening
Price notes:	Single occupancy premium 150 percent to 190 percent. Single Partners Program: agree to share a stateroom with another nonsmoking guest of the same sex, and you pay only the per-person, double-occupancy rate.
Tipping suggestions:	No tipping required

The flagship of the Holland America line, the *Rotterdam* is the sixth company ship to bear the name.

The onboard art collection includes artifacts related to the voyages of seventeenth century mariners for the Dutch East and West Indies Companies.

The two-deck, 747-seat La Fontaine Dining Room features a giant mural reminiscent of the wall treatment of the previous Rotterdam's much-loved Ritz Carlton room.

The ship's top cruising speed is 25 knots, faster than many other ships, allowing a greater range and longer port stops.

Westerdam

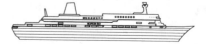

Econoguide rating:	★★★
Ship size:	**Grand**
Category:	**Top of the Line**
Price range:	**Premium $$$**
Registry:	Netherlands
Year built:	1986 (Built as *Homeric*. Lengthened by 130 feet in 1989.)
Itinerary:	Alaska, Caribbean, Central America, Mexico, South America, Panama Canal
Information:	(206) 283-2687, (800) 426-0327
Website:	www.hollandamerica.com
Passenger capacity:	1,494 (double occupancy)
Crew:	642
Passenger-to-Crew Ratio:	1:2.33
Tonnage:	53,872
Passenger Space Ratio:	36
Length:	798 feet
Beam:	95 feet
Draft:	23.6 feet
Cruising speed:	20.5 knots
Guest decks:	9
Total cabins:	747
Outside:	489
Inside:	252
Suites:	6
Wheelchair cabins:	4
Cuisine:	International
Style:	Elegantly casual to formal in evening
Price notes:	Single occupancy premium 150 percent to 190 percent. Single Partners Program: agree to share a stateroom with another nonsmoking guest of the same sex, and you pay only the per-person, double-occupancy rate.
Tipping suggestions:	No tipping required

The *Westerdam* was built in 1986 in West Germany as the *Homeric*, with a capacity of 1,000 passengers. After Holland America bought the ship in 1988, it was renamed and sent back to the shipyard for an $84 million expansion and redesign. The project included the insertion of a 130-foot section, increasing the ship's size by 13,872 tons to 53,872 tons. The capacity was increased to 1,494 passengers, and the ship's length from 668 to 798 feet. A highlight was the creation of the 800-seat, two-deck Admiral's Lounge in the new section.

The art collection onboard the ship includes seventeenth and eighteenth century art and antiques themed to Dutch worldwide exploration. One significant piece is a bronze cannon, cast in Rotterdam in 1634, which once graced a Dutch admiral's warship.

Nieuw Amsterdam

Econoguide rating:	★★★
Ship size:	**Medium**
Category:	**Top of the Line**
Price range:	**Moderate $$**
Registry:	Netherlands

Year built:	1983
Sister ship:	*Noordam*
Itinerary:	Caribbean
Information:	(206) 283-2687, (800) 426-0327
Website:	www.hollandamerica.com
Passenger capacity:	1,214 (double occupancy)
Crew:	542
Passenger-to-Crew Ratio:	2.2:1
Tonnage:	33,930
Passenger Space Ratio:	27.9
Length:	704.2 feet
Beam:	89.4 feet
Draft:	24.6 feet
Cruising speed:	21 knots
Guest decks:	9
Total cabins:	605
Outside:	391
Inside:	194
Suites:	20
Wheelchair cabins:	4
Cuisine:	International
Style:	Elegantly casual to formal in evening
Price notes:	Single occupancy premium 150 percent to 190 percent. Single Partners Program: agree to share a stateroom with another nonsmoking guest of the same sex, and you pay only the per-person, double-occupancy rate
Tipping suggestions:	No tipping required

The *Nieuw Amsterdam,* sister ship to the *Noordam,* will leave the Holland America Line fleet in October of 2000 to become the *Patriot,* flagship of the reborn United States Line operating out of Honolulu.

Until then, though, the classy ship sails in the Caribbean, carting around an art collection related to the exploration of the New World and early Dutch exploration, including the travels of Henry Hudson in Nieuw Amsterdam, the first Dutch trading settlement in America. Today, that settlement is better known as New York.

Display cases on the ship contain artifacts such as authentic navigation instruments, an exquisite Delft tile riverscape, and other items related to the Dutch West India Company.

Noordam

Econoguide rating:	**★★★**
Ship size:	**Medium**
Category:	**Top of the Line**
Price range:	**Premium $$$**
Registry:	Netherlands
Year built:	1984
Sister ship:	*Nieuw Amsterdam*
Itinerary:	Alaska, Caribbean, Central America, Mexico, Panama Canal
Information:	(206) 283-2687, (800) 426-0327
Website:	www.hollandamerica.com
Passenger capacity:	1,214 (double occupancy)
Crew:	605
Passenger-to-Crew Ratio:	2:1
Tonnage:	33,930
Passenger Space Ratio:	27.9

Length:	704.2 feet
Beam:	89.4 feet
Draft:	24.2 feet
Cruising speed:	21 knots
Guest decks:	10
Total cabins:	605
Outside:	391
Inside:	194
Suites:	20
Wheelchair cabins:	4
Cuisine:	International
Style:	Elegantly casual to formal in evening
Price notes:	Single occupancy premium 150 percent to 190 percent. Single Partners Program: agree to share a stateroom with another nonsmoking guest of the same sex, and you pay only the per-person, double-occupancy rate
Tipping suggestions:	No tipping required

Sister ship to the *Nieuw Amsterdam,* half of her sun deck is given over to cabins, limiting views from up top. The *Noordam's* theme is the Dutch East India Company, established in Amsterdam in 1603 for trade between Holland and the Far East and East Indies.

NORWEGIAN CRUISE LINE

Norwegian Cruise Line
7665 Corporate Center Drive
Miami, FL 33126
Information: (800) 327-7030
www.ncl.com

Norwegian Cruise Line Fleet

Norwegian Sky. (1999) 2,400 passengers. 78,000 tons

Norway. (1962, rebuilt 1980) 2,032 passengers. 76,049 tons

Norwegian Wind. (1993) 1,748 passengers. 50,760 tons

Norwegian Dream. (1992) 1,748 passengers. 46,000 tons

Norwegian Sea. (1988) 1,518 passengers. 42,000 tons

Norwegian Majesty. (1992, to NCL in 1997) 1,460 passengers. 38,000 tons

Norwegian Crown. (1988) 1,050 passengers. 34,250 tons. Redeployed to NCL's Orient Lines in Spring of 2000 to sail as *Crown Odyssey.*

Future Ships

Norwegian Sun. (September 2001). 2,400 passengers. 80,000 tons

Norwegian Cruise Line is a fleet on the move, growing rapidly and expanding its reach from its Caribbean roots to include Alaska, Hawaii, the Mexican Riviera, and a subsidiary operation out of Australia. The line will add a big new ship in 1999; in recent years, two of its ships were stretched to add the equivalent of another vessel in the fleet.

The flagship of the line is the venerable *Norway*, the longest cruise ship afloat at 1,035 feet. The *Norwegian Sky* joined the fleet in the summer of 1999, and in May of 2000, that ship will be based in Seattle for a series of week-long cruises to Alaska.

The *Norwegian Dynasty*, a smaller ship that had been operated by NCL under lease left the fleet in late 1999; the *Leeward* departed about the same time. The *Norwegian Crown* was transferred to NCL's Orient Line to sail in Asia.

In late 1999, NCL fought off a hostile takeover bid by Carnival Cruise Lines, but in the process ended up with controlling interest in the company going to Singapore and Malaysian-based Star Cruises Plc with a 40 percent stake held by Carnival.

It appears that the new owners intend to maintain NCL's identity and fleet. One new direction was apparent: the company's new president said he expected the line to add Megaships to its fleet.

The Norwegian Story

NCL, originally named Norwegian Caribbean Lines, began in 1966 as a partnership between the Norwegian shipping company Klosters and entrepreneur Ted Arison; that arrangement lasted until 1972 when Arison left to form Carnival Cruise Lines.

NCL's first vessel was the *Sunward*. Part ocean liner and part ferryboat, the ship was built to take British vacationers and their cars to Spain. That itinerary became less attractive because of political issues, and the ship was transferred to the then-obscure Port of Miami. A company named Norwegian Caribbean Lines was formed.

The *Sunward* was an instant success, contributing to Miami's tremendous growth as a cruise ship port. NCL brought out a line of new "white ships," beginning with the *Starward* in 1968.

In 1979, NCL rescued the nearly forgotten *France* from retirement for $18 million; the ship was towed to Bremerhaven, Germany and rebuilt for Caribbean cruising at a cost of $130 million. The flagship of the NCL fleet, renamed as the *Norway*, is the longest cruise ship afloat. It was recently refurbished again.

In 1984, the line's parent company purchased another Norwegian company, the Royal Viking Line, integrating it into NCL operations. Five years later, Royal Cruise line was also brought into NCL. Of the RVL and Royal ships, only the *Norwegian Star* (born as the *Royal Viking Sea* and renamed for a while as *Royal Odyssey*) remains in the fleet.

In 1997 and 1998, the *Windward* and *Dreamward* were stretched with the insertion of a 130-foot midsection, increasing each vessel's capacity by 40 percent; they were reborn as the *Norwegian Wind* and *Norwegian Dream*.

In the summer of 1998, NCL completed the acquisition of Orient Lines, including the 845-guest cruise ship *Marco Polo*. Orient Lines will continue to be marketed as an independent premium brand. The cruise line offers five- to 25-day itineraries onboard the *Marco Polo* to exotic destinations in Africa, Antarctica, Australia, Egypt, India, Southeast Asia, and the Mediterranean, including the Greek Isles.

In April of 1999, the *Norwegian Majesty* received a 100-foot stretch, with the new midsection adding 202 new staterooms and increasing capacity from 1,056 to 1,460 guests. Also in 1999, the *Norwegian Star* was redeployed to Australia, sailing for NCL's joint venture company, Norwegian Capricorn Line on seven- to 14-day cruises in Australia and New Zealand. The company's *Aida* sails under charter in Europe.

The line's newest ship, the *Norwegian Sky*, joined the fleet in the summer of 1999. NCL acquired the unfinished hull of the *CostaOlympia* in 1997 when a German shipyard went bankrupt; the hull was towed to another shipyard and recast as the *Norwegian Sky*, allowing completion within a speedy 20 months.

The *Norwegian Sun*, sister ship to the *Norwegian Sky*, is expected in September of 2001. The company also holds an option to build three additional ships for delivery in 2001, 2002, and 2003—all in the range of 2,000 guests— at an average price of $332 million.

The NCL Experience

The *Norway*, a gracefully maintained oldster, has been assigned to year-round duty in the Caribbean. Beginning with the *Norway*, and later on other ships in the fleet, look for The Sports Illustrated Café, a themed bistro featuring a collection of classic *Sports Illustrated* photography from the past 40 years, as well as sports memorabilia. Some of the exhibitions will tie in with sports-theme cruises.

NCL has rededicated its attention to the quality of food service, one of the knocks against the line in recent years. Menus have been completely redesigned, offering a wider variety of international and regional dishes. In the evening, six of the NCL ships offer Le Bistro, an informal European-style dining alternative. And then there's the infamous "Chocoholic" dessert buffet, served near midnight once each cruise.

The line also offers an energetic cast of performers on each of its ships, presenting Broadway shows on larger vessels and cabaret nights on smaller ships.

Recent theme cruises have included country music, rock oldies, big bands at sea, blues and Dixieland, and a two-week floating jazz festival. Sports theme cruises include football, hockey, basketball, baseball, Olympic and national champions, fitness and volleyball; passengers can mingle with athletes from various pro sports teams on "Sports Afloat" cruises.

The Kids Crew children's program for ages 3 to 17 offers games, parties, scavenger hunts, T-shirt painting, visits to the bridge and autograph-signing sessions with professional athletes during sports theme cruises.

Norway

Econoguide rating:	★★★★
Ship size:	**Megaship**
Category:	**Vintage**
Price range:	**Premium $$$**
Registry:	Bahamas
Year built:	1962 (As the *France* for the French Line. Purchased and renamed as *Norway*, returning to service in 1980. Rebuilt in 1980.)
Itinerary:	Eastern and Western Caribbean from Miami
Information:	(800) 327-7030
Website:	www.ncl.com
Passenger capacity:	2,032 (double occupancy)
Crew:	920 International
Passenger-to-Crew Ratio:	2.2:1
Tonnage:	76,049
Passenger Space Ratio:	37.4
Length:	1,035 feet
Beam:	110 feet
Draft:	35 feet
Cruising speed:	18 knots
Guest decks:	12
Total cabins:	1,061
Outside:	473
Inside:	423
Suites:	165
Wheelchair accessible:	9
Cuisine:	Contemporary
Style:	Informal with two formal nights per cruise
Price notes:	150 percent to 200 percent single surcharge
Tipping suggestions:	$9 pp/pd

A grand classic, remade and maintained for the modern era. The *Norway*, born as the *France*, is the longest ship now afloat. She is just a bit too long to squeeze through the Panama Canal; in 1999 she was assigned to year-round patrol in the Caribbean, operating out of Miami. You can read about a trip on the *Norway* in the cruise diaries of this book.

The great ocean liner *France* was rescued from oblivion by Norwegian Cruise Line and rebuilt for cruising. Her public rooms are old-world elegant, and other remnants of her original incarnation include the two separate (but now equal) dining rooms, a holdover from the days of cabin classes.

The ship's deep draft may make the *Norway* more stable in high seas, although that same draft often requires the ship to anchor out in the harbor instead of pulling into a dock in shallow waters.

Notable public rooms include the Saga Theatre, a two-story showplace with proscenium stage; the room is used for full-scale Broadway productions and special events.

The large Monte Carlo Casino on the Pool Deck includes 236 slot and poker machines, as well as gaming tables.

Kids can romp in the Trolland playroom and the Port Hole activity center. The Kids Crew program is available for youngsters from ages 3 to 17.

Norwegian Sky

Econoguide rating:	★★★★★
Ship size:	**Megaship**
Category:	**Top of the Line**
Price range:	**Premium to Opulent $$$–$$$$**
Registry:	Bahamas
Year built:	1999
Itinerary:	Caribbean in winter, Panama Canal, Alaska in summer
Information:	(800) 327-7030
Website:	www.ncl.com
Passenger capacity:	2,002 (double occupancy)
Crew:	800 International
Passenger-to-Crew Ratio:	2.5:1
Tonnage:	78,000
Passenger Space Ratio:	39
Length:	848 feet
Beam:	105.8 feet
Draft:	26 feet
Cruising speed:	20 knots
Guest decks:	12
Total cabins:	1,001
Outside:	317
Inside:	427
Suites:	257
Wheelchair cabins:	6
Cuisine:	Contemporary
Style:	Informal with two formal nights per cruise
Price notes:	150 percent to 200 percent single supplement
Tipping suggestions:	$9 pp/pd

The *Norwegian Sky* entered service in August of 1999, sailing from the shipyard to Boston to begin her service with a series of cruises to Canada. Unfortunately, the spectacular new ship made a most spectacular debut on her first passage in the St. Lawrence River, running aground at the juncture with the Saguenay River.

The ship was stuck in the mud for several hours, and at one point it appeared that guests would have to be taken off before it could be freed; the return of high tide, though, refloated her. The mishap damaged one of the rudders and a propeller, and cut a large gash in her side. There were no reported injuries (except perhaps to the resumé of the captain and the two river pilots aboard), but the brand-spanking new ship had to limp back to Quebec City and enter into dry dock for more than a month of repairs.

The ship missed three 10-day itineraries from Boston to Canada, emerging from the body shop just in time to steam south to Miami to arrive for her official christening for the winter Caribbean season.

After her first season in the Caribbean, she moved in May of 2000 to a home port at Seattle's new cruise terminal for summer cruises to Alaska. In the fall, she will reverse the schedule, heading back to Florida.

NCL acquired an unfinished hull in 1997 when the Bremer Vulkan shipyard in Germany went bankrupt. Intended as the *CostaOlympia* flagship of the Costa line, the ship was recast as the *Norwegian Sky,* allowing completion within a speedy 20 months.

Most of the cabins are on decks 8, 9, and 10, well above the lifeboats on deck 7; a bit more than 200 others are spread among the lower decks. About a quarter of the ship's 1,000 staterooms have a private teak-floored balcony, and four owners' suites also have private outdoor hot tubs.

Up top are three pools, including one with a waterfall.

The focus of the interior is a pair of glass-domed atria. Aft, there's Neptune's Court with a grand stair tower. Midships is The Atrium, eight decks high with four panoramic lifts.

There are two major restaurants on the Atlantic Deck: the Four Seasons and Seven Seas dining rooms. The Horizons Restaurant on the Atlantic Deck offers intimate dining for 84. The Stardust Lounge on the Promenade and International Decks seats 1,000 in a two-story show lounge that has a proscenium stage. The Sports Bar on Pool Deck serves as a teen disco during the day; also onboard is The Zone teenage disco, which has a soft drink bar. The Starlight Lounge is a two-story show lounge that has a proscenium stage.

The Kids Crew program is available for children from ages 3 through 17.

Norwegian Dream

Econoguide rating:	★★★★
Ship size:	**Grand**
Category:	**Top of the Line**
Price range:	**Premium to Opulent $$$–$$$$**
Registry:	The Bahamas
Year built:	1992 (As *Dreamward.* Stretched by 130 feet in 1998 and renamed)
Sister ships:	*Norwegian Wind*
Itinerary:	Caribbean in winter, Europe for Summer
Information:	(800) 327-7030
Website:	www.ncl.com
Passenger capacity:	1,760 (double occupancy)
Crew:	614 International
Passenger-to-Crew Ratio:	2.9:1
Tonnage:	46,000
Passenger Space Ratio:	26.1
Length:	758 feet
Beam:	94 feet
Draft:	23 feet
Cruising speed:	21 knots
Guest decks:	10
Total cabins:	870
Outside:	505
Inside:	212
Suites:	153
Wheelchair cabins:	13
Cuisine:	Continental
Style:	Informal with two formal nights per cruise
Price notes:	150 percent to 200 percent single supplement
Tipping suggestions:	$9 pp/pd

The *Norwegian Dream* and her sister ship the *Norwegian Wind* were reborn in 1998 after they were stretched and refurbished, growing from nice medium-sized vessels to even nicer grand ships.

You don't really "stretch" a ship—that brings to mind a Medieval torture rack. Instead, each ship was cut in half and a matching 130-foot midsection was installed. As a result, passenger capacity was increased by 40 percent, with the addition of 502 new berths, several new public rooms, and a few interesting amenities, including a swim-up pool bar.

On the *Dream*, the Stardust Lounge is a two-story main show lounge that has a proscenium stage, used for a full production of Broadway shows.

In August of 1999, the *Norwegian Dream* inexplicably collided with a large freighter in the English Channel, sustaining major damage and shaking up passengers, though none were seriously injured. The ship continued to England under her own power, but was disabled for more than a month.

Norwegian Wind

Econoguide rating:	★★★★
Ship size:	**Grand**
Category:	**Top of the Line**
Price range:	**Moderate-Premium $$–$$$**
Registry:	The Bahamas
Year built:	1992 (As *Windward*. Renamed as *Norwegian Wind* in 1998. Stretched by 130 feet in 1998)
Sister ships:	*Norwegian Dream*
Itinerary:	Caribbean, Panama Canal, Hawaii, Alaska
Information:	(800) 327-7030
Website:	www.ncl.com
Passenger capacity:	1,760 (double occupancy)
Crew:	614 International
Passenger-to-Crew Ratio:	2.9:1
Tonnage:	50,760
Passenger Space Ratio:	28.8
Length:	754 feet
Beam:	94 feet
Draft:	22 feet
Cruising speed:	21 knots
Guest decks:	10
Total cabins:	870
Outside:	505
Inside:	212
Suites:	153
Wheelchair cabins:	13
Cuisine:	Continental
Style:	Informal with two formal nights per cruise
Price notes:	150 percent to 200 percent single supplement
Tipping suggestions:	$9 pp/pd

Like the *Norwegian Dream*, the *Windward* was stretched by 130 feet in 1998 and renamed the *Norwegian Wind*. The two sisters are now nearly identical.

The Sports Bar and Grill on the Sports Deck features a wall of multiple televisions that display videotaped and live broadcasts of major sports events. The Stardust Lounge on the Star Deck is a two-story main show lounge used for full-scale productions of Broadway shows.

Norwegian Sea

Econoguide rating:	★★★
Ship size:	**Grand**
Category:	**Vintage**
Price range:	**Premium $$$**
Registry:	Bahamas
Year built:	1988 (As the *Seaward*)
Itinerary:	Caribbean from Houston
Information:	(800) 327-7030
Website:	www.ncl.com
Passenger capacity:	1,518 (double occupancy)
Crew:	630 International
Passenger-to-Crew Ratio:	2.4:1
Tonnage:	42,000
Passenger Space Ratio:	27.7
Length:	700 feet
Beam:	93 feet
Draft:	22 feet
Cruising speed:	20 knots
Guest decks:	9 decks
Total cabins:	747
Outside:	494
Inside:	246
Suites:	7
Wheelchair cabins:	4
Cuisine:	Contemporary
Style:	Informal with two formal nights per cruise
Price notes:	150 percent to 200 percent single supplement
Tipping suggestions:	$9 pp/pd

A veteran of the Caribbean, and on a comparative basis, a relatively homely member of the NCL fleet. The ship nevertheless has some nice touches in public areas, enhanced by a recent redecoration; the ship was also renamed from *Seaward* to add a reference to its owner's Scandinavian heritage.

In 2000, the *Norwegian Sea* sailed out of the Port of Houston on a Texaribbean itinerary of Cancun, Cozumel, and Roatan, Bay Island, Honduras. Beginning in January of 2001, she will be redeployed to Miami to offer three- and four-day cruises to Nassau and Great Stirrup Cay; four-day cruises will add a stop at Key West.

The Cabaret Lounge is used for full-scale Broadway productions; in recent years the show has been "Grease."

The Kids Crew program is available to youngsters from 3 to 17.

Norwegian Majesty

Econoguide rating:	★★★★
Ship size:	**Medium**
Category:	**Top of the Line**
Price range:	**Moderate-Premium $$–$$$**
Registry:	Bahamas
Year built:	1992 (As *Royal Majesty* of former Majesty Cruise Line. Purchased by NCL and renamed in 1997). Stretched by 112 feet and 203 cabins in 1999.)
Itinerary:	Boston to Bermuda spring and summer of 1999, Panama Canal
Information:	(800) 327-7030

Website:	www.ncl.com
Passenger capacity:	1,462 (double occupancy)
Crew:	550 International
Passenger-to-Crew Ratio:	2.65:1
Tonnage:	38,000
Passenger Space Ratio:	26
Length:	680 feet
Beam:	91 feet
Draft:	19 feet
Cruising speed:	21 knots
Guest decks:	9 decks
Total cabins:	731
Outside:	481
Inside:	249
Suites:	16
Wheelchair cabins:	4
Cuisine:	Contemporary
Style:	Informal with two formal nights per cruise
Price notes:	150 percent to 200 percent single supplement
Tipping suggestions:	$9 pp/pd

The *Norwegian Majesty* was stretched by 112 feet and 203 staterooms in early 1999; addition of the new midsection increased the guest capacity from 1,056 to 1,462 guests and boosted the crew size by 25 percent.

The new midsection contains a second swimming pool and dining room, a new casino, the intimate 58-seat Le Bistro restaurant, more deck space, and 203 new staterooms. Also included in the new section were two new elevators and a third set of stairs to improve movement throughout the ship.

An entirely new space, the Sky Deck, was added above the lengthened Sun Deck to add sunning areas and to create a ring of shaded areas around the two pools and whirlpools below.

Existing staterooms on the ship will be upgraded to match the new staterooms in upcoming refurbishments.

Installation of the new midsection took about three months. According to engineers, the new midsection actually helped the ship's underwater profile, allowing it to maintain its 21-knot speed without changes to the powerplant. And added buoyancy from the new midsection reduced the vessel's draft about 18 inches.

Norwegian Crown/Crown Odyssey

Econoguide rating:	★★★★
Ship size:	**Medium**
Category:	**Top of the Line**
Price range:	**Premium to Opulent $$$–$$$$**
Registry:	Bahamas
Year built:	1988 (As the *Crown Odyssey* of the Royal Viking Line and Royal Cruise Line. Renamed as *Norwegian Crown* for NCL in 1996. Renamed again as *Crown Odyssey* in 2000 for Orient Lines.)
Itinerary:	Asia
Information:	(800) 333-7300 (Orient Lines)

Website:	www.ncl.com
Passenger capacity:	1,050 (double occupancy)
Crew:	470 International
Passenger-to-Crew Ratio:	2.3:1
Tonnage:	34,250
Passenger Space Ratio:	32.6
Length:	614 feet
Beam:	92.5 feet
Draft:	24 feet
Cruising speed:	22 knots
Guest decks:	10
Total cabins:	526
Outside:	322
Inside:	114
Suites:	90
Wheelchair cabins:	4
Cuisine:	Contemporary
Style:	Informal with two formal nights per cruise
Price notes:	Single occupancy premium about 150 percent for guaranteed single room
Tipping suggestions:	$9/person/day

In the Spring of 2000, the *Norwegian Crown* was due to transfer to the Orient Line in Asia; in the process she will regain her original name of *Crown Odyssey*. Orient Lines, owned by the same company that owns NCL, also operates the 800-guest *Marco Polo*.

Built as an upper-ranks cruise ship, she has held up well as one of the smaller and somewhat more luxurious members of the NCL fleet.

The Seven Continents Restaurant on the Marina Deck is built on two levels with a central sunken section beneath a domed Tiffany-style glass ceiling.

In the Yacht Club/Midnight Sun Café, photos of America's Cup yachts and other sailing vessels decorate the poolside lounge, which is used for breakfast and lunch buffets and snacks, and in the evening it's used as a nightclub.

PRINCESS CRUISES

Princess Cruises
10100 Santa Monica Blvd.
Los Angeles, CA 90067
Information: (800) 421-0522, (800) 774-6237
www.princesscruises.com

Princess Cruises Fleet

Grand Princess. (1998) 2,600 passengers. 109,000 tons

Ocean Princess. (2000) 1,950 passengers. 77,000 tons

Sea Princess. (1998) 1,950 passengers. 77,000 tons

Dawn Princess. (1997) 1,950 passengers. 77,000 tons

Sun Princess. (1995) 1,950 passengers. 77,000 tons

Crown Princess. (1990) 1,590 passengers. 70,000 tons

Regal Princess. (1991) 1,590 passengers. 70,000 tons

Sky Princess/Pacific Sky. (1984) 1,200 passengers. 46,000 tons

Royal Princess. (1984) 1,200 passengers. 45,000 tons

Future Ships
Unnamed. (2002) 2,600 passengers. 110,000 tons

Unnamed. (2004) 2,600 passengers. 110,000 tons

Unnamed. (2003) 1,950 passengers. 88,000 tons

Unnamed. (2004) 1,950 passengers. 88,000 tons

All right, let's get it over with right up front: This is the company that tied its fortunes to "The Love Boat" as an advertising slogan and a television series, and it has hardly looked back since.

Today, Princess sails to six continents and calls at more than 230 ports around the world. Princess owns a big piece of Alaska, too, with six cruise ships in those waters, four riverside wilderness lodges, a fleet of deluxe motor-coaches, and eight luxury Midnight Sun Express rail cars.

The flagship of the fleet is the *Grand Princess.* Built at a cost of nearly $450 million, the 2,600-passenger, 109,000-ton ship is 951 feet long, and its hull is 118 feet wide—a few feet wider than the Panama Canal.

Princess itself was founded in 1965 with a single chartered ship cruising from Los Angeles to Mexico; within a few years, Princess Cruises had a small fleet of ships on the West Coast. London-based Peninsular and Orient Steam Navigation Company came to the same waters in the early 1970s but could not compete against Princess' head start.

P&O purchased Princess in 1974.

A year later a television producer approached Princess Cruises with an idea for a series about cruising, and "The Love Boat" was the result—the successful show became a weekly prime-time advertisement for cruising in general, and Princess in particular. The cruise company continued to market itself as The Love Boat well after the original series left the airwaves.

In 1988, P&O bought out another competitor, Sitmar Cruises of Los Angeles, and merged its operations and ships into the Princess fleet.

P&O dates back to 1822 to a fleet of small sailing ships; among their destinations was a link between Great Britain and Spain and Portugal—the Iberian Peninsula. To demonstrate their appreciation for the services provided during the Portuguese and Spanish civil wars of the early 1830s, the Royal Houses of both countries granted the company the right to fly their colors—the Portuguese blue and white, and the Spanish red and gold. Those colors continue to this day in the P&O flag.

In 1836, the partners began a regular steamer service to the Iberian Peninsula under the name "Peninsular Steam Navigation Company." Within a few years, the steamer company added routes to India and Egypt (with an overland route across Egypt until the opening of the Suez Canal in 1869). By 1845, the steamers reached to Malay and China, and "Orient" was added to the company's name.

P&O began offering leisure cruises in 1844 and eventually became known for its "big white ships."

In the spring of 2000, the *Ocean Princess* joins the fleet, a sister ship to *Sun Princess, Sea Princess,* and *Dawn Princess.*

In 1999, Princess placed an order for four more ships to be delivered between October 2002 and May 2004. Mitsubishi Heavy Industries of Japan will build two 110,000-ton, 2,600-passenger sisters to the *Grand Princess.* Chantioers de L'Atlantique in France will build a pair of 88,000-ton, 1,950-passenger vessels.

The new French-built ships will include an unusual combination of diesel and gas turbine engines. The design will have only 10 percent of staterooms inside, and 80 percent of the outside cabins will have balconies.

Beginning in 2001, Princess will maintain a year-round presence in the Caribbean for the first time; the *Grand Princess* will sail from Fort Lauderdale from the end of April through late September; in prior years, the huge ship had summered in the Mediterranean.

The Princess Experience

"The Love Boat" lives on in the hearts and minds of Princess executives and many of the company's passengers. In 1998, another go-round of the television show took to the airwaves. "Love Boat: The Next Wave" was in part filmed aboard the $300 million, 77,000-ton *Sun Princess,* one of Princess Cruises' newest ships.

The original "Love Boat" was set aboard the smaller 20,000-ton *Pacific Princess*; that ship, recently refurbished, sails in the Mediterranean. Its twin sister, the *Island Princess,* was sold in 1999 to a South Korean company.

"Love Boat" aside, Princess actually offers a pretty refined experience with Continental cuisine and a mostly Italian dining room staff. Add in sushi restaurants on all ships in the fleet during lunch hours. At the same time, you can expect a full regime of parties, games, and other cruise entertainment.

Princess was the first major cruise line to add live cameras on most of its ships; BridgeCams can be viewed on the Internet at www.princess.com, offering views from the bridge from seven of the ships in the fleet.

The company operates the Denali Princess Wilderness Lodge just outside the Denali National Park in Alaska, with a total of 353 rooms in 2000. The company also owns and operates the Kenai Princess Wilderness Lodge, the Mount McKinley Princess Wilderness Lodge, and the Fairbanks Princess Lodge. Princess has expanded the number of excursions it offers from its Alaskan cruises to Denali.

Ten-day voyages from Los Angeles to the Mexican Riviera include stops at Acapulco, Cabo San Lucas, Mazatlan, Puerto Vallarta, and Zihuatanejo/Ixtapa. The new Costa Rica eco-cruisetours include a 10-day trip to the Mexican Riviera plus an additional call in Guatemala to visit the Mayan ruins of Tikal and inland tours of Costa Rica.

Grand Princess

Econoguide rating:	★★★★★
Ship size:	**Colossus**
Category:	**Top of the Line**
Price range:	**Opulent $$$$**
Registry:	Liberia
Year built:	Entered service September 1998
Itinerary:	Eastern Caribbean from Ft. Lauderdale; Summer European cruises
Information:	(800) 774-6237
Website:	www.princesscruises.com
Passenger capacity:	2,600 (double occupancy)
Crew:	1,100 International
Passenger-to-Crew Ratio:	2.4:1
Tonnage:	109,000 tons
Passenger Space Ratio:	41.9
Length:	951 feet
Beam:	159 feet, including bridge wing; 118 feet, excluding bridge wing
Draft:	26 feet
Cruising speed:	22 knots; 24 knots, maximum
Guest decks:	12
Total cabins:	1,300
Outside:	720
Inside:	372
Suites:	208
Wheelchair cabins:	28 (18 outside/10 inside)
Cuisine:	International
Style:	Casual or semi-formal and occasionally formal
Price notes:	Single occupancy premium 160 percent to 200 percent
Tipping suggestions:	$7.75 pp/pd

At the start of 1999, The *Grand Princess* was the Colossus of the Oceans, the largest cruise ship afloat. (It's a title she held until midway through the year, when she was trumped by Royal Caribbean's *Voyager of the Seas*.)

How big? More than three football fields long, too wide to fit through the Panama Canal, and at 201 feet tall, the ship is 50 feet taller than the Statue of Liberty and higher than Niagara Falls. She's home to 3,700 or so close friends and crew members. The *Pacific Princess*, the original "Love Boat," could fit within the *Grand Princess'* Horizon Court dining and lido areas.

As befits the queen of the Love Boat line, the *Grand Princess* features the first ocean-going wedding chapel, including a program that allows passengers to be married by the ship's captain—something that despite the common conception, is not often permitted. Marriages are performed under the authority of the ship's registry—in the case of the *Grand Princess*, Liberia—and are legally recognized in most jurisdictions.

A disco/observation lounge is suspended 150 feet above water and accessible only by a glass-enclosed, moving "skywalk."

There's also the first ocean-going virtual reality game center and a bluescreen digital studio to permit guests to star in their own shipboard epic.

The *Grand Princess* sports five swimming pools, including a lap pool that allows you to swim against the current. Princess Links offers simulated play on the world's greatest courses as well as a 9-hole putting green.

The ship features the greatest number of cabins with private balconies (710 total) of any ship, and it has the largest casino at sea.

The *Grand Princess* is also the first major commercial ship built with fully redundant operational and technical systems. There are two separate engine rooms. Power supplies are duplicated, and cooling systems are split into two separate circuits, with pumps and coolers in separate spaces.

There are eight dining areas, including an Italian trattoria and a Southwestern restaurant.

The Horizon Court on the Lido Deck is a 24-hour café with 620 seats. On the Promenade Deck are two of the three main dining rooms, the Da Vinci with 486 seats and the Botticelli with 508 seats. Nearby is The Painted Desert, a 92-seat Southwestern restaurant also available to passengers.

The Plaza Deck is home to the third major restaurant, the 486-seat Michelangelo Dining Room. Nearby is Sabatini's Trattoria, a 90-seat bistro for casual Italian dining that serves fresh pasta and pizza.

On the health front, the ship includes a "telemedicine" setup that allows the ship's doctors to consult electronically with emergency physicians at Cedars Sinai Medical Center in Los Angeles.

The *Grand Princess* sails from Fort Lauderdale to the eastern Caribbean during the fall and winter, crossing over to the Mediterranean for a series of summer cruises—the first Megaship or Colossus to regularly cruise in Europe. She returns to the Caribbean in the fall of 2000. In 2001, she will stay in the Caribbean for the summer, sailing alternating week-long Eastern Caribbean itineraries to St. Thomas, St. Maarten, and Princess Cays with a Western Caribbean tour to Cozumel, Grand Cayman, and Princess Cays.

The *Grand Princess* is the first of a line of at least three similar ships, with two more under construction and expected in 2001.

Ocean Princess

Econoguide rating:	★★★★
Ship size:	**Megaship**
Category:	**Top of the Line**
Price range:	**Premium to Opulent $$$–$$$$**
Registry:	Liberia
Year built:	Spring 2000
Sister ships:	*Dawn Princess, Sea Princess, Sun Princess*
Itinerary:	Caribbean, Mexico, Alaska

Information:	(800) 774-6237
Website:	www.princesscruises.com
Passenger capacity:	1,950 (double occupancy)
Crew:	900 Italian officers
Passenger-to-Crew Ratio:	2.2:1
Tonnage:	77,000
Passenger Space Ratio:	39.5
Length:	856 feet
Beam:	105.8 feet
Draft:	26 feet
Cruising speed:	N/A
Guest decks:	14
Total cabins:	1,050
Outside:	646
Inside:	398
Suites:	6
Wheelchair accessible:	20
Cuisine:	Contemporary
Style:	Casual or semi-formal and occasionally formal
Price notes:	Single occupancy premium 160 percent to 200 percent
Tipping suggestions:	$7.75 pp/pd

The latest Grand Class ship, sister to the *Sun Princess, Dawn Princess,* and *Sea Princess.*

In her first season, she sails the Mexican Riviera in late Spring, moving on to Alaska from Vancouver for the summer, returning to the Caribbean for the winter.

Dawn Princess

Econoguide rating:	★★★★
Ship size:	**Megaship**
Category:	**Top of the Line**
Price range:	**Premium to Opulent $$$–$$$$**
Registry:	Liberia
Year built:	1997
Sister ships:	*Ocean Princess, Sea Princess, Sun Princess*
Itinerary:	Southern Caribbean, Panama Canal, Mexico, Alaska (Gulf), Mexico
Information:	(800) 774-6237
Website:	www.princesscruises.com
Passenger capacity:	1,950 (double occupancy)
Crew:	900 Italian officers
Passenger-to-Crew Ratio:	2.2:1
Tonnage:	77,000
Passenger Space Ratio:	39.5
Length:	856 feet
Beam:	105.8 feet
Draft:	26 feet
Guest decks:	14
Total cabins:	1,050
Outside:	646
Inside:	398
Suites:	6
Wheelchair cabins:	20
Cuisine:	Contemporary

Style:	Casual or semi-formal and occasionally formal
Price notes:	Single occupancy premium 160 percent to 200 percent
Tipping suggestions:	$7.75 pp/pd

A member of Princess' Grand Class of ships, the *Dawn Princess* is sister ship to the *Sun Princess, Sea Princess,* and *Ocean Princess.* For a while after the *Sun Princess* was launched, she was the largest cruise ship afloat.

There are more than 400 verandas among the cabins. Public areas include the impressive Princess Theatre. A teak promenade deck encircles the entire ship. Within is a $2.5 million art collection.

She sails in the Caribbean from San Juan in the winter, crossing through the Panama Canal in the spring and making her way to Alaska for the summer; she reverses the schedule in the fall.

Sea Princess

Econoguide rating:	★★★★
Ship size:	**Megaship**
Category:	**Top of the Line**
Price range:	**Premium $$$**
Registry:	Liberia
Year built:	1998
Sister ships:	*Dawn Princess, Ocean Princess, Sun Princess*
Itinerary:	Caribbean, Vancouver, Alaska
Information:	(800) 774-6237
Website:	www.princesscruises.com
Passenger capacity:	1,950 (double occupancy)
Crew:	900 Italian officers
Passenger-to-Crew Ratio:	2.2:1
Tonnage:	77,000
Passenger Space Ratio:	39.5
Length:	856 feet
Beam:	105.8 feet
Draft:	26 feet
Guest decks:	14
Total cabins:	1,050
Outside:	652
Inside:	398
Suites:	6
Wheelchair cabins:	20
Cuisine:	Contemporary
Style:	Casual or semi-formal and occasionally formal
Price notes:	Single occupancy premium 160 percent to 200 percent
Tipping suggestions:	$7.75 pp/pd

The *Sea Princess* joined the Princess fleet in late 1998, sister to the *Sun Princess, Dawn Princess,* and *Ocean Princess.*

Her schedule covers the Western Caribbean from Fort Lauderdale in the winter, moving through the Panama Canal to Vancouver for summer in Alaska.

Sun Princess

Econoguide rating:	★★★★
Ship size:	**Megaship**
Category:	**Top of the Line**
Price range:	**Premium to Opulent $$$–$$$$**
Registry:	Liberia
Year built:	1995
Sister ships:	*Dawn Princess, Ocean Princess, Sea Princess*
Itinerary:	Western Caribbean, Panama Canal, Mexico, Alaska (Gulf)
Information:	(800) 774-6237
Website:	www.princesscruises.com
Passenger capacity:	1,950 (double occupancy)
Crew:	900 Italian officers, international crew
Passenger-to-Crew Ratio:	2.2:1
Tonnage:	77,000
Passenger Space Ratio:	39.5
Length:	856 feet
Beam:	105.8 feet
Draft:	26 feet
Guest decks:	14
Total cabins:	1,050
Outside:	652
Inside:	398
Suites:	6
Wheelchair cabins:	19
Cuisine:	Contemporary
Style:	Casual or semi-formal and occasionally formal
Price notes:	Single occupancy premium 160 percent to 200 percent
Tipping suggestions:	$7.75 pp/pd

Sister ship to *Dawn Princess, Sea Princess,* and *Ocean Princess.* The *Sun Princess* sails a series of cruises from San Juan to Costa Rica through the Panama Canal, spends winters in the Caribbean, crossing the Panama Canal in the spring and moving to Alaska for the summer.

Crown Princess

Econoguide rating:	★★★★
Ship size:	**Megaship**
Category:	**Top of the Line**
Price range:	**Premium to Opulent $$$–$$$$**
Registry:	Liberia
Year built:	Crown entered service 1990
Sister ships:	Regal Princess
Itinerary:	Alaska, Hawaii, Hawaii/Tahiti, Costa Rica, Mexico, Panama Canal, Canada
Information:	(800) 774-6237
Website:	www.princesscruises.com
Passenger capacity:	1,590 (double occupancy)
Crew:	696 Italian officers, international crew
Passenger-to-Crew Ratio:	2.3:1
Tonnage:	69,845
Passenger Space Ratio:	43.9
Length:	811 feet
Beam:	105.8 feet
Draft:	26.5 feet
Guest decks:	12

Total cabins:	795
Outside:	610
Inside:	171
Suites:	14
Wheelchair cabins:	10
Cuisine:	Contemporary
Style:	Casual or semi-formal and occasionally formal
Price notes:	Single occupancy premium 160 percent to 200 percent
Tipping suggestions:	$7.75 pp/pd

Twin to the *Regal Princess,* the *Crown Princess* sails Panama Canal trips from Fort Lauderdale, moving to Europe for the summer, and returning to the East Coast in the fall for a series of trips in Canada and New England from New York and Montréal.

Public rooms include a domed observation lounge that has an entertainment complex and casino.

Regal Princess

Econoguide rating:	★★★★
Ship size:	**Megaship**
Category:	**Top of the Line**
Price range:	**Premium to Opulent $$$–$$$$**
Registry:	Liberia
Year built:	Entered service 1991
Sister ships:	*Crown Princess*
Itinerary:	Alaska in summer, Panama Canal from Fort Lauderdale remainder of year
Information:	(800) 774-6237
Website:	www.princesscruises.com
Passenger capacity:	1,590 (double occupancy)
Crew:	696 Italian officers, international crew
Passenger-to-Crew Ratio:	2.3:1
Tonnage:	69,845
Passenger Space Ratio:	43.9
Length:	811 feet
Beam:	105.8 feet
Draft:	26.5 feet
Guest decks:	12 total decks
Total cabins:	795
Outside:	610
Inside:	171
Suites:	14
Wheelchair cabins:	10
Cuisine:	Contemporary
Style:	Informal with one or more semi-formal nights
Price notes:	Single occupancy premium 160 percent to 200 percent
Tipping suggestions:	$7.75 pp/pd

Sister to the *Crown Princess,* she embarked on a new schedule in 2000. In the spring she moved to the West Coast to sail a series of cruises from Mexico to Hawaii, and Hawaii on to Vancouver for a summer in Alaska. Beginning in October of 2000, she was due to head for the Far East, visiting China, Thailand, Australia, New Zealand, the South Pacific, and other ports. In April of 2001 she was due to return to Vancouver for the Alaskan summer.

Royal Princess

Econoguide rating:	★★★
Ship size:	**Medium**
Category:	**Golden Oldie**
Price range:	**Moderate $$**
Registry:	Great Britain
Year built:	1984
Itinerary:	World Cruise, South America, Europe
Information:	(800) 774-6237
Website:	www.princesscruises.com
Passenger capacity:	1,200 (double occupancy)
Crew:	520 British officers, international crew
Passenger-to-Crew Ratio:	2.3:1
Tonnage:	46,000
Passenger Space Ratio:	38.3
Length:	789 feet
Beam:	95.8 feet
Draft:	25.5 feet
Guest decks:	11
Total cabins:	586
Outside:	586
Inside:	0
Suites:	14
Wheelchair cabins:	4
Cuisine:	Contemporary
Style:	Casual with one or more formal nights
Price notes:	Single occupancy premium 160 percent to 200 percent
Tipping suggestions:	$7.75 pp/pd

A gracefully aging pioneer of cruising, among the first ships to offer verandas on many of her cabins. All 586 staterooms are in prime outside, upper-deck locations; public rooms are located on lower decks. (Some of the outside cabins, though, have restricted views because of low-hanging lifeboats.)

In the winter of 2000, the *Royal Princess* cruised South America, crossing over to Europe for the summer. In June and July, she was to visit the Norwegian and Scandinavian fjords. In November, she is due to return to South America. In February of 2001, the vessel is to embark on a 72-day world cruise from Fort Lauderdale.

Sky Princess/Pacific Sky

Econoguide rating:	★★★
Ship size:	**Medium**
Category:	**Golden Oldie**
Price range:	**Premium $$$**
Registry:	Liberia
Year built:	1984 (As Sitmar's *Fairsky*)
Itinerary:	South Pacific from Sydney.
Information:	(800) 774-6237
Website:	www.princesscruises.com
Passenger capacity:	1,200 (double occupancy)
Crew:	550
Passenger-to-Crew Ratio:	2.2:1

Tonnage:	46,000
Passenger Space Ratio:	38.3
Length:	789 feet
Beam:	91.3 feet
Draft:	26.7 feet
Guest decks:	11 total decks
Total cabins:	600
Outside:	375
Inside:	215
Suites:	10
Wheelchair cabins:	19
Cuisine:	Contemporary
Style:	Casual with one or more formal nights.
Price notes:	Single occupancy premium 160 percent to 200 percent
Tipping suggestions:	$7.75 pp/pd

One of the last turbine steamships built, with touches of her original French design, including silk and leather.

In 2000, the *Sky Princess* sails in Australia and New Zealand, moving on to China in April of 2000, and then sailing in Alaska from San Francisco for the summer.

In September of 2000, she is to be transferred out of the Princess fleet and into another division of P&O to sail from Australia under a new name of *Pacific Sky.*

RADISSON SEVEN SEAS
CRUISES

Radisson Seven Seas Cruises
600 Corporate Drive, Suite 410
Fort Lauderdale, FL 33334
Information: (800) 333-3333, (800) 285-1835
www.rssc.com

Radisson Seven Seas Fleet

Radisson Seven Seas Navigator. (1999) 490 passengers. 33,000 tons

Radisson Diamond. (1992) 350 passengers. 20,295 tons

Paul Gauguin. (1998) 320 passengers. 18,800 tons

Hanseatic. (1993) 188 passengers. 9,000 tons

Future Ships
Radisson Seven Seas Mariner. (March 2001) 708 passengers. 48,000 tons

Radisson Seven Seas Cruises has an eclectic collection of small luxury cruise ships and a pair of Sybaritic adventure ships. The tony ships are managed by the upscale hotel chain of the same name.

They claim to be the only cruise line whose vessels reach all of the continents on earth, including the two polar regions.

Seven Seas Cruises operates and markets the cruise ships *Radisson Diamond, Song of Flower,* and *Paul Gauguin,* as well as the *Hanseatic,* one of the most luxurious adventure cruise ships afloat.

The line's newest and largest vessel, the *Seven Seas Navigator,* brings luxury cruising to Alaska's Inside Passage from May to August of 2000, sailing out of San Francisco and Vancouver. In the fall, she will move across the Pacific to Sydney, sailing in and around Australia, New Zealand, Indonesia, and Hong Kong for the rest of the year. In December of 2000, she will return to the U.S. West Coast and then pass through the Panama Canal to take up winter residence in Fort Lauderdale for Caribbean cruises.

A newer and larger ship, the *Seven Seas Mariner,* joins the fleet in March of 2001.

The *Diamond* alternates between the Caribbean and Europe. From May through of October, she will sail in the Mediterranean, Scandinavia, and in and around Turkey and Greece. She returns to San Juan in October for Caribbean and Panama Canal itineraries. Special theme cruises include "The Imperial House of Fabergé and the Tsars" in August, a tour in the baltic with its very own archduke/historian onboard. Also in the summer is the Royal Music Festival series with tickets to performances at sites such as the Hermitage Theater in St. Petersburg, Russia, and the Stockholm Royal Palace.

Hanseatic cruises from Antartica to the Americas, the Russian Far East and the Far North including Iceland and Greenland.

The *Song of Flower* and the *Paul Gauguin* live in Europe and the South Seas. In the summer of 2000, guests on the *Song of Flower* can enjoy a seven-night Grand Imperial Dinner cruise from Stockholm to Copenhagen, as the ship's chefs recreate the lavish meal enjoyed by Kaiser Wilhelm I of Germany, Tsar Alexander II of Russia, and the Tsarvitch (later Alexander III) at a celebrated Paris restaurant in 1867.

The company is part of Carlson Hospitality Worldwide, which includes amongst its holdings the Radisson and Regent hotel chains, Country Inns & Suites by Carlson, and TGI Friday's.

The *Seven Seas Navigator* gives 490 passengers an all-suite 33,000-ton luxury cruise ship with 245 ocean view suites; 90 percent feature private balconies. The ship will cruise the world, with a regular circuit including the Americas and a series of Panama Canal transits.

The 20,295-ton *Radisson Diamond* is one of the most readily identifiable ships afloat with its one-of-a-kind, twin-hull design intended to cut down on pitch and roll movements. Of her 177 outside staterooms, 123 feature private balconies. She sails in the winter on a trans-Panama Canal itinerary, including port calls in Costa Rica and the Caribbean islands; she moves to the Mediterranean for the summer.

The 9,000-ton *Hanseatic* boasts the highest ice-class rating for a passenger vessel, but hardly looks like an icebreaker within. The ship all but circumnavigates the globe with exploration cruises in the Arctic and Antarctic and seasonal operations in lesser-visited regions such as the Spitsbergen Archipelago, Iceland and Greenland.

Gratuities are neither expected nor accepted. The ship's staff is made up of Norwegian officers and Scandinavian stewardesses.

This is a cruise line that is definitely oriented toward adults; no infants under 1 year of age are allowed on Radisson ships, and there is a limit on the number of children onboard younger than 3 years of age. Older kids are allowed, but will be pretty much on their own for entertainment and minding.

In early 2001, the company will welcome the *Seven Seas Mariner*, the largest vessel in the fleet. The all-suite, all-balcony ship will accommodate 708 passengers. The new ship will be approximately 48,000 tons in size and about 713 feet long. The *Seven Seas Mariner* will use a "pod" propulsion system, which eliminates the traditional shaft and rudder system. The pods have forward-facing propellers that can be turned in a complete circle, optimizing maneuverability, fuel efficiency, and speed.

The ship will offer four dining venues, including a main dining room that is capable of seating the entire passenger load at once.

Hanseatic

Econoguide rating:	★★★★★
Ship size:	**Medium**
Category:	**Ultra-Luxury**
Price range:	**Beyond Opulent $$$$$**
Registry:	Bahamas
Year built:	1993
Itinerary:	Antarctica
Information:	(800) 285-1835
Website:	www.rssc.com
Passenger capacity:	188 (double occupancy)
Crew:	125 European
Passenger-to-Crew Ratio:	1:1.5
Tonnage:	9,000
Passenger Space Ratio:	47.9
Length:	403 feet
Beam:	59 feet
Draft:	15.4 feet
Cruising speed:	17 knots
Guest decks:	4
Total cabins:	90
Outside:	90
Inside:	0
Suites:	4
Wheelchair accessible:	2
Cuisine:	International. Single seating dining in Marco Polo restaurant
Style:	Resort casual, with occasional semi-formal nights
Price notes:	Single occupancy premium about 125 percent to 150 percent
Tipping suggestions:	Gratuities are included

A joint venture between Radisson Seven Seas Cruises and Hanseatic Tours of Hamburg, the ultra-deluxe cruise vessel includes visits to some of the more obscure parts of the world, including the Far North, Greenland, the Northwest Passage, the Galapagos Islands, Patagonia and Antarctica. She earns mention in this book because of occasional itineraries that include Alaska, Canada, and New England.

The *Hanseatic* is the most luxurious adventure ship in the world to have an ice classification of 1A1 Super, the highest rating for a passenger cruise ship. The only higher classification is reserved for commercial icebreakers.

Distinguished lecturers and naturalists take the podium on each journey with presentations in Darwin Hall. A fleet of 14 Zodiac landing craft provide access to some of the world's most remote locations.

The Observation Deck features a 180-degree panoramic view and includes a "Passenger Bridge" with ocean charts and a radar monitor. Passengers are also welcome on the Navigational Bridge.

The 170-seat Marco Polo Restaurant welcomes all passengers at one seating.

Paul Gauguin

Econoguide rating:	★★★★★
Ship size:	**Medium**
Category:	**Ultra-Luxury**
Price range:	**Beyond Opulent $$$$**
Registry:	France
Year built:	1998
Itinerary:	Sails from Tahiti
Information:	(800) 333-3333
Website:	www.rssc.com
Passenger capacity:	320 (double occupancy)
Crew:	206 European officers, international crew
Passenger-to-Crew Ratio:	1.6:1
Tonnage:	18,800
Passenger Space Ratio:	58.8
Length:	513 feet
Beam:	71 feet
Draft:	17 feet
Guest decks:	7
Total cabins:	161
Outside:	142
Inside:	0
Suites:	19
Wheelchair cabins:	1
Cuisine:	Inventive, international cuisine by 2-star Michelin chef Jean-Pierre Vigato
Style:	Resort casual with occasional semi-formal nights
Price notes:	Single occupancy premium up to 200 percent
Tipping suggestions:	Gratuities are included

An elegant resident of Polynesia, among recreational facilities is a retractable watersports platform that brings guests to sea level for windsurfing, kayaking, water skiing, snorkeling, and more. Original works by Gauguin in the 1890s and a gallery of vintage black-and-white photographs of French Polynesia are part of the ship's decor.

Radisson Diamond

Econoguide rating:	★★★★★★
Ship size:	**Medium**
Category:	**Ultra-Luxury**
Price range:	**Opulent and Beyond $$$$–$$$$$**
Registry:	Bahamas
Year built:	1992
Itinerary:	Panama Canal, Costa Rica, Caribbean, Mediterranean
Information:	(800) 333-3333
Website:	www.rssc.com
Passenger capacity:	354 (double occupancy)
Crew:	192 International
Passenger-to-Crew Ratio:	1.8:1
Tonnage:	20,295
Passenger Space Ratio:	57.3
Length:	420 feet
Beam:	103 feet
Draft:	23 feet
Cruising speed:	12.5 knots
Guest decks:	12
Total cabins:	177
Outside:	177
Inside:	0
Suites:	2 master suites, Deck 9
Wheelchair cabins:	2
Cuisine:	Inventive, international cuisine. Single,open-seating dining. Indoor/outdoor specialty restaurant and lounge offering Northern Italian cuisine
Style:	Resort casual with occasional semi-formal evenings
Price notes:	Single occupancy premium 125 percent to 200 percent
Tipping suggestions:	Gratuities are included

A luxury hotel afloat, the *Radisson Diamond* is also one of the most unusual seagoing vessels. She is the world's first major cruise ship to use a submerged twin hull; there are only a handful of other passenger-carrying twin-hull vessels, all considerably smaller.

The SWATH (Small Waterplane Area Twin Hull) design utilizes a narrow hull area in contact with the waves and computer-controlled fins to counteract the effects of the sea. According to the company, the resulting degree of vessel roll is only one-fifth that of a monohull cruise vessel and the vibration level is one-tenth that of a conventional ship.

By placing the propulsion machinery in the hulls beneath the water line, the ship's 26-foot draft adds to the ship's stability, and also greatly reduces engine noise and vibration. The ship features a wind-resistant nose cone on the bow, and a computerized control center.

In a traditional single-hull ship, stabilizers are only effective in reducing side-to-side rolling. By contrast, the *Radisson Diamond* has stabilizer fins on the front and back of each submerged hull, thus reducing pitching and rolling.

The space ratio of 58.0 is among the highest of any cruise ship in its class. About the only downside to the design—besides its most untraditional profile that makes it look like an overgrown houseboat—is the relatively poky speed of the ship. The *Diamond* can eke out a top speed of approximately 12.5 knots.

The five-story entry atrium features a grand staircase and glass-enclosed elevators. The 230-seat Windows Lounge, located at the bow of the ship on the eighth deck, offers a breathtaking view. The elegant Grand Dining Room offers individualized seating at times convenient to passengers.

Recreational facilities include a jogging track, swimming pool, a golf driving range with nets and putting green, and a hydraulic marina for such activities as windsurfing and wave runners.

Radisson Seven Seas Navigator

Econoguide rating:	★★★★★★
Ship size:	**Medium**
Category:	**Ultra Luxury**
Price range:	**Beyond Opulent $$$$$**
Registry:	Bahamas
Year built:	1999
Itinerary:	Caribbean, Panama Canal and Costa Rica, South America, Bermuda, Transatlantic, Europe, Australia, Asia, South Pacific
Information:	(800) 333-3333
Website:	www.rssc.com
Passenger capacity:	490
Crew:	325. Italian officers, international crew
Passenger-to-Crew Ratio:	1.5:1
Tonnage:	33,000
Passenger Space Ratio:	67.3
Length:	560 feet
Beam:	81 feet
Draft:	21 feet
Cruising speed:	20 knots
Guest decks:	12
Total cabins:	245
Outside:	245
Inside:	0
Suites:	All
Cuisine:	International. Open single-seating dining in main restaurant
Style:	Jackets required for men on occasion; suitable resort wear or dresses for women
Price notes:	Single occupancy premium expected to be up to 200 percent
Tipping suggestions:	Gratuities are included in cruise fare. No tips are expected onboard.

The all-suite *Seven Seas Navigator,* the fastest and largest ship in the fleet, began operations in the fall of 1999. The smallest accommodations on the ship are a spacious 301 square feet, about twice the size of a typical small cabin on a cruise ship. The Passenger Space Ratio is 67.3, the highest of any cruise ship afloat.

The ship's ice-strengthened hull permits operation around the world.

The first major cruise for the ship was a 50-night circumnavigation of South America, with stops at a variety of Caribbean islands and French Guinea. From there she went to Brazil, Argentina, Uruguay, Chilean fjords, around the southernmost tip of the Americas at Cape Hope, then up the western coast to Peru and Ecuador, through the Panama Canal to Mexico and the Cayman Islands, arriving back in Fort Lauderdale.

There is open seating in the main restaurant with sufficient space to seat the entire passenger complement, plus an alternative restaurant featuring Italian cuisine.

Radisson Seven Seas Mariner (Preview)

Econoguide rating:	★★★★★★
Ship size:	**Grand**
Category:	**Ultra Luxury**
Price range:	**Beyond Opulent $$$$$**
Registry:	French
Year built:	2001 (February)
Itinerary:	Worldwide
Information:	(800) 333-3333
Website:	www.rssc.com
Passenger capacity:	720
Crew:	440
Passenger-to-Crew Ratio:	1.6:1
Tonnage:	46,000 (estimated)
Passenger Space Ratio:	63.9(estimated)
Length:	713 feet
Beam:	95 feet
Draft:	21.4 feet
Cruising speed:	NA
Guest decks:	NA
Total cabins:	360
Outside:	360
Inside:	0
Suites:	All
Cuisine:	Inventive, international cuisine. Open, single-seating dining in main restaurant
Style:	Jackets required for men on occasion; suitable resort wear or dresses for women
Price notes:	Single occupancy premium expected to be up to 200 percent
Tipping suggestions:	Gratuities are included in cruise fare. No tips are expected onboard.

The newest ship in the fleet will be its first all-balcony, all-suite vessel. Another new feature will be a pod propulsion system; slung below the ship are a pair of pods with forward-facing propellers that can be turned 360 degrees to drive the ship in any direction.

The ship will include four dining areas, including a main dining room capable of accommodating her entire guest contingent in one seating.

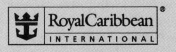

Royal Caribbean International
1050 Caribbean Way
Miami, FL 33132-2096
Information: (800) 327-6700
www.royalcaribbean.com

Royal Caribbean Fleet

Voyager of the Seas. (1999) 3,114 passengers. 142,000 tons.

Vision of the Seas. (1998) 2,435 passengers. 78,491 tons

Rhapsody of the Seas. (1997) 2,435 passengers. 78,491 tons

Enchantment of the Seas. (1997) 2,446 passengers. 74,140 tons

Grandeur of the Seas. (1996) 2,446 passengers. 74,140 tons

Majesty of the Seas. (1992) 2,744 passengers. 73,941 tons

Monarch of the Seas. (1991) 2,744 passengers. 73,941 tons

Sovereign of the Seas. (1988) 2,850 passengers. 73,192 tons

Splendour of the Seas. (1996) 2,076 passengers. 69,130 tons

Legend of the Seas. (1995) 2,076 passengers. 69,130 tons

Nordic Empress. (1990) 2,020 passengers. 48,563 tons

Viking Serenade. (1982, rebuilt 1991) 1,863 passengers. 40,132 tons

Future Ships

Explorer of the Seas. (Fall of 2000) 3,114 passengers. 142,000 tons

Radiance of the Seas. (June 2001) 2,100 passengers. 88,000 tons

Brilliance of the Seas. (April 2002) 2,100 passengers. 88,000 tons

Adventure of the Seas. (Spring of 2002) 3,114 passengers. 142,000 tons

Unnamed Eagle-class. (June 2002) 3,114 passengers. 142,000 tons

Unnamed Eagle-class. (June 2003) 3,114 passengers. 142,000 tons.

Unnamed Vantage-class. (June 2003) 2,100 passengers. 88,000 tons

Unnamed Vantage-class. (June 2004) 2,100 passengers. 88,000 tons.

Think Royal Caribbean, and think large. As 2000 began, the line owns and operates the largest cruise ship afloat—the 142,000-ton *Voyager of the Seas*. And just in case that's not enough, there are two more sister ships in the Eagle class under construction. The second, *Explorer of the Seas*, is due in the fall of 2000 and *Adventure of the Seas* is expected for the spring of 2002.

But wait: There is also a pair of svelte 88,000-ton Vantage Class ships under way, as well as two more sisters, due in 2003 and 2004. Vantage-class ships are powered by gas turbines, claimed to reduce airborne emissions, noise, and vibration. The turbines provide power to electric propulsion motors that turn the propellers mounted in rotating pods beneath the ship's hull. Exhaust heat from the turbines is captured to spin turbines for lighting, air conditioning, and water heating.

The *Voyager of the Seas* took the mantle as the largest cruise ship when she debuted in November of 1999, at 1,019 feet long, 157.5 feet wide, and 206.5 feet above the waterline. The behemoth is thus about 20 feet too long and 50 feet too wide to fit through the Panama Canal. It has to be that big, you see, to fit the skating rink, twin 11-story atria, and the Royal Promenade shopping district with its own version of Mardi Gras onboard.

The *Voyager of the Sea* will sail 7-night Western Caribbean cruises from Miami year-round, stopping at the cruise line's private resort Labadee in Haiti, Ocho Rios in Jamaica, and Cozumel Mexico.

Six older ships in the fleet are members of the Vision Class: *Vision of the Seas, Enchantment, Grandeur, Legend, Rhapsody,* and *Splendour.* They were among the first cruise ships to open up large portions of the public areas with glass windows and skylights.

The RCI Story

Royal Caribbean Cruise Line was founded in 1969 by three Norwegian shipping companies: Anders Wilhelmsen & Co., I.M. Skaugen & Company, and later, Gotaas Larsen. The company's first ship, *Song of Norway,* entered service in 1970, claimed as the first passenger ship built specifically for warm-weather cruising rather than point-to-point transport. The *Song of Norway* was also the first ship to have a cocktail lounge cantilevered from its smokestack; the Viking Crown Lounge has since become the hallmark of every Royal Caribbean vessel.

The *Nordic Prince* followed the next year and the *Sun Viking* a year later.

The cruise company pioneered air/sea vacations, flying cruise guests to meet the ships in their first port, Miami.

In 1978, the *Song of Norway* became the first major passenger cruise ship to be "stretched" by being cut in two and having an 85-foot mid-section added, increasing guest capacity from 700 to just over 1,000; the *Nordic Prince* underwent a similar conversion in 1980. The *Nordic Prince* and the *Song of Norway* were sold in 1995 and 1997 respectively to the British leisure company, Airtours plc.

In 1988, Royal Caribbean merged its operations with Admiral Cruises, and Anders Wilhelmsen & Company bought out its original partners. That same year, the massive *Sovereign of the Seas* debuted, introduced a five-deck atrium known as The Centrum with glass elevators, sweeping staircases, and fountains in marble pools; the first time such a central atrium had been constructed in a passenger ship.

Royal Caribbean became a publicly traded company in 1993. The line sold *Song of America* in early 1999 to Airtours. The 1,400-passenger ship, introduced in 1982, most recently sailed 7-night Mexican Riviera cruises in the winter and Bermuda itineraries in the summer.

The RCI Experience

Royal Caribbean goes for headlines—an ice skating rink on *Voyager of the Seas,* an 18-hole miniature golf course on *Splendour of the Seas* and *Legend of the Seas,* and cantilevered cocktail lounges up high on the smokestacks.

RCI delivers a high-quality product aimed at the middle of the cruise market. A corporate goal is to make the experience pretty much the same across all of its ships, even though they may differ in size and configuration.

Royal Caribbean offers two private spots just for its guests in the Caribbean and the Bahamas. Labadee is a 260-acre wooded peninsula at Pointe Ste. Honore, about six miles from Cap Haitien on the mountainous and secluded north coast of Haiti. There are five beaches, an outdoor performance area, an open air dining area, nature trails, shaded hammocks, and a coral reef that includes a sunken airplane. Recreational highlights include paddleboats, watercycles, para-sailing, sailboats, and snorkeling with underwater cameras.

CocoCay is a 140-acre island in the Bahamas' Berry Island chain between Freeport and Nassau, offering similar facilities to those of Labadee.

In 1997, Royal Caribbean made a small but interesting change in its age guidelines. The company said it would no longer accept student group bookings, and no guest under 21 will be booked in a stateroom unless accompanied by an adult 25 years or older. The age limit will be waived for under-21-year-old married couples, or when families or guardians sailing together with minor children share adjacent staterooms.

The Adventure Ocean children's program has offerings for Aquanauts (3–5), Explorers (6–8), Voyagers (9–12), and Navigators (13–17).

Programs include finger painting and dress-up for the very young to arts and crafts, sports and pool activities, karaoke, talent shows, and special parties. Island activities include beach parties and games, sand castle building, seashell collecting, and more.

During summers and holidays, Adventure Science classes are conducted by specially trained science staff. The program blends science and entertainment—rockets, slime, and bubbling potions included.

Voyager of the Seas

Econoguide rating:	★★★★★	
Ship size:	**Colossus**	
Category:	**Top of the Line**	
Price range:	**Premium $$$**	
Registry:	Liberia	

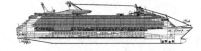

Year built:	1999
Sister ship:	*Explorer of the Seas*
Itinerary:	Western Caribbean from Miami
Information:	(305) 539-6000, (800) 327-6700
Website:	www.royalcaribbean.com
Passenger capacity:	3,114 (double occupancy)
Crew:	1,181 Norwegian/International
Passenger-to-Crew Ratio:	2.6:1
Tonnage:	142,000
Passenger Space Ratio:	45.6 (estimated)
Length:	1,021 feet
Beam:	157.5 feet
Draft:	29 feet
Cruising speed:	22 knots
Guest decks:	14
Total cabins:	1,557
Outside:	939
Inside:	618, including 138 Promenade View staterooms
Suites:	119
Wheelchair accessible:	Call (305) 539-4440 for special assistance
Cuisine:	International
Style:	Resort casual with occasional formal nights
Price notes:	Single occupancy premium 150 percent to 200 percent. Single Guarantee Program guests add $250 or $500. Special Share Program pairs you with a person of same sex and smoking preference.
Tipping suggestions:	$7.50 pp/pd

The world's largest cruise ship entered service in November of 1999. The first of Royal Caribbean's Eagle-class ships, the *Voyager of the Seas* came in at about 142,000 tons, about twice the capacity of a typical large cruise ship and half again as capacious as a Megaship. Her twin, *Explorer of the Seas*, arrived in the fall of 2000.

On December 26, 1999, its millennium cruise, the ship gathered together 3,537 guests, claiming the world's record for a cruise ship. The theoretical limit for the vessel, if all of its third and fourth berths were filled, is 3,838.

In 2000, *Voyager of the Seas* sails all year from Miami on a seven-night Western Caribbean itinerary. Ports of call include Labadee, Hispaniola; Ocho Rios, Jamaica, and Cozumel, Mexico. Royal Caribbean also debuted the world's largest passenger cruise terminal as home base in Miami. The building has to be large; on turnaround day as many as 8,400 guests may be getting off or on the ship, more or less at the same time. The roof features a replica of Royal Caribbean's signature Viking Crown Lounge as an observation point on top.

This is not your typical cruise ship: It includes an ice-skating rink with its own Zamboni machine, a wedding chapel in the sky, and an Aquarium Bar that has a $1 million, 50-ton set of tanks. There's also a Peek-A-Boo Bridge above the wheelhouse, which allows guests to watch the team that is "driving" and navigating the ship.

The Royal Promenade runs most of the length of the ship, four decks high, punctuated by two atria (The Centrums) up to 11 decks high. The core of the ship offers shops, restaurants, and entertainment areas fronting on a winding "street." Special lighting effects allow the promenade to change in ambiance from day to night.

The Royal Promenade includes street festivities and performers, including *Voyager*'s own version of Mardi Gras. Spinners is a revolving gaming arcade with what is claimed to be the world's largest interactive roulette wheel, activated by a four-deck-high roulette ball tower. Arching over the promenade is The Captain's Balcony, a podium for the captain.

The Royal Promenade also features inside staterooms that offer a view of the atrium and street scene. The cabins—representing about 10 percent of the staterooms on the ship—have bay windows, the first such inside views on a cruise ship.

Almost half of the cabins offer balconies, and rooms are generally larger than those on other ships.

Voyager of the Seas includes a three-level main dining room with separate and distinct themed dining areas: "Carmen," "La Boheme," and "Magic Flute," all connected by a dramatic three-deck grand staircase. Smaller dining rooms, Seville and Granada, adjoin the Carmen area. Casual eateries include the Sea-Side Diner, a 1950s-style, 24-hour spot; Island Grill, a casual restaurant; and Portofino, an upscale Euro-Italian retaurant.

Entertainment areas include the La Scala Theater, a 1,350-seat theater that spans five decks and offers a hydraulic orchestra pit and stage area and above-stage fly space for full productions.

Studio B is a 900-seat arena for variety shows, ice shows, game shows, and rock 'n' roll performances. The seating and floor can be retracted and the area used as an ice skating rink for guests.

Casino Royale is the largest casino on a cruise ship, with slot machines, table gaming, and sports betting.

The *Voyager*'s outdoor sports deck includes a golf course, driving range, and golf simulator. Also onboard is a rock-climbing wall, an in-line skating track, and regulation-sized basketball, paddle ball, and volleyball courts.

A full range of youth facilities for Aquanauts (3- to 5-year-olds), Explorers (6–8), and Voyagers (9–12) include Mission Control with interactive virtual rockets and a space theater. There's a computer lab that has games and educational software, and a large arcade. Optix, for teens, is a clubhouse that has computers, a soda bar, and a dance area with a DJ.

Explorer of the Seas (Preview)

Econoguide rating:	★★★★★
Ship size:	**Colossus**
Category:	**Top of the Line**
Price range:	**Premium $$$**
Registry:	Liberia
Year built:	Fall 2000
Sister ship:	*Voyager of the Seas*
Itinerary:	Eastern Caribbean from Miami
Information:	(305) 539-6000, (800) 327-6700
Website:	www.royalcaribbean.com
Passenger capacity:	3,114 (double occupancy)

Crew:	1,181 Norwegian/International
Passenger-to-Crew Ratio:	2.6:1 (estimated)
Tonnage:	142,000
Passenger Space Ratio:	45.6 (estimated)
Length:	1,020 feet
Beam:	157.5 feet
Draft:	29 feet
Cruising speed:	22 knots
Guest decks:	14
Total cabins:	1,557
Outside:	939
Inside:	618, including 138 Promenade View staterooms
Suites:	119
Wheelchair accessible:	Call (305) 539-4440 for special assistance
Cuisine:	International
Style:	Resort casual with occasional formal nights
Price notes:	Single occupancy premium 150 percent to 200 percent. Single Guarantee Program guests add $250 or $500. Special Share Program pairs you with a person of same sex and smoking preference.
Tipping suggestions:	$7.50 pp/pd

In her first year, *Explorer of the Seas* will sail a seven-night Eastern Caribbean itinerary. Departing Miami, ports of call include Labadee, Hispaniola; San Juan, Puerto Rico; and St. Thomas, USVI.

Explorer of the Seas is the first cruise ship to boast a state-of-the-art atmospheric and marine laboratory, with an interactive environmental classroom. More ordinary amenities include an ice skating rink, an inline skating track, and a rock-climbing wall.

Rhapsody of the Seas

Econoguide rating:	★★★★
Ship size:	**Megaship**
Category:	**Top of the Line**
Price range:	**Moderate to Premium $$$–$$$$**
Registry:	Norwegian
Year built:	1997
Sister ship:	*Vision of the Seas*
Itinerary:	Panama Canal, Alaska, Hawaii, Mexico
Information:	(305) 539-6000, (800) 327-6700
Website:	www.royalcaribbean.com
Passenger capacity:	2,000 (double occupancy)
Crew:	765 International
Passenger-to-Crew Ratio:	2.6:1
Tonnage:	78,491
Passenger Space Ratio:	39.2
Length:	915 feet
Beam:	105.6 feet
Draft:	25 feet
Cruising speed:	22 knots
Guest decks:	11
Total cabins:	1,000
Outside:	496
Inside:	407
Suites:	97

Wheelchair cabins:	14
Cuisine:	International
Style:	Resort casual with occasional formal nights
Price notes:	Single occupancy premium 150 percent to 200 percent. Single Guarantee Program guests add $250 or $500. Special Share Program pairs you with a person of same sex and smoking preference
Tipping suggestions:	$7.50 pp/pd

Twin to *Vision of the Seas,* and close sister to *Enchantment, Grandeur, Legend,* and *Splendour of the Seas.* The sprawling Edelweiss Dining Room seats an astounding 1,200 passengers.

In 2000, she sails out of Vancouver to Alaska in the summer, returning to San Diego by way of Hawaii in September; for the remainder of the year she will sail out of Los Angeles to the Mexican Riviera.

Vision of the Seas

Econoguide rating:	★★★★
Ship size:	**Megaship**
Category:	**Top of the Line**
Price range:	**Premium $$$**
Registry:	Liberia
Year built:	1998
Sister ship:	*Rhapsody of the Seas*
Itinerary:	Alaska, Hawaii, Mexican Riviera, Panama Canal
Information:	(305) 539-6000, (800) 327-6700
Website:	www.royalcaribbean.com
Passenger capacity:	2,000 (double occupancy)
Crew:	765
Passenger-to-Crew Ratio:	2.6:1
Tonnage:	78,491
Passenger Space Ratio:	39.2
Length:	915 feet
Beam:	105.6 feet
Draft:	25 feet
Cruising speed:	22 knots
Guest decks:	11
Total cabins:	1,000
Outside:	496
Inside:	407
Suites:	97
Wheelchair cabins:	14
Cuisine:	International
Style:	Resort casual with occasional formal nights
Price notes:	Single occupancy premium 150 percent to 200 percent. Single Guarantee Program guests add $250 or $500. Special Share Program pairs you with a person of same sex and smoking preference
Tipping suggestions:	$7.50 pp/pd

Twin to *Rhapsody of the Seas,* and close sister to *Enchantment, Grandeur, Legend,* and *Splendour of the Seas.* The Aquarius Dining Room sets the tables for 1,200 passengers per seating.

In May 2000, Seattle was to become the seasonal home to the *Vision of the Seas,* sailing five three- and four-night itineraries with ports of call at Vancouver and Victoria, British Colombia. Beginning in June, she will sail week-long trips from Vancouver to Alaska. In September, the vessel moves to Mexico by way of Honolulu, sailing to the Mexican Riviera and through the Panama Canal to Fort Lauderdale and back in the winter.

Enchantment of the Seas

Econoguide rating:	★★★★
Ship size:	**Megaship**
Category:	**Top of the Line**
Price range:	**Premium $$$**
Registry:	Norwegian
Year built:	1997
Sister ship:	*Grandeur of the Seas*
Itinerary:	Western and Eastern Caribbean from Fort Lauderdale
Information:	(305) 539-6000, (800) 327-6700
Website:	www.royalcaribbean.com
Passenger capacity:	1,950 (double occupancy)
Crew:	760 International
Passenger-to-Crew Ratio:	2.6:1
Tonnage:	74,140
Passenger Space Ratio:	38
Length:	916 feet
Beam:	105.6 feet
Draft:	25 feet
Cruising speed:	22 knots
Guest decks:	11
Total cabins:	975
Outside:	554
Inside:	399
Suites:	22
Wheelchair cabins:	14
Cuisine:	International
Style:	Resort casual with occasional formal nights
Price notes:	Single occupancy premium 150 percent to 200 percent. Single Guarantee Program guests add $250 or $500. Special Share Program pairs you with a person of same sex and smoking preference
Tipping suggestions:	$7.50 pp/pd

The *Enchantment of the Seas* and her near-identical twin sister *Grandeur of the Seas,* are members of Royal Caribbean's six-ship Project Vision series, a group of vessels that are aflood with light from acres of windows. Their seven-deck-high central atrium is topped off with a glass skylight and nearly every other public room is open to the sunsets, sunrises, daylight, and moonlight of a voyage at sea.

In April of 2000, *Enchantment of the Seas* moved her base to Port Everglades near Fort Lauderdale, sailing alternating Eastern and Western Caribbean itineraries. The move opened space at the Port of Miami for Royal Caribbean's two new 142,000-ton Eagle-class vessels.

The Vision series, which also includes the *Legend of the Seas, Rhapsody of the Seas, Splendour of the Seas,* and the namesake *Vision of the Seas* are big ships, but well below the size of the Megaships and Colossuses that are now becoming common.

Royal Caribbean is known for its shipboard entertainment as well, presenting Broadway-style revues, musicals, comedians, movies, discos, limbo competitions, Country line dancing, and just about anything to draw a crowd.

The free Adventure Ocean program for children from ages 3 through 17 includes a professional staff, play facilities, science demonstrations, a video game room, arts and crafts and a teen disco.

The massive My Fair Lady Dining Room seats 1,171 close friends; the Orpheum Theater can hold 870 for shows.

Grandeur of the Seas

Econoguide rating:	★★★★	
Ship size:	**Megaship**	
Category:	**Top of the Line**	
Price range:	**Premium $$$**	
Registry:	Liberia	
Year built:	1996	
Sister ship:	*Enchantment of the Seas*	
Itinerary:	Eastern Caribbean/Southern Caribbean from Miami and San Juan	
Information:	(305) 539-6000, (800) 327-6700	
Website:	www.royalcaribbean.com	
Passenger capacity:	1,950 (double occupancy)	
Crew:	760 International	
Passenger-to-Crew Ratio:	2.6:1	
Tonnage:	74,140	
Passenger Space Ratio:	38	
Length:	916 feet	
Beam:	105.6 feet	
Draft:	25 feet	
Cruising speed:	22 knots	
Guest decks:	11	
Total cabins:	975	
Outside:	554	
Inside:	399	
Suites:	22	
Wheelchair cabins:	14	
Cuisine:	International	
Style:	Resort casual with occasional formal nights	
Price notes:	Single occupancy premium 150 percent to 200 percent. Single Guarantee Program guests add $250 or $500. Special Share Program pairs you with a person of same sex and smoking preference	
Tipping suggestions:	$7.50 pp/pd	

The slightly older near-twin to *Enchantment of the Seas* and member of Royal Caribbean's Project Vision series. The balconied Great Gatsby Dining Room spans the Main and Promenade decks and seats 1,171 guests.

In October 2000, the ship was due to move from Miami to San Juan to replace *Majesty of the Seas* on seven-night Southern Caribbean itineraries.

Majesty of the Seas

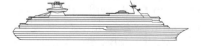

Econoguide rating:	★★★	
Ship size:	**Megaship**	
Category:	**Top of the Line**	
Price range:	**Moderate $$**	
Registry:	Norwegian	

Year built:	1992
Sister ships:	*Monarch of the Seas* and *Sovereign of the Seas*
Itinerary:	Bahamas from Miami
Information:	(305) 539-6000, (800) 327-6700
Website:	www.royalcaribbean.com
Passenger capacity:	2,744 (double occupancy)
Crew:	822 International
Passenger-to-Crew Ratio:	2.9:1
Tonnage:	73,941
Passenger Space Ratio:	31.5
Length:	880 feet
Beam:	106 feet
Draft:	25 feet
Cruising speed:	22 knots
Guest decks:	14
Total cabins:	1,177
Outside:	669
Inside:	445
Suites:	63
Wheelchair cabins:	4
Cuisine:	International
Style:	Resort casual with occasional formal nights
Price notes:	Single occupancy premium 150 percent to 200 percent. Single Guarantee Program guests add $250 or $500. Special Share Program pairs you with a person of same sex and smoking preference
Tipping suggestions:	$7.50 pp/pd

Sister to the *Monarch of the Seas*. The design of these ships puts most of the cabins forward and the public rooms aft, allowing passengers to move vertically by elevator or stairs from lounge to restaurant or showroom without having to traverse hallways of cabins.

The massive A Chorus Line Lounge seats 1,050 intimate strangers.

In May of 2000, *Majesty of the Seas* was due to move to Miami to replace *Sovereign of the Seas* on three- and four-night Bahamas sailings.

Monarch of the Seas

Econoguide rating:	**★★★**
Ship size:	**Megaship**
Category:	**Top of the Line**
Price range:	**Moderate $$**
Registry:	Norwegian
Year built:	1991
Sister ships:	*Majesty of the Seas* and *Sovereign of the Seas*
Itinerary:	Southern Caribbean from San Juan
Information:	(305) 539-6000, (800) 327-6700
Website:	www.royalcaribbean.com
Passenger capacity:	2,744 (double occupancy)
Crew:	822 International
Passenger-to-Crew Ratio:	2.9:1
Tonnage:	73,941
Passenger Space Ratio:	31.5
Length:	880 feet
Beam:	106 feet
Draft:	25 feet
Cruising speed:	22 knots
Guest decks:	14
Total cabins:	1,177

Outside:	669
Inside:	445
Suites:	63
Wheelchair cabins:	4
Cuisine:	International
Style:	Resort casual with occasional formal nights
Price notes:	Single occupancy premium 150 percent to 200 percent. Single Guarantee Program guests add $250 or $500. Special Share Program pairs you with a person of same sex and smoking preference
Tipping suggestions:	$7.50 pp/pd

Twin to the *Majesty of the Seas,* and like her sister, she has most passenger cabins in the forward portion of the ship with most public rooms aft.

The *Monarch of the Seas* suffered an unpleasant encounter with an underwater shoal off the coast of St. Maarten in mid-December of 1998 and began taking on water. Her captain was able to steer the ship back to port where it was beached; all 2,557 passengers were evacuated from the ship in the middle of the night without injury. After a few weeks of repairs, the ship was returned to service.

In recent years, the ship has operated out of San Juan with ports of call in St. Thomas, USVI; Castries, St. Lucia; Bridgetown, Barbados; St. John's, Antigua, and Philipsburg, St. Maarten.

Sovereign of the Seas

Econoguide rating:	★★★
Ship size:	**Megaship**
Category:	**Top of the Line**
Price range:	**Moderate $$**
Registry:	Norwegian
Year built:	1988
Sister ships:	*Majesty of the Seas, Monarch of the Seas*
Itinerary:	Bahamas from Port Canaveral
Information:	(305) 539-6000, (800) 327-6700
Website:	www.royalcaribbean.com
Passenger capacity:	2,250 (double occupancy)
Crew:	840 International
Passenger-to-Crew Ratio:	2.7:1
Tonnage:	73,192
Passenger Space Ratio:	32.5
Length:	880 feet
Beam:	106 feet
Draft:	25 feet
Cruising speed:	19 knots
Guest decks:	14
Total cabins:	1,140
Outside:	710
Inside:	418
Suites:	12
Wheelchair cabins:	6
Cuisine:	International
Style:	Resort casual with occasional formal nights
Price notes:	Single occupancy premium 150 percent to 200 percent. Single Guarantee Program guests add $250 or $500. Special Share Program pairs you with a person of same sex and smoking preference
Tipping suggestions:	$7.50 pp/pd

This is the older, slightly smaller sister to the *Majesty of the Seas* and the *Monarch of the Seas.*

On the five lowest decks—Tween, Showtime, Main, A, and B—there are as many as nine cabins shoehorned across the beam of the ship. There is a pair of outside cabins, of course, with five or more cross-width hallways serving rows of seven inside cabins. Put another way, on this class of ship some inside cabins are as far as four cabins away from the nearest outside window; that's really inside.

The ship's home base moved to Port Canaveral in the Spring of 2000, as Royal Caribbean opened up room at the Port of Miami for its two massive new 142,000-ton Eagle-class vessels. The ship will offer three- and four-night trips with stops at Nassau and CocoCay in the Bahamas.

Legend of the Seas

Econoguide rating:	★★★
Ship size:	**Grand**
Category:	**Top of the Line**
Price range:	**Moderate to Premium $$–$$$**
Registry:	Liberia
Year built:	1995
Sister ship:	*Splendour of the Seas*
Itinerary:	Panama Canal, Mexico, Hawaii. Europe and Africa in 2000 and 2001
Information:	(305) 539-6000, (800) 327-6700
Website:	www.royalcaribbean.com
Passenger capacity:	1,800 (double occupancy)
Crew:	720
Passenger-to-Crew Ratio:	2.5:1
Tonnage:	69,130
Passenger Space Ratio:	38.4
Length:	867 feet
Beam:	105 feet
Draft:	24 feet
Cruising speed:	24+ knots
Guest decks:	11
Total cabins:	902
Outside:	488
Inside:	327
Suites:	87
Wheelchair cabins:	17
Cuisine:	International
Style:	Resort casual with occasional formal nights
Price notes:	Single occupancy premium 150 percent to 200 percent. Single Guarantee Program guests add $250 or $500. Special Share Program pairs you with a person of same sex and smoking preference
Tipping suggestions:	$7.50 pp/pd

Along with her near-twin the *Splendour of the Seas,* this is the slightly smaller and oldest sister in the Project Vision series for Royal Caribbean.

Among the *Legend of the Seas'* claims to fame is the first miniature golf course at sea, a nine-hole challenge 10 decks up on the Compass Deck, just below the cruise line's signature Viking Crown Lounge.

In April of 2000, *Legend of the Seas* will relocate to Barcelona for a series of Mediterranean cruises, moving again in November to Piraeus for cruises in

Greek and Italian waters. It is unclear whether the *Legend of the Seas* will return to U.S. waters after then.

In 2000 and 2001, *Legend of the Seas* will lead the Royal Journeys program, which includes voyages in Europe and on the continent of Africa. The ship will sail to 14 countries, and more than 30 cities in 172 days. The program will feature safari adventures in Kenya, and overnight excursions in Israel, Egypt, India, Australia, and New Zealand. Guests will be able to disembark the ship in a port-of-call, travel to an alternative destination, and then rejoin the vessel in another port.

Splendour of the Seas

Econoguide rating:	★★★★
Ship size:	**Grand**
Category:	**Top of the Line**
Price range:	**Moderate $$**
Registry:	Norwegian
Year built:	1996
Itinerary:	Caribbean from Miami for winter, Europe for summer, Canada, New England in fall
Sister ship:	*Legend of the Seas*
Information:	(305) 539-6000, (800) 327-6700
Website:	www.royalcaribbean.com
Passenger capacity:	1,800 (double occupancy)
Crew:	720
Passenger-to-Crew Ratio:	1:2.5
Tonnage:	69,130
Passenger Space Ratio:	38.4
Length:	867 feet
Beam:	105 feet
Draft:	24 feet
Cruising speed:	24+ knots
Guest decks:	11
Total cabins:	902
Outside:	488 (231 with balconies)
Inside:	327
Suites:	87
Wheelchair cabins:	17
Cuisine:	International
Style:	Resort casual with occasional formal nights
Price notes:	Single occupancy premium 150 percent to 200 percent. Single Guarantee Program guests add $250 or $500. Special Share Program pairs you with a person of same sex and smoking preference
Tipping suggestions:	$7.50 pp/pd

A slightly smaller and older sister in the Project Vision series for Royal Caribbean, twin to the *Legend of the Seas.*

Splendour of the Seas offers a nine-hole miniature golf course at sea, circled by the jogging track on the Compass Deck.

The ship was repositioned to Barcelona in April of 2000 for tours throughout Europe, the Mediterranean, and Scandinavia.

Among itineraries are a series of trips from Harwich, England to Oslo,

Helsinki, St. Petersburg, Russia, and Copenhagen. Another trip departs Harwich for cruising in and around the Arctic Circle and Norway.

Beginning in December 2000, *Splendour of the Seas* will sail a first-time series of South American cruises, with stops in Brazil, Argentina, and Uruguay.

Nordic Empress

Econoguide rating:	★★★
Ship size:	**Grand**
Category:	**Top of the Line**
Price range:	**Moderate $$**
Registry:	Liberia
Year built:	1990
Itinerary:	Caribbean from San Juan in winter, Bermuda from New York in summer
Information:	www.royalcaribbean.com
Website:	(305) 539-6000, (800) 327-6700
Passenger capacity:	1,600 (double occupancy)
Crew:	671 International
Passenger-to-Crew Ratio:	2.4:1
Tonnage:	48,563
Passenger Space Ratio:	30.4
Length:	692 feet
Beam:	100 feet
Draft:	25 feet
Cruising speed:	19 knots
Guest decks:	12
Total cabins:	800
Outside:	467
Inside:	329
Suites:	4
Wheelchair accessible:	4
Cuisine:	International
Style:	Resort casual with occasional formal nights
Price notes:	Single occupancy premium 150 percent to 200 percent. Single Guarantee Program guests add $250 or $500. Special Share Program pairs you with a person of same sex and smoking preference
Tipping suggestions:	$7.50 pp/pd

The *Nordic Empress* is a classy, newer version of the short-cruise ship, a segment of the market usually delegated to Oldies But Goodies and Vintage ships serving out their final days.

The ship is organized around the dramatic Centrum atrium, with access to most other parts of the ship branching off from there.

Viking Serenade

Econoguide rating:	★★★
Ship size:	**Grand**
Category:	**Top of the Line**
Price range:	**Moderate $$**
Registry:	Liberia
Year built:	1982 (As the *Scandinavia* ferry, then the *Stardancer*. Rebuilt in 1991 as a cruiseship.)

Itinerary:	Los Angeles to Mexico
Information:	(305) 539-6000, (800) 327-6700
Website:	www.royalcaribbean.com
Passenger capacity:	1,500 (double occupancy)
Crew:	612 International
Passenger-to-Crew Ratio:	2.5:1
Tonnage:	40,132
Passenger Space Ratio:	26.8
Length:	623 feet
Beam:	89 feet
Draft:	24 feet
Cruising speed:	21 knots
Guest decks:	11
Total cabins:	756
Outside:	470
Inside:	278
Suites:	8
Wheelchair cabins:	4
Cuisine:	International
Style:	Resort casual with occasional formal nights
Price notes:	Single occupancy premium 150 percent to 200 percent. Single Guarantee Program guests add $250 or $500. Special Share Program pairs you with a person of same sex and smoking preference
Tipping suggestions:	$7.50 pp/pd

Built in 1981 as the *Scandinavia,* a car-carrying ferry, she later operated as the *Stardancer,* a ferry in Alaska for the short-lived Sundance Cruises. In 1991, she was born again as the *Viking Serenade* after a major rebuilding for cruising, with a whole block of new cabins inserted into the former car deck.

Overcoming her humble beginnings, the *Viking Serenade* is now an attractive, popular ship for getaways from Los Angeles to the Mexican Riviera.

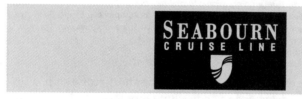

Seabourn Cruise Line
6100 Blue Lagoon Drive, Suite 400
Miami, FL 33126
Information: (800) 929-9391
www.seabourn.com

Seabourn Cruise Line Fleet

Seabourn Sun. **(Formerly Cunard *Royal Viking Sun.)* (1988) 758 passengers. 38,000 tons**

Seabourn Legend. (1993) 200 passengers. 10,000 tons

Seabourn Spirit. (1989) 200 passengers. 10,000 tons

Seabourn Pride. (1988) 200 passengers. 10,000 tons

*Seabourn Goddess I. (*Formerly Cunard *Sea Goddess I.)* (1984) 116 passengers. 4,250 tons

*Seabourn Goddess II. (*Formerly Cunard *Sea Goddess II.)* (1985) 116 passengers. 4,250 tons

Seabourn is a floating home for the rich and famous, the rich and private, and others for whom price is of little object. The only real question is whether these are very large yachts or relatively small cruise ships.

Seabourn, with its sister operation Cunard line, is one of the anchors of the luxury cruise ship business. Seabourn operates three all-suite sister ships: the *Seabourn Pride, Seabourn Spirit,* and *Seabourn Legend.* Each is a 200-passenger all-suite vessel, with a crew of 150. Over the course of 2000, all three of the ships were due to be upgraded to replace picture windows with French Balconies: sliding doors and mini-balconies in 44 suites.

In 2000, the fleet was augmented with a trio of luxury ships formerly part of the Cunard Line, sister company to Seabourn. The *Seabourn Goddess I* and *II* are 116-passenger twins; the *Seabourn Sun* is larger but still sumptious.

The company's first vessel, the *Seabourn Pride,* set sail in 1988 and today includes itineraries that enter North American waters and the Caribbean. The other ships cruise the Mediterranean, Western Europe, Scandinavia, the British Isles, South America, Southeast Asia, India, Africa, and the Red Sea.

The *Seabourn Sun* will sail its first world cruise in the winter of 2001, a 99-day journey departing San Francisco on January 9, 2001 and ending in Fort Lauderdale on April 19, 2001 with stops at 31 ports in 21 countries.

In 1998, Seabourn became a division of Cunard Line Limited, which also owns and operates Cunard Line. Cunard is in turn owned by Carnival Corporation and a consortium of Norwegian investors.

The Seabourn Experience

The basic idea of Seabourn can be summed up like this: This is about as close as you can get to owning your own luxury yacht without having to go out and hire yourself a captain and crew.

The three Seabourn sisters, cut from the same pattern and nearly identical inside, feature large outside suites with all the amenities.

Passengers can dine when they please, with whom they please, and pretty much where they please in the formal dining room, the indoor/outdoor Veranda Café, the Sky Grill on deck, or in your cabin. And where appropriate, you can even pick up some "take out" to bring with you to shore. You'll travel in no ordinary tender, either; guests are chauffeured from anchorage to shore in a mahogany-paneled water taxi. Somewhere on the beach, the staff will also set up a catered barbecue, served on fine china and crystal.

The 440-foot-long vessels carry about half the number of passengers of comparably sized ships. Standard suites offer 277 square feet of space, with walk-in closets, marble-clad bathrooms, and large picture windows.

The cuisine on the ships is described as a mixture of classic and eclectic offerings. Dishes are prepared "a la minute" (as they are ordered) as they

would be in a fine restaurant. The Veranda Café offers alternative casual dining. A selection of wines and spirits are included in the fare, but the ship also
carries a more specialized wine cellar for those who just have to spend more.

The crew is drilled to learn the names of all passengers, and keep up-to-
speed on their preferences in food, entertainment, and comfort.

Each ship features a marina at the stern that opens out into the ocean to
provide a dock for watersports. An enclosed steel mesh pool allows passengers to swim without fear of interruption by unpleasant marine creatures.

All this comes at a price, of course. Per-person rates for Seabourn's suites
average about $761 per day; there is a strict no-tipping policy aboard ship.
According to the company, on any cruise as many as half the passengers are
repeat customers, which says a lot about satisfaction with the product.

If you become a regular, the Seabourn Club offers a complimentary cruise
of up to 14 days after you have sailed 140 days.

Seabourn Legend

Econoguide rating:	★★★★★★
Ship size:	**Medium**
Category:	**Ultra Luxury**
Price range:	**Beyond Opulent $$$$$**
Registry:	Norway
Year built:	1993 (Acquired 1996)
Sister ships:	*Seabourn Pride, Seabourn Spirit*
Itinerary:	Caribbean, South America, TransAtlantic, Mediterranean, Scandinavia, Russia
Information:	(800) 929-9391
Website:	www.seabourn.com
Passenger capacity:	208 (double occupancy)
Crew:	150
Passenger-to-Crew Ratio:	1.3:1
Tonnage:	10,000
Passenger Space Ratio:	50
Length:	440 feet
Beam:	63 feet
Draft:	16.4 feet
Cruising speed:	18 knots
Guest decks:	4
Total cabins:	104
Outside:	104
Inside:	0
Suites:	104
Wheelchair accessible:	4
Cuisine:	International cuisine and eclectic offerings; alternative casual dining in Veranda Café. The onboard wine cellar features boutique wines from the vineyards of Italy, France and the United States.
Style:	Semi-formal to formal
Price notes:	Single occupancy premium 175 percent to 200 percent, with some special offers available
Tipping suggestions:	Strict no-tipping policy

The *Seabourn Legend* is one of the super-yachts of the Seabourn Cruise Line.
Every stateroom is a suite, each with a large picture window that has an elec-

trically operated blackout curtain. A marina opens out into the ocean from the stern of the ship providing a launch for watersports. An enclosed steel mesh pool allows for swimming right in the ocean (weather permitting).

Seabourn Pride

Econoguide rating:	★★★★★★
Ship size:	**Medium**
Category:	**Ultra Luxury**
Price range:	**Beyond Opulent $$$$$**
Registry:	Norway
Year built:	1988
Sister ships:	*Seabourn Legend, Seabourn Spirit*
Itinerary:	Caribbean, South America, Transatlantic, Western Europe, Scandinavia, Russia, British Isles, New England, Canada, Colonial America
Information:	(800) 929-9391
Website:	www.seabourn.com
Passenger capacity:	208 (double occupancy)
Crew:	150
Passenger-to-Crew Ratio:	1.3:1
Tonnage:	10,000
Passenger Space Ratio:	50
Length:	440 feet
Beam:	63 feet
Draft:	16.4 feet
Cruising speed:	18 knots
Guest decks:	4
Total cabins:	100
Outside:	100
Inside:	0
Suites:	100
Wheelchair cabins:	4
Cuisine:	International cuisine and eclectic offerings; alternative casual dining in Veranda Café
Style:	Semi-formal to formal
Price notes:	Single occupancy premium 175 percent to 200 percent, with some special offers available
Tipping suggestions:	Strict no-tipping policy

Near-identical twin to the *Seabourn Legend,* about as close as most of us will get to having our own super-yacht.

Seabourn Spirit

Econoguide rating:	★★★★★★
Ship size:	**Medium**
Category:	**Ultra Luxury**
Price range:	**Beyond Opulent $$$$$**
Registry:	Norway
Year built:	1988
Sister ships:	*Seabourn Legend, Pride*
Itinerary:	Southeast Asia, Indian Ocean, Arabian Sea, Mediterranean
Information:	(800) 929-9391
Website:	www.seabourn.com
Passenger capacity:	208 (double occupancy)
Crew:	150

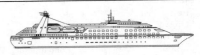

Passenger-to-Crew Ratio:	1.3:1
Tonnage:	10,000
Passenger Space Ratio:	50
Length:	440 feet
Beam:	63 feet
Draft:	16.4 feet
Guest decks:	4
Total cabins:	100
Outside:	100
Inside:	0
Suites:	100
Wheelchair cabins:	4
Cuisine:	International cuisine and eclectic offerings; alternative casual dining in Veranda Café
Style:	Semi-formal to formal
Price notes:	Single occupancy premium 175 percent to 200 percent
Tipping suggestions:	Strict no-tipping policy

Near-identical twin to the *Seabourn Legend,* about as close as most of us will get to having our own super-yacht.

Seabourn Goddess I

Econoguide rating:	★★★★★★
Ship size:	**Small**
Category:	**Ultra-Luxury**
Price range:	**Beyond Opulent $$$$$**
Registry:	Bahamas
Year built:	1984 as *Cunard Sea Goddess I* (Refurbished 1997)
Sister ship:	*Seabourn Goddess II*
Itinerary:	Caribbean and Mediterranean
Information:	(800) 929-9391
Website:	www.seabourn.com
Passenger capacity:	116 (double occupancy)
Crew:	90 European and American
Passenger-to-Crew Ratio:	1.3:1
Tonnage:	4,253 tons
Passenger Space Ratio:	36.7
Length:	334 feet
Beam:	47 feet
Draft:	14 feet
Cruising speed:	15 knots
Guest decks:	5
Total cabins:	58
Outside:	58
Inside:	0
Suites:	58
Wheelchair cabins:	0
Cuisine:	Contemporary. Complimentary wine at lunch and dinner
Style:	Casual with several formal nights per cruise.
Price notes:	Single occupancy premium 125 percent to 200 percent
Tipping suggestions:	Included

The two near-identical sisters, *Seabourn Goddess I* and *Seabourn Goddess II,* are like very large private yachts (or very small ultra-luxury cruise ships.) Either way, you'll be just one of just 100 or so passengers in a world of elegance and indulgence.

Recreational facilities include a stern platform for water sports, directly from ship.

Seabourn Goddess II

Econoguide rating:	★★★★★★
Ship size:	**Small**
Category:	**Ultra-Luxury**
Price range:	**Beyond Opulent $$$$$**
Registry:	Bahamas
Year built:	1985 as *Cunard Sea Goddess II* (Refurbished 1998)
Sister ship:	*Seabourn Goddess I*
Itinerary:	Caribbean and Mediterranean
Information:	(800) 929-9391
Website:	www.seabourn.com
Passenger capacity:	116 (double occupancy)
Crew:	90 European and American
Passenger-to-Crew Ratio:	1.3:1
Tonnage:	4,253 tons
Passenger Space Ratio:	36.7
Length:	334 feet
Beam:	47 feet
Draft:	14 feet
Cruising speed:	15 knots
Guest decks:	5
Total cabins:	58
Outside:	58
Inside:	0
Suites:	58
Wheelchair cabins:	0
Cuisine:	Contemporary. Complimentary wine at lunch and dinner
Style:	Informal with several formal nights per cruise
Price notes:	Single occupancy supplement 125 percent to 200 percent
Tipping suggestions:	Included

Seabourn Sun

Econoguide rating:	★★★★★★
Ship size:	**Medium**
Category:	**Ultra-Luxury**
Price range:	**Beyond Opulent $$$$$**
Registry:	Bahamas
Year built:	1988 as Cunard's *Royal Viking Sun*. (Refurbished 1995 and 1999.)
Itinerary:	South America, Caribbean, Mediterranean, Scandinavia, Russia, British Isles, Greenland, Canada, Colonial America, South Pacific, Mexico, Panama Canal
Information:	(800) 929-9391
Website:	www.seabourn.com
Passenger capacity:	758 (double occupancy)
Crew:	460 Norwegian officers, international crew
Passenger-to-Crew Ratio:	1.6:1
Tonnage:	37,845 tons
Passenger Space Ratio:	49.9
Length:	669 feet
Beam:	95 feet
Draft:	23 feet
Cruising speed:	21.4 knots

Guest decks:	8
Total cabins:	384
Outside:	336
Inside:	25
Suites:	19
Wheelchair cabins:	4
Cuisine:	Contemporary. Complimentary wine at lunch and dinner
Style:	Informal with several formal nights per cruise
Price notes:	Single occupancy premium 110 percent to 200 percent
Tipping suggestions:	Included

An understatedly elegant ship, designed for the Royal Viking Line and now in the Cunard fleet. The ship's public rooms were completely refitted in 1999; a Roman-style health spa and expanded golf facilities were added. Improvements to the spa on the Scandinavia Deck began at the entrance to the beauty salon, which was enlarged to add a reception area; an outdoor pool previously there was covered and enclosed to become a gymnasium. The center of the deck was extended to accommodate a new lap pool and two whirlpools.

In January of 2001, the Seabourn Sun will embark on its first world cruise under its new name, a 99-day cruise from San Francisco to Fort Lauderdale, with 31 stops in 21 countries including South Pacific islands, Australia, New Guinea, the Phillipines, Hong Kong, Vietnam, Singapore, Malaysia, Sri Lanka, India, Dubai, Oman, Jordan, Egypt, through the Suez Canal, Rome, Barcelona, Cadiz, and then transatlantic to Florida. The entire tour can be booked, or selected segments.

Theme cruises include Theatre at Sea with Broadway and Hollywood stars including Eli Wallach, Lynn Redgrave, and Gena Rowlands.

The *Royal Viking Sun's* two pools are filled with heated salt water; the pool on the Bridge Deck includes a swim-up bar.

Four modern catamaran tenders have sloping bows for beach landings. The especially splendiferous Owner's Suite includes an oceanview whirlpool on a private veranda.

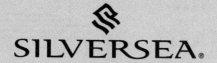

Silversea Cruises
110 East Broward Blvd.
Ft. Lauderdale, FL 33301
Information: (800) 722-9955, (954) 522-4477
Fax-on-demand information service: (888) 704-7447
www.silversea.com

Silversea Cruises Fleet

Silver Cloud. (1994) 296 passengers. 16,800 tons

Silver Wind. (1994) 296 passengers. 16,800 tons

Future Ships

Silver Shadow. (September 2000) 396 passengers. 25,000 tons

Silver Mirage. (June 2001) 396 passengers. 25,000 tons

Guests are greeted by white-gloved attendants offering perfectly chilled flutes of champagne; they are then escorted to their suites where a private bottle awaits. Need we say more?

Life aboard the *Silver Cloud* and *Silver Wind,* a pair of near-identical luxury twins, is pretty rarified: Limoges china, Christofle silverware, Frette linens, and soft down pillows. Guests who can afford the fare can keep abreast of their wealth with personalized daily stock market reports.

They also make a big deal about wine onboard a Silversea vessel, offering selected wines as part of a cruise package, and carrying a seagoing wine cellar and a staff of sommeliers for guests who insist on spending even more. So, too, with caviar and other gastronomic specialties. Some of the cruises are conducted in partnership with the renowned Le Cordon Bleu Culinary Academy.

The dining room is simply called The Restaurant, although it is less than simple. There's a single sitting with open seating. On formal nights, the ship's orchestra provides dancing music; if you don't feel like wearing a tuxedo or dinner jacket, you can have dinner served in your cabin—course by course.

A small troupe of performers, from cabaret singers and dancers to musical ensembles and magicians is onboard each ship.

The Silversea Story

Silversea is owned by the Lefebvre family of Rome, former owners of Sitmar Cruises. The company was founded in the early 1990s with a concept for "ultra-luxury" ships with the largest Passenger-Space Ratio of any ship at sea.

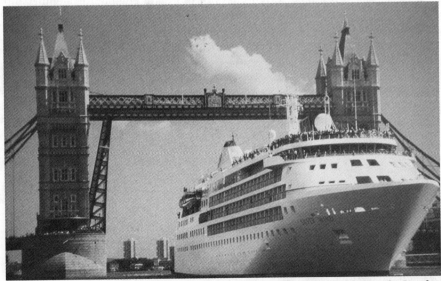

Silver Wind arrives in London
Silversea Cruises

All cabins are outside, and most feature private verandas. There's an open, single-seating dining room and a show lounge for nightly entertainment.

Silversea has ordered a pair of new luxury ships for delivery in mid-2000 and mid-2001, with an option for two additional ships in following years.

The new vessels are planned to be 597 feet long and 25,000 tons in size, with 198 outside suites for 396 passengers. The resulting Passenger-Space Ratio of 63 places the ships among the most spacious afloat.

New aboard each ship will be The Grill, a poolside dining area. The main dining room will be The Restaurant, an elegant single-seating room.

All-inclusive prices wrap up accommodations, roundtrip economy air transportation, deluxe pre-cruise hotel stay, all gratuities, all beverages including select wines and spirits, all port charges, and The Silversea Experience, a complimentary shore event on selected sailings.

Prices for Silversea cruises are appropriately high-floating, with a typical seven-day voyage priced between $6,300 and $12,000 per person, including airfare; for the Millennium, a lucky few will cruise to Tahiti, with basic room rates beginning at $25,665 per person for a 15-day voyage.

The Silversea Experience

The Silversea ships visit 280 ports worldwide, including the Mediterranean, Northern Europe and the Baltic, Africa, India, and the Far East, South Pacific including Australia and New Zealand, Canada and New England, South America and the Mexican Riviera. Cruises vary from 7 to 21 days with air/sea fares that range from $3,995 to $26,095 per person.

The relatively shallow 18-foot draft of the *Silver Cloud* and *Silver Wind* permit the ships to enter some smaller harbors where larger vessels would have to stand offshore.

Guests who have sailed for 100 days or more are eligible for membership in the Silversea Venetian Society; they are also eligible to receive a 5 percent discount. At 250 days or more the discount rises to 10 percent, and guests will also receive a free 7-day cruise; at the 500-day milestone, the company offers a complimentary 14-day cruise.

Silver Cloud

Econoguide rating:	★★★★★★	
Ship size:	**Medium**	
Category:	**Ultra Luxury**	
Price range:	**Beyond Opulent $$$$$**	
Registry:	Bahamas	
Year built:	1994	
Sister ships:	*Silver Wind*	
Itinerary:	Mexico, Caribbean, Colonial America, Canada, South Pacific and Australia, South America, U.S. Pacific Coast	
Information:	(800) 722-9955	
Website:	www.silversea.com	
Passenger capacity:	296 (double occupancy)	
Crew:	209 Italian officers, international crew	
Passenger-to-Crew Ratio:	1.4:1	

Tonnage:	16,800
Passenger Space Ratio:	56.8
Length:	514 feet
Beam:	70 feet
Draft:	18 feet
Cruising speed:	20.5 knots
Guest decks:	6
Total cabins:	148
Outside:	148
Inside:	0
Suites:	148
Wheelchair cabins:	2
Cuisine:	Regional, American, Continental cuisine. Select wines, spirits and champagnes from around the world included
Style:	Casual to formal. Sailings of 8 days or less have 2 formal nights; longer cruises usually have 3 or 4 formal nights
Price notes:	Single occupancy premium from 110 percent to 200 percent. Venetian Society discounts of 5 percent to 15 percent for past customers
Tipping suggestions:	All gratuities included

A luxurious cruising experience, with opulent appointments and service within and a wide range of interesting ports of call without, helped by the shallow draft of the yacht-like ship.

The *Silver Cloud* and her near-twin *Silver Wind* have itineraries including Canada and Colonial America, cruising the St. Lawrence Seaway from Montreal to Québec, heading into quiet coves of Nova Scotia, then calling on New York City, Boston, Yorktown, Charleston, Savannah, Key West, and Nassau en route to a season in the Caribbean.

This is a classy, pricey world of Limoges china, Christofle silverware, Frette bed linens monogrammed with the Silversea logo, down pillows and brand-name bath amenities.

The Restaurant offers open-seating for the entire passenger complement; on select formal nights, there's an orchestra for dancing. Terrace Café offers alternate dining with Italian regional specialties on a reservation basis. Items from the restaurant menu can be delivered to your suite.

Visiting chefs from Le Cordon Bleu Culinary Academy on select sailings prepare delicacies to complement the menu selections, including Regional, American and Continental cuisine.

In recent years, Silversea also offered a series of National Geographic Traveler Cruises, hosted by photographers and journalists. In 1998, Silversea hired Walter Painter, a 3-time Emmy Award-winning producer to produce and stage new entertainment for each of the ships.

In 1999, the line banned smoking in all dining areas. The new ships, *Silver Shadow* and *Silver Mirage* feature Cigar Bars as designated smoking areas.

Silver Wind

Econoguide rating:	★★★★★
Ship size:	**Medium**
Category:	**Ultra Luxury**
Price range:	**Beyond Opulent $$$$$**

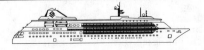

Registry:	Italy
Year built:	1994
Sister ship:	*Silver Cloud*
Itinerary:	Mexico, Caribbean, Colonial America, Canada, South Pacific and Australia, South America, U.S. Pacific Coast
Information:	(800) 722-9955
Website:	www.silversea.com
Passenger capacity:	296 (double occupancy)
Crew:	209 Italian officers, international crew
Passenger-to-Crew Ratio:	1.4:1
Tonnage:	16,800
Passenger Space Ratio:	56.8
Length:	514 feet
Beam:	70 feet
Draft:	18 feet
Cruising speed:	20.5 knots
Guest decks:	6
Total cabins:	148
Outside:	148
Inside:	0
Suites:	148
Wheelchair cabins:	2
Cuisine:	Regional, American, Continental cuisine. Select wines, spirits and champagnes from around the world included
Style:	Casual to formal. Sailings of 8 days or less have 2 formal nights; longer cruises usually have 3 or 4 formal nights
Price notes:	Single occupancy premium 110 percent to 200 percent
Tipping suggestions:	All gratuities included

In January of 2001, the luxurious *Silver Wind* will embark on Silversea's first world cruise, a 126-day journey from Los Angeles to London including visits to Hawaii, the South Pacific, the Far East, India and the Red Sea, and the Mediterranean.

Silver Shadow (Preview)

Econoguide rating:	★★★★★★
Ship size:	**Medium**
Category:	**Ultra Luxury**
Price range:	**Beyond Opulent $$$$$**
Registry:	Bahamas
Year built:	Fall 2000
Sister ships:	*Silver Mirage*
Itinerary:	Mediterranean, Northern Europe and the Baltic, Africa, India and the Far East, South Pacific and Australia, Canada and New England, South America, and the Panama Canal
Information:	(800) 722-9955
Website:	www.silversea.com
Passenger capacity:	388 (double occupancy)
Crew:	295 Italian officers, international crew
Passenger-to-Crew Ratio:	1.3:1
Tonnage:	25,000
Passenger Space Ratio:	64.4
Length:	597 feet
Beam:	81.8 feet
Draft:	19.6 feet
Cruising speed:	21 knots

Guest decks:	11
Total cabins:	194
Outside:	194
Inside:	0
Suites:	194
Wheelchair cabins:	NA
Cuisine:	Regional, American, Continental cuisine. Select wines, spirits and champagnes from around the world included
Style:	Casual to formal. Sailings of 8 days or less have 2 formal nights; longer cruises usually have 3 or 4 formal nights
Price notes:	Single occupancy premium 110 percent to 200 percent
Tipping suggestions:	All gratuities included

The inaugural season of Silversea's most luxurious ship is planned for the fall of 2000 in Europe, a transatlantic voyage to New York, and a trip down the East Coast of the United States to the Caribbean and South America for the winter.

Silver Mirage (Preview)

Econoguide rating:	★★★★★★
Ship size:	**Medium**
Category:	**Ultra Luxury**
Price range:	**Beyond Opulent $$$$$**
Registry:	Bahamas
Year built:	2001
Sister ships:	*Silver Shadow*
Itinerary:	Mediterranean, Northern Europe and the Baltic, Africa, India and the Far East, South Pacific and Australia, Canada and New England, South America, and the Panama Canal
Information:	(800) 722-9955
Website:	www.silversea.com
Passenger capacity:	388 (double occupancy)
Crew:	295 Italian officers, international crew
Passenger-to-Crew Ratio:	1.3:1
Tonnage:	25,000
Passenger Space Ratio:	64.4
Length:	597 feet
Beam:	81.8 feet
Draft:	19.6 feet
Cruising speed:	21 knots
Guest decks:	11
Total cabins:	194
Outside:	194
Inside:	0
Suites:	194
Wheelchair cabins:	NA
Cuisine:	Regional, American, Continental cuisine. Select wines, spirits and champagnes from around the world included
Style:	Casual to formal. Sailings of 8 days or less have 2 formal nights; longer cruises usually have 3 or 4 formal nights
Price notes:	Single occupancy premium 110 percent to 200 percent
Tipping suggestions:	All gratuities included

Chapter 14
Other Cruise Lines

American Hawaii Cruises
Cape Canaveral Cruise Line
Commodore Cruise Line
Crown Cruise Line
Great Lakes Cruise Company
Imperial Majesty Cruise Line
Mediterranean Shipping Cruises
Premier Cruise Lines
Regal Cruises
United States Line
World Explorer Cruises

AMERICAN HAWAII CRUISES®

American Hawaii Cruises
Robin Street Wharf
1380 Port of New Orleans Place
New Orleans, LA 70130-1890
Information: (800) 765-7000
www.cruisehawaii.com

American Hawaii Cruises Fleet

Independence. (1951) 867 passengers. 20,221 tons

American Hawaii Cruises operates the *Independence*, a classic cruise liner built in 1951, on week-long cruises in the Hawaiian Islands. As a U.S.-flagged ship, the vessel is permitted to operate entirely in American waters.

Parent company American Classic Voyages Co. (also the owner of the Delta Queen Steamboat Co.) will introduce a second cruise line in Hawaii in late 2000 with the reborn United States Line, sailing the *Patriot*.

The American Hawaii Story

The *Independence* and her sister ship the *Constitution* were built at the Beth-lehem Steel Shipyard in Quincy, Mass. In the 1950s, she sailed between New York and the Mediterranean.

Intended for use as a trans-Atlantic passenger liner, the *Independence* was designed to U.S. Navy specifications that would permit rapid conversion into a troop ship,with the capacity of carrying a mind-boggling 5,000 men and their equipment. It was constructed entirely of non-combustible or fire-resis-tant materials, equipped with extra hull plating, and outfitted with two engine rooms so if one were damaged, the other could keep the ship moving.

The *Independence* was the first U.S. ship to feature fully air-conditioned pas-senger and crew cabins. Its original design allowed it to carry 1,000 passen-gers, more than 100 beyond the current configuration.

In the 1950s, the ship sailed the "Sun Lane" route between New York and the Mediterranean. With the decline of liner service in the 1960s, the ship was repositioned in the Caribbean.

In 1968, the ship was refurbished and repainted with a sunburst mural and Jean Harlow eyes above water level; the new look did not go over well, and six months later the hull was repainted white. Another unsuccessful experi-ment was a Modified American Plan cruise, with all meals extra. Within a year, the ship was laid up, remaining out of service for more than 10 years.

In 1978, a group of American investors began planning for the resumption of passenger service under the American flag; thus was born American Hawaii Cruises. After a refurbishment that included the addition of bow thrusters to facilitate maneuvering in Hawaii's harbors, the *Independence* returned to ser-vice in 1980.

In 1993, American Hawaii Cruises was acquired by The Delta Queen Steam-boat Co., the oldest U.S. flag cruise line and the only operator of authentic, steam-powered paddlewheelers.

The American Hawaii Experience

There is no getting around the fact that the *Independence* is an older lady. Her owners have spent a good deal of money maintaining the ship in recent years, but she cannot compete against newer and larger ships on the basis of glitz and size.

Instead, American Hawaii Cruises emphasizes the America and Hawaii in its name. This is the only ship that can make a tour of the Hawaiian islands in a week's time because she does not have to make a detour to a foreign port to meet the requirements of the Jones Act; the standard itinerary touches five ports on four islands. And the line also works to create a Hawaiian feeling onboard the ship with décor, meals, and presentations.

The line also offers theme cruises that include whale watching, Big Band, and Hawaiian heritage motifs. In 2000, featured musicians included the Glenn Miller Orchestra, the Harry James Orchestra, the Jimmy Dorsey Orchestra, the Sammy Kaye Orchestra, The Four Freshmen, the Ink Spots, and the Platters.

Independence

Econoguide rating:	★★★
Ship size:	**Medium**
Category:	**Vintage**
Price range:	**Moderate to Premium $$–$$$**
Registry:	United States
Year built:	1951 (Refurbished 1994 and 1997)
Itinerary:	Hawaiian islands from Honolulu until November 2000, then from Maui
Information:	(800) 765-7000
Website:	www.cruisehawaii.com
Passenger capacity:	867 (double occupancy)
Crew:	320 American
Passenger-to-Crew Ratio:	2.7:1
Tonnage:	20,221 tons
Passenger Space Ratio:	23.3
Length:	682 feet
Beam:	89 feet
Draft:	26.5 feet
Cruising speed:	17 knots
Guest decks:	10 decks
Total cabins:	446
Outside:	169
Inside:	240
Suites:	37
Wheelchair accessible:	2
Cuisine:	Pacific Rim
Style:	Attire for dinner is semi-formal
Price notes:	Single supplement 160 percent to 200 percent
Tipping suggestions:	$10 pp/pd

The *Independence* and her corporate cousin the *Patriot* of United States Lines represent the entire U.S.-flagged major cruise ship industry, soldiering on as the only ships making year-round circuits of the Hawaiian islands. The basic itinerary for the *Independence* is a seven-night cruise from Honolulu, with stops in Kauai on Maui, and Hilo and Kona on Hawaii. The line also sells three- and four-day segments of the trip.

Beginning in November of 2000, the *Independence* will change her home port to Maui, sailing week-long itineraries from there. The move will make room for the arrival of the *Patriot*, which will begin service from Honolulu in December.

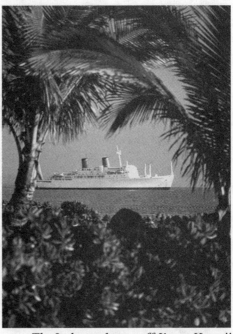

The Independence *off Kona, Hawaii*
American Hawaii Cruises

The *Independence* was refurbished in 1994 to add more of a Hawaiian ambiance, and again in 1997 to add 25 new passenger cabins. Safety and emergency systems were also modernized. The interior features traditional Hawaiian themes, natural woods, rattan, and wicker.

An onboard kumu (Hawaiian teacher) shares the myths, legends, and culture of the islands. In Hawaiian tradition, kumus are designated at birth by their grandparents, and raised apart from their siblings by older relatives or other kumus, who tutor them daily in the ancient ways.

Throughout the day, the kumu gathers people together on deck and in the Kumy Study to tell ghost tales, stories of Hawaiian royalty, and the mythical menehue (little people), or the legend of "Haleakala, the House of the Sun." On Thursday evenings, passengers on deck can also hear of "Pele, the fire goddess" as they view the Kilaueau crater's dramatic lava flow into the sea.

There are childrens' programs for ages 5–17. The ship's cuisine mingles fresh Hawaiian and Pacific Rim ingredients, including fresh fish from local waters, including mahi mahi (dolphin), ahi (tuna), opah (moonfish), and a'u (marlin.) Specialties include Seared Fresh Island Sashimi with Pickled Ginger and Wasabi, Seared Sea Scallops with Gingered Black Bean Sauce, and Black Tiger Shrimp sauteed with lemon grass, elephant garlic, and fresh island herbs.

Each day's lunch menu includes a traditional Hawaiian "plate lunch," a chicken, pork, or fish entrée served with salad and rice. One example is the laulau: beef, pork, butterfish, and taro tops, wrapped and steamed in ti leaves.

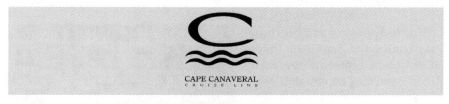

CAPE CANAVERAL
C R U I S E   L I N E

Cape Canaveral Cruise Line
7099 Atlantic Ave.
Cape Canaveral, FL 32920
Information: (800) 910-7447, (321) 783-4052
www.capecanaveralcruise.com

Cape Canaveral Cruise Line Fleet

Dolphin IV. (1956) 718 passengers. 13,650 tons

Cape Canaveral Cruise Line is a toe in the water aimed at first-timers and bargain hunters. As such, it delivers a decent product for a reasonable price.

The *Dolphin IV* sails from Port Canaveral, competing directly against the much more expensive—and considerably fancier—Disney Cruise Line ships and others from major lines.

The ship is a classic, small liner that has traveled all over the world in various roles and with a fascinating history that began with the birth of the State of Israel; few ships have sailed under a more interesting collection of flags.

This is definitely not a luxury cruise; cabins and public spaces on the ship, now in its fifth decade, are small and somewhat Spartan and a full load of passengers will often find lines for buffets and shows.

But this is also not just a party line, a "cruise to nowhere." The ship makes two-night cruises from Port Canaveral to Grand Bahama Island, and four-night cruises every other week that also include a stop at Key West, Florida.

As I've said, this is an old ship, one of the most elderly cruise ships still in service. Though it cannot possibly stand up against the glitz and flash of a newer ship like those put to sea by the much larger cruise lines, the *Dolphin IV* still holds a bit of elegance and charm from her original role as a long distance cruise ship.

Happily, prices are definitely at a relative bargain level, working out to less than $100 per person per night for double occupancy in a cabin. Third and fourth persons in the cabin are charged even less, and during the low seasons, the line offers sales that reduce the cost even more.

You'll see billboards advertising the cruise on the roads along the Florida coast and as far inland as Orlando. It's possible to work a three-day, two-night cruise into a week-long visit to one of the other attractions of Central Florida, including the Space Coast and Orlando areas.

I have also seen some less-than-wonderful direct mail come-ons tied into a timeshare offering; I'd pass on those supposed deals.

Dolphin IV

Econoguide rating:	★★
Ship size:	**Medium**
Category:	**Vintage**
Price range:	**Budget $**
Registry:	Panama
Year built:	1956 (*Zion, Amelia do Mello, Ithaca.* Refurbished 1973, 1998, 1999)
Itinerary:	Freeport, Bahamas and Key West from Port Canaveral
Information:	(800) 910-7447
Website:	www.capecanaveralcruise.com
Passenger capacity:	718 (double occupancy)
Crew:	300 International
Passenger-to-Crew Ratio:	2.4:1
Tonnage:	13,650
Passenger Space Ratio:	19
Length:	503 feet
Beam:	65 feet
Draft:	26 feet
Cruising speed:	17 knots
Guest decks:	5 passenger decks plus promenade deck
Total cabins:	294
Outside:	208
Inside:	77
Suites:	9
Wheelchair accessible:	Boat/Atlantis deck or forward section of the Barbizon deck
Cuisine:	Classical dining with a contemporary flair
Style:	Resort casual/ dresses, sport coat with tie for Captain's dinner
Price notes:	Single supplement 150 percent. Reduced rates for third and fourth person
Tipping suggestions:	$9.50 pp/pd

The *Dolphin IV* made her maiden voyage in 1956 as the *Zion* of Israel's Zim Lines; a combination passenger and cargo ship built for Israel as part of a German war reparations package. The *Zion* spent about a decade carrying passengers in First and Tourist Class cabins on a route from Haifa, Piraeus, Naples, Lisbon and Brooklyn.

In 1966, the *Zion* and her sister ship *Israel* were sold to a Portuguese carrier, trading from Lisbon to Guinea and Angola and operating under the name *Amelia do Mello*. In 1971, the *Zion* was sold to a Greek company that carried out a conversion to a full-time cruise ship; the ship was extensively rebuilt, with new public areas shoehorned into place and cabins improved with private bathrooms for the first time. Now called the *Ithaca*, the ship sailed for Ulysses Cruises and was under charter to a British tour operator and later a Canadian company, Strand Cruises, which operated in the Mediterranean.

The ship's next incarnation was under ownership of Paquet Lines, which renamed her as the *Dolphin IV* in 1979 and put her on a schedule from Miami to the Bahamas. Paquet is credited with upgrading the food service.

Since her maiden voyage she has been rebuilt, refitted, refurbished and redecorated no less than 10 times. Public rooms include a casino, disco, and a theater. Limited supervised children's activities are available.

The ship sails a mixed schedule of two-night cruises from Port Canaveral to Freeport in the Bahamas, and four-night itineraries that also make a port call in Key West.

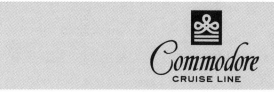

Commodore Cruise Line
4000 Hollywood Blvd., Suite 385 South
Hollywood, FL 33021
Information: (800) 237-5361
www.commodorecruise.com

Commodore Cruise Line Fleet

Enchanted Isle. (1957, refurbished 1997) 725 passengers. 23,395 tons

Enchanted Capri. (1975, refurbished 1998) 637 passengers. 15,410 tons

Universe Explorer. (1958) Under charter to World Explorer Cruises for most of the year; see World Explorer section for details.

Commodore Cruise Line sails out of the Big Easy across the Gulf of Mexico to the Western Caribbean, Mexico, and Central America. The company's flagship is the *Enchanted Isle,* a classic old liner. Also in the fleet is the *Enchanted Capri*, a more recent small cruise ship.

Commodore operates what the company calls "classic traditional midsize ships that offer great value." That's a fair appraisal of the fleet; these are well-maintained, well-traveled senior citizens, a description that also applies to many of the passengers, although you'll also find many first-time cruisers and families looking for a good deal.

In late 1999, Commodore established Crown Cruise Line. The first ship is the *Crown Dynasty,* a classy mid-sized cruise ship most recently operated by Norwegian Cruise Line as the *Norwegian Dynasty.* See her listing under Crown Cruise Lines later in this chapter.

Commodore's *Universe Explorer* operates in the summer months as a joint venture with World Explorer Cruises and sails to Alaska. During the fall and spring the ship is used by Semester at Sea, a program administered by the Institute for Shipboard Education and academically affiliated with the University of Pittsburgh. And from time to time, she rejoins the Commodore fleet for special sailings, as she did for the millennium celebration.

The *Enchanted Isle, Enchanted Capri,* and *Universe Explorer* are modest ships, but they are priced accordingly. As long as you are not expecting modern appointments and luxury, Commodore's offerings represent some of the best bargains in cruising.

The *Enchanted Isle* sails from New Orleans to Mexico, Jamaica, and the Cayman Islands for much of the year, switching over to a Mexico and Central America itinerary for several cruises each year.

The *Enchanted Capri* operates alternating two- and five-day cruises; the shorter voyage is basically a party-and-casino cruise to nowhere. The five-day voyage visits Cancun and Cozumel, Mexico.

In 2000, both ships will sail a series of longer special cruises in the fall and winter. In September, the *Enchanted Isle* will sail a two-week itinerary from New Orleans to the Panama Canal, and 10- and 11-day cruises from New Orleans to San Juan, or the reverse. In December, *Enchanted Capri* will sail from New Orleans deep into the Caribbean to San Juan, and then make a return journey to the same ports.

Commodore was founded in 1966, offering cruises from Miami; the company was a pioneer of theme cruises, including "Remember When" music motifs. In 1987, Commodore was acquired by the Effoa and Johnson Line, which subsequently became the Scandinavian-based EffJohn International. In 1989, EffJohn purchased the Bermuda Star Line; and in 1990, merged the two companies. In 1995, the company was acquired by JeMJ Financial Services of Miami and is now operated by Commodore Holdings Ltd.

A Tale of Two Sisters

In 1958, Moore McCormack Lines' *Brasil* and *Argentina* were launched from the yards at Pascagoula, Mississippi, considered at the time among the most luxurious and advanced ocean liners. They were designed with powerful engines and extra-thick hull plating for the New York to South America run, on month-long roundtrip cruises to Trinidad, Rio de Janeiro, Santos, Montevideo, and Buenos Aires.

Eventually, the two ships were found to be too large and expensive to operate on the long South American rounds, and in 1963 both were rebuilt. They spent the next few years sailing to Bermuda, the Caribbean, Scandinavia, the Mediterranean, and around Africa before they were taken out of service in Baltimore in 1969.

The pair was sold to the Holland America Line in 1971 and rebuilt in Bremerhaven, West Germany. The *Brasil* became the *Volendam,* and the *Argentina* the *Veendam.* After just a few cruises, Holland America chartered both ships to the Panama-flagged Monarch Cruise Line, sailing from 1976 to 1978 as the *Monarch Sun* and the *Monarch Star* respectively.

In 1978, the ships returned to service for Holland America and retook their Dutch names, adding cruises from New York to Bermuda to their schedules.

In 1984, both ships were sold once more, this time to the C. Y. Tung Group, a Taiwan-based shipping conglomerate. The *Volendam* was leased to the Banstead Shipping Co., and was then used for a while as the hotel-ship *Island Sun* before undergoing a full refit in Japan; she was next chartered by American Hawaiian Cruises sailing as the *Liberte* on seven-day cruises from Papeete, Tahiti. After only a year, the ship was laid up in San Francisco and then sold to the Bermuda Star Line and renamed *Canada Star.* In the spring of 1988, she acquired her eighth name, *Queen of Bermuda.*

The *Veendam* was chartered to Bermuda Star Line in 1984 and renamed the *Bermuda Star.* In 1990, Bermuda Star Line was merged with Commodore Cruise Line, bringing the two classic sister ships together once again as the *Enchanted Isle* (the former *Argentina/Veendam,* etc.) and the *Enchanted Seas* (the former *Brasil, Volendam,* etc.)

In April of 1993, the *Enchanted Isle* went to St. Petersburg, Russia to serve as a hotel-ship, while the *Enchanted Seas* sailed seven-night itineraries from New Orleans to the Caribbean.

In 1995, the *Enchanted Seas* began service as a floating classroom for the Semester at Sea, a program administered by the University of Pittsburgh. She was renamed once again, this time as the Universe Explorer. Currently, the *Universe Explorer* sails the globe twice yearly on the Semester at Sea itinerary, and for the rest of the year is operated by World Explorer Cruises on Alaskan and Caribbean routes. The *Enchanted Isle* returned from Russia to New Orleans to sail as a cruise ship once more.

Enchanted Isle

Econoguide rating:	★★★	
Ship size:	**Medium**	
Category:	**Vintage**	
Price range:	**Moderate $$**	
Registry:	Panama	
Year built:	1958 (*Argentina* (Moore McCormick); *Veendam* (Holland America); *Monarch Star* (Monarch); *Veendam* (Holland America); *Bermuda Star* (Bermuda Star); *Enchanted Isle* (Commodore); Hotel Commodore, Russia; *Enchanted Isle.* Refurbished 1994 and 1997)	
Sister ship:	*Universe Explorer*	

Itinerary:	From New Orleans to Montego Bay, Jamaica, Mexico, Cayman Islands
Information:	(800) 237-5361
Website:	www.commodorecruise.com
Passenger capacity:	725 (double occupancy)
Crew:	350 Officers, European and American; international crew
Passenger-to-Crew Ratio:	2:1
Tonnage:	23,395
Passenger Space Ratio:	32.3
Length:	617 feet
Beam:	84 feet
Draft:	28 feet
Cruising speed:	18 knots
Guest decks:	9
Total cabins:	361
Outside:	280
Inside:	72
Suites:	9
Wheelchair accessible:	0
Cuisine:	Continental
Style:	Informal with one or more semi-formal evenings
Price notes:	Single occupancy 150 percent to 200 percent premium for most cabins; reduced rates for third and fourth persons in cabin
Tipping suggestions:	$12 pp/pd

An old lady of the sea, pretty well kept for a ship now in her fifth decade. Her well-traveled passport includes stints in South America, the Mediterranean, the Caribbean, and a job as a floating hotel in Russia.

In 1997, the *Enchanted Isle* underwent renovations to update and upgrade many of her public areas. Forty cabins were fitted with double beds and nine suites were added; cabins throughout were given fresh carpeting, drapes, bedspreads, wall coverings and other new appointments. The Riviera Dining Room was given a major facelift with the installation of new carpeting, mirrored walls, lighting, and dining room upholstery. The ship's informal dining area, the Bistro, now has a Caribbean feel.

In 1998, the ship sailed from New Orleans to Gulf of Mexico resorts and made several trips to Key West, Florida.

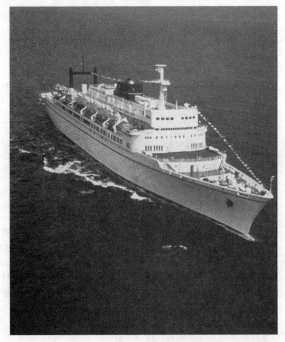

Enchanted Isle
Courtesy of Commodore Cruise Line

Enchanted Capri

Econoguide rating:	★★★
Ship size:	**Medium**
Category:	**Vintage**
Price range:	**Budget $**
Registry:	Bahamas
Year built:	1975 (In Finland. *Arkadya, Azerbajian, Island Holiday.* Refurbished 1984, 1997, and 1998)
Itinerary:	New Orleans to Mexico and Playa del Carmen/Cozumel
Information:	(800) 237-5361
Website:	www.commodorecruise.com
Passenger capacity:	488 (double occupancy)
Crew:	275 European and American officers; international crew
Passenger-to-Crew Ratio:	1.8:1
Tonnage:	15,410
Passenger Space Ratio:	31.6
Length:	515 feet
Beam:	71 feet
Draft:	20 feet
Cruising speed:	18 knots
Guest decks:	7
Total cabins:	244
Outside:	131
Inside:	113
Suites:	8
Wheelchair accessible:	No
Cuisine:	Continental. One seating
Style:	Casual, with one semi-formal evening
Price notes:	Reduced rates for third and fourth persons in cabin
Tipping suggestions:	$12 pp/pd

Born as a small Russian cruise ship, her odyssey has brought her to New Orleans for two-night weekend cruises sailing the Mississippi River and the Gulf of Mexico, and five-night cruises to Cancun and Cozumel. There are also a few week-long trips to Jamaica and Grand Cayman.

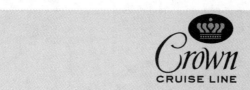

Crown Cruise Line
4000 Hollywood Boulevard
Suite 385, South Tower
Hollywood, FL 33021
Information: (877) 276-9621 or (954) 967-2100
www.crowncruiseline.com

Crown Cruise Line Fleet

Crown Dynasty. (1993) 800 passengers. 20,000 tons

A new premium cruise company, an offshoot of Commodore, Crown Cruise Line took to the seas at the end of 1999 with the debut of *Crown Dynasty*, an elegant mid-sized ship.

The company is seeking to position itself a notch above the middle, delivering guests to destinations in the southern Caribbean from Aruba in the winter and, at least in its first year, offering a full slate of cruises from Philadelphia and Baltimore to Bermuda in the summer. In October of 2000, the Crown Dynasty was due from Baltimore to New York and on to Halifax, Sydney, and Quebec City; from there she will return down the St. Lawrence River to the Gaspé Peninsula, Prince Edward Island, Newport, and back to Baltimore. The trip can be booked as a two-week roundtrip or as individual weeks.

According to the company, Crown's plan is to offer a premium product at a moderate price, priced about 10 percent to 15 percent below rates charged by Celebrity and Holland America. In its initial years, half of the staterooms in Aruba and all of the capacity to Bermuda was being marketed by Apple Vacations, a major travel packager.

We sailed on the still-young *Crown Dynasty* on one of the first journeys under her new banner from Aruba to Barbados and four other Caribbean ports. A few years back we spent 10 days in the South Pacific when she was dressed in the colors of Norwegian Cruise Line as the *Norwegian Dynasty*. She is a ship well-suited for veteran cruisers who don't need to be constantly entertained, enjoying instead refined and elegant surroundings and service.

You can read about our trip in the cruise diaries section of this book.

Crown Dynasty

Econoguide rating:	★★★★
Ship size:	**Medium**
Category:	**Top of the Line**
Price range:	**Moderate-Premium $$–$$$**
Registry:	Panama
Year built:	1993 (As *Crown Dynasty* of Crown Cruise Line, then *Cunard Dynasty*, then *Crown Majesty*. Leased by NCL in 1997 and renamed *Norwegian Dynasty*. Refurbished for Crown Cruise Line in 1999 and renamed *Crown Dynasty*.)
Itinerary:	Caribbean from Aruba in winter, Bermuda from Philadelphia in summer.
Information:	(800) 327-7030
Website:	www.crowncruiseline.com
Passenger capacity:	800 (double occupancy)
Crew:	339 International
Passenger-to-Crew Ratio:	2.4:1
Tonnage:	20,000
Passenger Space Ratio:	25
Length:	537 feet
Beam:	74 feet
Draft:	18 feet
Cruising speed:	19 knots
Guest decks:	7 decks
Total cabins:	400
Outside:	233
Inside:	124
Suites:	43
Wheelchair cabins:	4

Cuisine:	Continental
Style:	Informal with two formal nights per cruise
Price notes:	200 percent single surcharge
Tipping suggestions:	$13.25 pp/pd

A relatively small gem of a ship; she lacks the large showrooms, movie theaters, and lounges of other members of the fleet but the public spaces are very pleasant and comfortable. There are but 10 balconies among the deluxe suites.

Some cruise travelers prefer the more intimate spaces and personalized service of a ship this size. Cabins are attractively furnished; there are only a handful of verandas on one upper deck.

The handsome ship has had a hard time finding a permanent home, apparently because she lacks the amenities and open space of the megaships. But some cruisers love the ship. In 1999, Norwegian Cruise Line did not renew its lease for the ship, and she moved to the new Crown Cruise Line.

The latest renovation applied a Bermudas theme to the ship, with public rooms including the Queen of Bermuda Bar, the Hamilton Dining Room, and the Gombey Lounge showroom.

The first year of service included a winter and spring of voyages from Aruba with stops at five "hidden harbors" of the southern Caribbean: Barbados, St. Lucia, Grenada, Bonaire, and Curaçao. After then, the ship was due to move to Philadelphia and Baltimore for summer sailings to Bermuda.

We sailed on the *Norwegian Dynasty* in 1998 from Honolulu to the South Pacific, a voyage recounted in the Cruise Diary section of the book. Then we journeyed on the Crown Dynasty from Aruba through the southern Caribbean; you can also read about that trip in the Cruise Diaries.

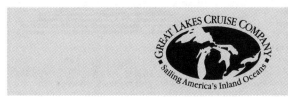

Great Lakes Cruise Company
3270 Washtenaw Avenue
Ann Arbor, MI 48104
Information: 888-891-0203
www.greatlakescruising.com

Great Lakes Cruise Company Fleet

Columbus. (1997) 418 passengers, 14,903 tons

Le Levant. (1998) 90 passengers, 3,500 tons

The Great Lakes, almost like inland oceans, were once served by many modest cruise ships. The Great Lakes Cruise Company, an offshoot of a Michigan travel agency, has updated the concept with a modest schedule of trips on a pair of not-so-modest modern ships under charter from their European operators, *Columbus* and *Le Levant*.

Columbus

Econoguide rating:	★★★★
Ship size:	**Medium**
Category:	**Top of the Line**
Price range:	**Premium $$$**
Registry:	Netherlands Antilles
Year built:	1997
Itinerary:	Great Lakes cruises under charter
Information:	(888) 891-0203
Passenger capacity:	418 (double occupancy)
Crew:	170
Passenger-to-Crew Ratio:	2.5:1
Tonnage:	14,903
Passenger Space Ratio:	35.7
Length:	473 feet
Beam:	71 feet
Draft:	16.8 feet
Cruising speed:	NA
Guest decks:	6
Total cabins:	207
Outside:	160
Inside:	47
Suites:	8
Wheelchair accessible:	Elevators
Cuisine:	International
Style:	Informal
Price notes:	Single cabins 175 percent premium
Tipping suggestions:	$7 pp/pd

Equipped with an ice-hardened hull, the ship is among the few substantial cruisers to venture into the Great Lakes in many years.

In the summer of 2000, one nine-night cruise began at Windsor, Ontario, continuing on through Georgian Bay and on to Sault Ste. Marie and Thunder Bay in Ontario, Duluth and Marquette, Michigan, and on to Manitowoc, Wisconsin. The cruise ended in Chicago.

Le Levant

Econoguide rating:	★★★★
Ship size:	**Medium**
Category:	**Top of the Line**
Price range:	**Premium $$$**
Registry:	N/A
Year built:	1998
Itinerary:	Great Lakes cruises under charter
Information:	(888) 891-0203
Passenger capacity:	90 (double occupancy)
Crew:	50
Passenger-to-Crew Ratio:	1.8:1
Tonnage:	3,500
Passenger Space Ratio:	38.9
Length:	328 feet
Beam:	46 feet
Draft:	14 feet
Cruising speed:	16 knots
Guest decks:	5
Total cabins:	45

Outside:	45
Inside:	0
Suites:	0
Wheelchair accessible:	Elevator
Cuisine:	French. Wine included at lunch and dinner
Style:	Informal
Price notes:	Single cabins at 175 percent of per-person rate
Tipping suggestions:	Gratuities included

This French luxury yacht offers eight-night cruises from Toronto on Lake Ontario, through the Welland Canal into Lake Erie and on to Windsor, Ontario and past Detroit, Michigan. From there, the ship enters into Lake Huron, to Manitoulin Island, Sault Ste. Marie, Mackinac Island, and into Lake Michigan, ending at Chicago's Navy Pier.

Imperial Majesty Cruise Line
2900 Gateway Blvd., Suite 200
Pompano Beach, FL 33069
Information: 800-511-5737

Imperial Majesty Cruise Line Fleet

OceanBreeze. (1955) 776 passengers, 21,486 tons

Now in her sixth decade, the *OceanBreeze* has seen the world, from long voyages from England to Australia in her early years to her most recent incarnation sailing two-night back-and-forths from Fort Lauderdale to Nassau.

In 1999, the *OceanBreeze* began a two-year charter by its owner, Premier Cruise Lines, to Imperial Majesty Cruise Line. The company has an option to extend the lease for another two years beginning in January of 2001, although no decision had been made as this book went to press. Imperial Majesty also says it is looking for additional ships to add to its fleet in coming years.

The short cruises are marketed for first-time cruisers, families, and for those looking for a quick getaway. Per-person rates run from as low as $150 for a minimal inside cabin to $400 for a suite for two nights. Peak season cruises in holiday periods are priced at more than double.

OceanBreeze

Econoguide rating:	★★	
Ship size:	**Medium**	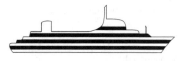
Category:	**Vintage**	
Price range:	**Moderate $$**	
Registry:	Liberia	
Year built:	1955 (Built as the *Southern Cross,* later the *Calypso* and *Azure Seas.* Refurbished 1992, 1997)	

Itinerary:	Fort Lauderdale to Nassau
Information:	(800) 511-5737
Passenger capacity:	776 (double occupancy)
Crew:	400
Passenger-to-Crew Ratio:	1.9:1
Tonnage:	21,486
Passenger Space Ratio:	27.7
Length:	604 feet
Beam:	78 feet
Draft:	29 feet
Cruising speed:	20 knots
Guest decks:	9
Total cabins:	388
Outside:	226
Inside:	150
Suites:	12
Cuisine:	American
Style:	Informal. Second night semi-formal optional
Price notes:	Third or fourth person in cabin $129. Child rate for ages 3–12.
Tipping suggestions:	$9.75 pp/pd

Born as the *Southern Cross* in 1954 (and christened by Queen Elizabeth II in the first full year of her reign), the ship's initial assignment was the long haul from Great Britain to Australia and New Zealand.

The liner was laid up in 1971, returning to service two years later as the refurbished cruise liner *Calypso,* sailing in the Mediterranean. In 1981, the vessel was sold to Western Steamship Lines and renamed the *Azure Seas* and used for three- and four-day cruises from Los Angeles to Mexico. The ship was renamed once again as the *OceanBreeze* and was purchased by Dolphin Cruise Line, now part of Premier.

A neat ship with little flash and sparkle, she is among the last steam turbine ocean liners still operating.

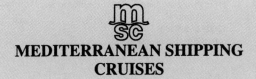

MEDITERRANEAN SHIPPING CRUISES

Mediterranean Shipping Cruises
420 Fifth Ave.
New York, NY 10018-2702
Information: 800-666-9333
www.msccruisesusa.com

Mediterranean Shipping Cruises Fleet

Melody. (1982) 1,076 passengers, 36,500 tons

Mediterranean Shipping Cruises operates a small fleet of cruise ships around the world, including the *Melody*, which sails in the Caribbean in the winter and Europe for the remainder of the year. The *Melody* is the former *Star/Ship Atlantic,* one of The Big Red Boats of Premier Cruise Line.

Other ships in the fleet include the *Rhapsody,* formerly the *Cunard Princess;* the *Symphony,* formerly the *Enrico Costa* of Costa Cruises, and the *Monterey,* a former U.S. flag liner. They serve European, South American, and South African ports.

Mediterranean Shipping Cruises began as Flotta Lauro, an Italian carrier little known outside its home waters until the 1985 terrorist attack on its cruise ship *Achille Lauro* off Egypt. The *Achille Lauro* later sank off Africa in 1994.

The company was purchased in 1990 by Mediterranean Shipping Cruises, part of the Swiss-based Mediterranean Shipping Company, which is one of the world's largest container carrier companies with a fleet of 74 freighters.

The MSC Experience

In 2001, the *Melody* plans alternating 11-night Western Caribbean/Costa Rica and West Indies itineraries out of Fort Lauderdale from January through April, returning to its base in Genoa, Italy for the remainder of the year.

The Western route includes stops at Montego Bay, Cartagena, a partial transit of the Panama Canal, and Key West. The West Indies route visits St. Thomas, Antigua, Grenada, St. Lucia, Guadeloupe, Tortola, and Nassau.

Transatlantic cruises between Fort Lauderdale and Genoa are offered in April and late December; the 17-day trip makes port calls in the Caribbean and Funchal, Gibraltar, or Barcelona.

Melody

Econoguide rating:	★★
Ship size:	**Medium**
Category:	**Vintage**
Price range:	**Budget $**
Registry:	Panama
Year built:	1982 (Former *Star/Ship Atlantic* of Premier Cruise Line. Refurbished 1996)
Itinerary:	From Port Everglades to West Caribbean and West Indies in winter, Europe in the summer
Information:	(800) 666-9333
Passenger capacity:	1,076 (double occupancy)
Crew:	535
Passenger-to-Crew Ratio:	2:1
Tonnage:	36,500
Passenger Space Ratio:	33.9
Length:	672 feet
Beam:	90 feet
Draft:	24.5 feet
Cruising speed:	21 knots
Guest decks:	8
Total cabins:	532
Outside:	381
Inside:	151
Suites:	78
Wheelchair accessible:	4 wheelchair cabins, but not up to modern standards for handicapped facilities
Cuisine:	Italian and International cuisine
Style:	Casual with two or more semi-formal evenings
Price notes:	Single occupancy premium 150 percent
Tipping suggestions:	$8 pp/pd

The *Melody* is a sturdy but undistinguished vessel that manages to pack a large number of guests onboard. There's a nice pool area with a retractable cover that allows use in any weather.

There are only three of the lowest-price staterooms on the ship, two on the bottom-most Bahamas deck and one on the Restaurant deck. The most plentiful outside cabins are Class 8 staterooms, primarily on the Oceanic deck, with some additional cabins scattered about the ship.

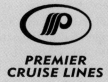

PREMIER CRUISE LINES

Premier Cruise Lines
400 Challenger Road
Cape Canaveral, FL 32920
Information: (800) 990-7770, (800) 327-9766
www.premiercruises.com

Premier Cruises Fleet

Big Red Boat I. (Formerly *Oceanic.*) (1965) 1,116 passengers, 38,772 tons

Big Red Boat II. (Formerly *Edinburgh Castle.*) (1966) 1,116 passengers, 35,000 tons

Big Red Boat III. (Formerly *IslandBreeze.*) (1961) 1,146 passengers, 31,793 tons

Big Red Boat IV. (Formerly *Rembrandt.*) (1959) 1,106 passengers, 38,000 tons

SeaBreeze. (1958) 840 passengers, 21,000 tons

Seawind Crown. (1961) 764 passengers, 24,000 tons

Despite its name, Premier Cruises is by no means the first home for its fleet of classic cruise ships; all are in their fourth or even fifth decade of service and each has a notable history. The ships are well-maintained ladies of a certain age—with hints of their original elegance; cabins and public rooms are smaller and considerably less flashy than you'll find on modern ships.

Premier was founded in 1997 when Dolphin Cruise Line, Seawind Cruise Line and Premier Cruise Lines were merged under new management.

In 2000, four of the line's ships will come under the Big Red Boat brand, sailing from four corners of the U.S. And the company promises a "Seven Star" upgrade in service and quality of food and cabin appointments.

The *Big Red Boat I,* formerly the *Oceanic,* features 3- and 4-night trips from Port Canaveral to the Bahamas. The *Big Red Boat II,* formerly the *Edinburgh Castle* and before then the *Eugenio Costa,* began service in May of 2000 with summer sailings from New York to New England and Canada. In the fall, she will move to Port Canaveral for cruises in the eastern and western Caribbean.

The *Big Red Boat III*, formerly the *IslandBreeze*, moves to Houston in June of 2000 for year-round cruises to Cozumel, Playa del Carmen, and Veracruz in Mexico. The *Big Red Boat IV*, formerly the *Rembrandt* and before then *Rotterdam V* of Holland America Line, moves to Los Angeles in November of 2000, adding Alaskan itineraries in the summer of 2001.

The *Seawind Crown* visits some of the less-traveled ports of the Caribbean. The *OceanBreeze*, which in recent years has journeyed in the Caribbean, is under a two-year charter to Imperial Majesty Cruises through January 2001.

The original Big Red Boat operated in the early 1990s under a license from the Walt Disney Company with appearances by Disney characters and tie-ins to the Disney theme park in Orlando. In 1998, the Disney Cruise Line began service from Port Canaveral to the Bahamas. The *Disney Magic* and the *Disney Wonder* are marketed toward families and first-time cruisers, and carry with them the endorsement of Mickey Mouse and his crew.

Big Red Boat I/Oceanic

Econoguide rating:	★★
Ship size:	**Medium**
Category:	**Vintage**
Price range:	**Moderate $$**
Registry:	Bahamas from Port Canaveral
Year built:	1965 (For Home Lines. Refurbished 1997)
Itinerary:	Bahamas from Port Canaveral
Information:	(800) 990-7770
Website:	www.premiercruises.com
Passenger capacity:	1,116 (double occupancy)
Crew:	565
Passenger-to-Crew Ratio:	2:1
Tonnage:	38,772 tons
Passenger Space Ratio:	34.7
Length:	782 feet
Beam:	96 feet
Draft:	28 feet
Cruising speed:	27 knots
Guest decks:	8
Total cabins:	574
Outside:	190
Inside:	335
Suites:	65
Wheelchair accessible:	1
Cuisine:	American
Style:	Informal with one or more semi-formal evenings
Price notes:	Single occupancy premium 125 percent to 200 percent. Single parent plan has 125 percent supplement for most cabins, with children sharing cabin charged at third guest rate. Senior discount 15 percent.
Tipping suggestions:	$11.75 pp/pd

Today's version of the Big Red Boat is a classic cruise liner built for Home Lines in 1965 and well-maintained over the years. Designed as a two-class North Atlantic liner, she never was used for that purpose; instead, the *Oceanic*'s first assignment was a weekly New York-to-Nassau run. After 20 years, she was sold to Premier Cruise Lines to sail from Port Canaveral to the Bahamas as the Big Red Boat.

It has been hard-worked in recent times, shuttling budget travelers on 3- or 4-day cruises. This is by no means a luxury ship, and most veterans of more modern and flashy ships will be disappointed by the small and simple cabins and public areas; first-time cruisegoers, though, will likely enjoy the experience of going to sea. Among her best features is a glass-roofed swimming pool.

From 1986 through the mid-1990s, the Big Red Boat was co-marketed with Walt Disney World, with Disney characters onboard and tie-ins with visits to the park. Of course, Disney now has its own cruise line, with a pair of ships that depart from a beautiful new terminal across the bay from the Big Red Boat's dock.

Big Red Boat II/Edinburgh Castle

Econoguide rating:	★★
Ship size:	**Medium**
Category:	**Vintage**
Price range:	**Moderate $$**
Registry:	Bahamas
Year built:	1966. Former *Edinburgh Castle, Eugenio Costa.*
Itinerary:	Summer New York to New England and Canada, winter Eastern Caribbean
Information:	(800) 990-7770
Website:	www.premiercruises.com
Passenger capacity:	1,116 (double occupancy)
Crew:	568
Passenger-to-Crew Ratio:	2:1
Tonnage:	35,000 tons
Passenger Space Ratio:	31.4
Length:	713 feet
Beam:	96 feet
Draft:	29 feet
Cruising speed:	24 knots
Guest decks:	9
Total cabins:	453
Outside:	265
Inside:	188
Suites:	N/A
Wheelchair accessible:	4
Cuisine:	American
Style:	Informal with one or more semi-formal evenings
Price notes:	Single occupancy premium 125 percent to 200 percent. Single parent plan has 125 percent supplement for most cabins, with children sharing cabin charged at third guest rate. Senior discount 15 percent.
Tipping suggestions:	$9.50 pp/pd

Big Red Boat III/IslandBreeze

Econoguide rating:	★★
Ship size:	**Medium**
Category:	**Vintage**
Price range:	**Moderate $$**

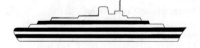

Registry:	Bahamas
Year built:	1961 (*Transvaal Castle, Vale, Festivale, IslandBreeze.* Refurbished 1997, 2000)
Itinerary:	Year-round from Houston to Vera Cruz, Cozumel, Playa del Carmen
Information:	(800) 990-7770
Website:	www.premiercruises.com
Passenger capacity:	1,146 (double occupancy)
Crew:	612
Passenger-to-Crew Ratio:	1.9:1
Tonnage:	31,793
Passenger Space Ratio:	27.7
Length:	760 feet
Beam:	90 feet
Draft:	32 feet
Cruising speed:	22 knots
Total cabins:	583
Outside:	268
Inside:	315
Cuisine:	American
Style:	Informal with one or more semi-formal nights
Price notes:	Single occupancy premium 125 percent to 200 percent. Single parent plan has 125 percent supplement for most cabins, with children sharing cabin charged at third guest rate. Senior discount 15 percent
Tipping suggestions:	$11.75 pp/pd

The ship entered service in 1961 as the *Transvaal Castle,* joining the Union-Castle Steamship Co. as a passenger and mail ship. Unusual at the time as a single-class ship, she was billed as "The Grand Hotel of the South Atlantic."

In 1965, she became the S.A. *Vaal* when the South African government became a major owner of the mail service. The *Vaal* made her last voyage as a mail ship in 1977. That year she was purchased by Carnival Cruise Line and rebuilt in Japan to re-emerge as the *Festivale.* In 1996, the *Festivale* joined Dolphin Cruise Line, which has since become part of Premier.

In recent years, the ship had been deployed in the Canary Islands on a loop to Funchal and Casablanca. The *IslandBreeze* was brought back to the Americas beginning in May of 2000, and will sail from Houston on week-long trips to Cozumel, Playa del Carmen, and Veracruz, Mexico.

Big Red Boat IV/Rembrandt

Econoguide rating:	★★★
Ship size:	**Medium**
Category:	**Vintage**
Price range:	**Moderate $$**
Registry:	Bahamas
Year built:	1959 (*Rotterdam V* for Holland America Line.) Refurbished 2000
Itinerary:	Eastern Caribbean, New York to Bar Harbor, Halifax, and Montreal. Moves to Los Angeles for West Coast cruising in November 2000.
Information:	(800) 990-7770
Website:	www.premiercruises.com
Passenger capacity:	1,106 (double occupancy)
Crew:	550
Passenger-to-Crew Ratio:	2:1
Tonnage:	38,645 tons
Passenger Space Ratio:	34.9
Length:	748 feet
Beam:	94 feet

Draft:	29.6 feet
Cruising speed:	17 knots
Guest decks:	11
Total cabins:	575
Outside:	280
Inside:	295
Suites:	N/A
Wheelchair accessible:	0
Cuisine:	American
Style:	Informal with one or more semi-formal evenings
Price notes:	Single occupancy premium 125 percent to 200 percent. Single parent plan has 125 percent supplement for most cabins, with children sharing cabin charged at third guest rate. Senior discount 15 percent.
Tipping suggestions:	$11.75 pp/pd

SeaBreeze

Econoguide rating:	★★
Ship size:	**Medium**
Category:	**Vintage**
Price range:	**Budget $**
Registry:	Panama
Year built:	1958 (As *Federico C* of Costa, later Premier's *Royale*. Refurbished 1997)
Itinerary:	Montego Bay to South America and Central America in winter. New York to New England and Halifax in spring and summer
Information:	(800) 990-7770
Website:	www.premiercruises.com
Passenger capacity:	840 (double occupancy)
Crew:	400 0
Passenger-to-Crew Ratio:	2.1:1
Tonnage:	21,000
Passenger Space Ratio:	25
Length:	605 feet
Beam:	79 feet
Draft:	29 feet
Cruising speed:	21 knots
Guest decks:	9
Total cabins:	421
Outside:	256
Inside:	158
Suites:	7
Wheelchair accessible:	0
Cuisine:	Continental
Style:	Informal with one or more semi-formal nights
Price notes:	Single occupancy premium 125 percent to 200 percent. Single parent plan has 125 percent supplement for most cabins, with children sharing cabin charged at third guest rate. Senior discount 15 percent. Combine Eastern and Western Caribbean itineraries at discount.
Tipping suggestions:	$11.75 pp/pd

Built in 1958 as Costa Line's flagship, *Federico C,* a two-class transatlantic liner, she was recommissioned by Premier Cruise Line in 1983 and became the *Royale.* The ship was refurbished and renamed as the *SeaBreeze* in 1989 when Dolphin Cruise Line purchased the ship.

She sails today as a well-maintained budget class ship. In 1999, she moved from her former base in Fort Lauderdale to take over the schedule of the *Ocean-Breeze,* sailing from Montego Bay to South and Central America.

Seawind Crown

Econoguide rating:	★★★
Ship size:	**Medium**
Category:	**Vintage**
Price range:	**Moderate $$**
Registry:	Panama
Year built:	1961 (As the *Infante dom Enrique,* later *Vasco de Gama.* Refurbished 1997)
Itinerary:	Out of fleet on charter in 2000
Passenger capacity:	764 (double occupancy)
Crew:	362
Passenger-to-Crew Ratio:	2.1:1
Tonnage:	24,000
Passenger Space Ratio:	31.4
Length:	641 feet
Beam:	81 feet
Draft:	27 feet
Cruising speed:	17 knots
Guest decks:	9 total decks
Total cabins:	367
Outside:	246
Inside:	121
Suites:	16
Wheelchair accessible:	2
Cuisine:	International
Style:	Informal with one or more semi-formal nights

Currently out of the fleet on charter, the *Seawind Crown* is one of the great postwar passenger liners, the former flagship of the Portuguese Merchant Marine. She entered service in 1961 as the largest passenger liner ever built for the 7,230-mile route from Portugal to Mozambique in East Africa, sailing around the Cape of Good Hope. She was laid up in 1976 after Mozambique was given its independence from Portugal. In 1988, she was refurbished and launched as the *Vasco de Gama,* converted from a two-class to a one-class ship.

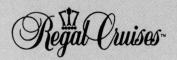

Regal Cruises
300 Regal Cruises Way
P.O. Box 1329
Palmetto, FL 34221
Information: (800) 270-7245, (941) 721-7300
www.regalcruises.com

The Regal Cruises Fleet

Regal Empress. (1953) 1,180 passengers. 21,909 tons

Regal Cruises is a one-ship cruise line, keeping afloat a very old lady with an ambitious schedule that moves from New England and Canada in the summer and fall to Mexico and the Caribbean in the winter and spring.

The line's fleet consists of the *Regal Empress,* born as the ocean liner *Olympia* for the Greek Line in 1953; she was recast as a cruise ship in 1983 as the *Caribe I* for Commodore Cruise Line. She moved on to Regal Cruises in 1993 when that company was founded by executives of two large travel agencies and tour packagers, Liberty Travel and GoGo Tours.

The ship is based in Port Manatee, near St. Petersburg for its Caribbean cruises, and from New York in the summer and fall; other summer ports include Mobile, Savannah, and Philadelphia.

Regal Empress

Econoguide rating:	★★
Ship size:	**Medium**
Category:	**Vintage**
Price range:	**Budget $**
Registry:	Bahamas
Year built:	1953 (*Olympia, Caribe I.* Refurbished 1993, 1999)
Itinerary:	Panama Canal, South America, New England, Canada, Mexico, Caribbean, Key West, New Orleans
Information:	(800) 270-7245
Website:	www.regalcruises.com
Passenger capacity:	900 (double occupancy)
Crew:	396
Passenger-to-Crew Ratio:	2.4:1
Tonnage:	21,909 tons
Passenger Space Ratio:	24.3
Length:	612 feet
Beam:	80 feet
Draft:	28 feet
Cruising speed:	17 knots
Guest decks:	8
Total cabins:	455
Outside:	227
Inside:	2287
Suites:	29
Wheelchair accessible:	0
Cuisine:	International and American
Style:	Informal with one or more semi-formal evenings
Price notes:	Single occupancy premium 150 percent
Tipping suggestions:	$9 pp/pd

Built in 1953 as the liner *Olympia* for the Greek Line. She went into involuntary retirement in 1974, emerging after a major refurbishment in 1983 as the *Caribe I* for Commodore Cruise Lines.

This is a fine old ship, a bit worn around the edges, but very appropriate for cruise virgins and travelers looking for an excellent deal and some less-visited ports of call. A renovation in 1999 added a new small and casual restaurant, computer café, and other amenities. The ship has been brought up to date with most SOLAS regulations, including fire safety sprinklers.

Note that, like many older liners, many of the "outside" cabins actually look out on an open or enclosed promenade along the rail.

Under her new flag, the *Regal Empress* sails an interesting, peripatetic schedule. In the summer, she cruises New England and Canada; the cruises from New York include stops in Newport, R.I.; Martha's Vineyard, Massachusetts, Portland, Maine, and St. John, New Brunswick.

In the winter, she sails out of Port Manatee, Florida to the Caribbean, Mexico, and the Panama Canal; several trips depart from Savannah, Georgia.

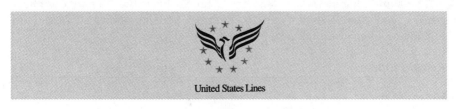

United States Lines

United States Lines
Robin Street Wharf
1380 Port of New Orleans Place
New Orleans, LA 70130
Information: (877) 330-6600
www.unitedstateslines.com

United States Lines Fleet

Patriot. (1983) 1,214 passengers. 33,930 tons

United States Lines was one of the best known names of the golden era of transatlantic liners, a period that ran from the beginning of the twentieth century through the early 1960s. The company's ships, including the *America, Manhattan, Leviathan,* and the *George Washington* were favorites of movie stars, royalty, and other celebrities of the time.

The last remaining passenger vessel of the United States Lines, the fabled *United States,* was retired in 1969. The fastest transatlantic passenger ship ever built, her four steam turbine engines allowed her to cruise at speeds of 32 to 33 knots; she retired with the Blue Riband trophy still in hand.

The line's name has been resurrected by American Classic Cruise Voyages, parent company to American Hawaii Cruises and the Delta Queen Steamboat Co., the only operator of American-flagged cruise ships.

The first ship to sail for the new United States Lines is the 1,214-passenger *Patriot,* originally the *Nieuw Amsterdam* of Holland America Line. Under terms of a special law passed by Congress, after renovations the ship will be allowed to sail under the American flag with an American crew.

The ship is scheduled to begin year-round 7-night cruise service among the Hawaiian Islands in December 2000, sailing from Honolulu.

The company has also contracted to build a pair of 1,900-passenger, 72,000 ton cruise ships. These vessels, to be built at the Ingalls yard in Pascagoula, Miss., are the first major, ocean-going passenger ships to be built in the United States in more than 40 years. The first of the ships is planned to enter service in winter 2003; one year later the second vessel will enter service. Preliminary plans call for the two new ships to join the *Patriot* in service in the Hawaiian islands.

In 2001, American Classic Cruise Voyages will launch Delta Queen Coastal Voyages with a fleet of new 226-passenger ships along the East and West Coasts of the United States, and to selected destinations in the Caribbean and Mexico.

Patriot

Econoguide rating:	★★★
Ship size:	**Medium**
Category:	**Top of the Line**
Price range:	**Moderate $$**
Registry:	United States
Year built:	1983 as HAL's *Nieuw Amsterdam.* Refurbished 2000.
Sister ships:	Holland America Line's *Noordam*
Itinerary:	Hawaii circle from Honolulu, beginning December 2000
Information:	(877) 330-6600
Website:	www.unitedstateslines.com
Passenger capacity:	1,214 (double occupancy)
Crew:	542 (estimated)
Passenger-to-Crew Ratio:	2.2:1 (estimated)
Tonnage:	33,930
Passenger Space Ratio:	27.9
Length:	704.2 feet
Beam:	89.4 feet
Draft:	24.6 feet
Cruising speed:	21 knots
Guest decks:	9
Total cabins:	605
Outside:	391
Inside:	194
Suites:	20
Wheelchair cabins:	4
Cuisine:	International
Style:	Elegantly casual to formal in evening
Price notes:	Single Guaranty Program provides single occupancy of staterooms as assigned by cruise line; to reserve specific staterooms for singles, premium of 160 to 200 percent applies
Tipping suggestions:	Approximately $10 pp/pd

The new flagship of the reborn United States Line, the *Patriot* was born as the *Nieuw Amsterdam* of the Holland America Line. The ship will offer 7-night cruise vacations throughout the Hawaiian Islands sailing every Saturday year-round from Honolulu, Oahu to Nawiliwili, Kauai; Kahului, Maui; Kona, Hawaii; and Hilo, Hawaii.

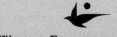

WORLD EXPLORER CRUISES

World Explorer Cruises
555 Montgomery St., Suite 1400
San Francisco, CA 94111-2544
Information: (800) 854-3835, (415) 820-9200
www.wecruise.com

World Explorer Cruises Fleet

Universe Explorer. (1957) 739 passengers. 23,500 tons

The *Universe Explorer* is one of the oldest cruise ships still in use, and lacks the glitz and glitter and some amenities today's guests may have come to expect, such as multiple restaurants and fancy health spas. But her classic lines and well-maintained interior evoke memories of the era of the ocean liners when she was new.

The real star here is the itinerary she follows, an extended tour of the Inside Passage of Alaska with side trips into glacier fjords and inlets. The *Universe Explorer* spends an average of nine hours in each port, more than most other cruise lines. And she carries onboard a mini-university of historians, anthropologists, sociologists, and artists on most cruises.

You can read about a cruise on the *Universe Explorer* in the Cruise Diaries of this book.

There's no casino; instead there's the largest library afloat with some 15,000 eclectic volumes.

The ship serves as a floating university every winter and spring for the Semester at Sea program operated by the University of Pittsburgh and the Institute for Shipboard Education.

A Classic Ship with a Complex History

The *Universe Explorer* has been around. The twin sisters *Brasil* and *Argentina* were launched from the yards at Pascagoula, Mississippi in 1957 and 1958; they were among the last major ocean liners built in the United States. They were designed for the difficult run from New York to South America, a route they both served until 1963 when they were rebuilt for cruising.

Eventually, the two ships were found to be too large and expensive to operate on the long South American rounds, and in 1963 both were rebuilt. They spent the next few years sailing to Bermuda, the Caribbean, Scandinavia, the Mediterranean, and around Africa before they were taken out of service in Baltimore in 1969.

The pair was sold to the Holland America Line in 1971 and rebuilt in Bremerhaven, West Germany. The *Brasil* became the *Volendam,* and the *Argentina* the *Veendam*. After just a few cruises, Holland America chartered both ships to the Panama-flagged Monarch Cruise Line, sailing from 1976 to 1978 as the *Monarch Sun* and the *Monarch Star* respectively.

In 1978, the ships returned to service for Holland America and retook their Dutch names, adding cruises from New York to Bermuda to their schedules. In 1984, both ships were sold once more, this time to the C. Y. Tung Group, a Taiwan-based shipping conglomerate.

The *Volendam* was leased to the Banstead Shipping Co., and was then used as the hotel-ship *Island Sun* for a while before undergoing a full refit in Japan; she was next chartered by American Hawaiian Cruises sailing as the *Liberte* on seven-day cruises from Papeete, Tahiti. After just a year, the ship was laid up in San Francisco and then sold to the Bermuda Star Line and renamed *Canada Star*. In the spring of 1988, she acquired her eighth name, *Queen of Bermuda*.

The *Veendam* was chartered to Bermuda Star Line in 1984 and renamed the *Bermuda Star*. In 1990, Bermuda Star Line was merged with Commodore Cruise Line, bringing the two classic sister ships together once again as the *Enchanted Isle* (the former *Argentina/Veendam*, etc.) and the *Enchanted Seas* (the former *Brasil, Volendam*, etc.)

In April of 1993, the *Enchanted Isle* went to St. Petersburg, Russia to serve as a hotel-ship, while the *Enchanted Seas* sailed seven-night itineraries from New Orleans to the Caribbean.

In 1995, the *Enchanted Seas* began service as a floating classroom for the Semester at Sea, a program administered by the University of Pittsburgh. She was renamed once again, as the *Universe Explorer*. The *Enchanted Isle* returned from Russia to New Orleans where she now sails for Commodore Cruises.

Currently, the *Universe Explorer* sails the globe twice yearly in the spring and fall on the Semester at Sea itinerary, and for the rest of the year is operated by World Explorer Cruises on Alaskan and Caribbean routes.

World Explorer Cruises is owned by the C. Y. Tung shipping conglomerate, which has a 10-year charter for the vessel from Commodore. The University of Pittsburgh has a similar relation to Commodore for its floating classroom program.

Universe Explorer

Econoguide rating:	★★★
Ship size:	**Medium**
Category:	**Vintage**
Price range:	**Moderate $$**
Registry:	Panama
Year built:	1957 (As the *Brasil*. Refurbished 1996, 1999)
Sister ships:	*Enchanted Isle* of Commodore Cruise Line
Itinerary:	Vancouver to Alaska in early May through September. Used for educational world cruises in fall and spring.
Information:	(800) 854-3835
Website:	www.wecruise.com
Passenger capacity:	731 (double occupancy)
Crew:	300 International

Passenger-to-Crew Ratio:	2.5:1
Tonnage:	23,500
Passenger Space Ratio:	31.8
Length:	617 feet
Beam:	84 feet
Draft:	27 feet
Cruising speed:	18 knots
Guest decks:	7
Total cabins:	364
Outside:	284
Inside:	74
Suites:	6
Wheelchair accessible:	2
Cuisine:	American and Continental
Style:	Casual
Price notes:	Single occupancy supplement 150 percent for categories 3–9
Tipping suggestions:	$8 pp/pd

Cabins onboard are plain and simple, but more than adequate. The ship is a bit outdated in some of its design features, operating under an exemption from some of the safety-at-sea requirements demanded of current vessels. A fire in the crew's quarters several years ago killed five members of the staff on a cruise in Alaskan waters.

To their credit, though, Commodore and the companies to which it leases the ship, have been working to keep the ship as up-to-date as possible and extend her life. At the end of 1998, the ship went into drydock for installation of fire sprinklers, one of the steps necessary to bring her closer to modern safety requirements.

Chapter 15
Adventure Cruise Lines

Alaska Sightseeing/Cruise West
American Canadian Caribbean Line
American Cruise Lines
Clipper Cruise Line
Delta Queen Coastal Voyages
Delta Queen Steamboat Co.
Glacier Bay Tours and Cruises
Lindblad Special Expeditions

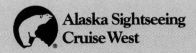

Alaska Sightseeing/Cruise West
2401 Fourth Ave., Suite 700
Seattle, WA 98121
Information: (206) 441-8687, (800) 888-9378
www.cruisewest.com

Alaska Sightseeing/Cruise West Fleet

Spirit of '98. (1984) 96 passengers. 96 tons

Spirit of Alaska. (1980) 78 passengers. 97 tons

Spirit of Columbia. (1979) 78 passengers. 98 tons

Spirit of Discovery. (1976) 84 passengers. 94 tons

Spirit of Endeavor. (1983) 102 passengers. 95 tons

Spirit of Glacier Bay. (1971) 52 passengers. 97 tons

Chuck West, a World War II pilot who returned home to start a bush flying service in Alaska, founded a small cruise company that eventually became

Open space on small ships. Most of the ships in this chapter do not have a passenger space ratio listed; smaller ships are usually configured differently from sprawling cruise ships, doing without open atriums and making multiple use of dining rooms and theaters.

Westours. That company was sold to Holland America Line, and he later began Alaska Sightseeing/Cruise West.

The company began with day cruises in the Inside Passage, and by 1990 had added overnight cruises on the Spirit of Glacier Bay. In 1991, the company introduced cruises from Seattle to Alaska, restoring a long-suspended U.S. flag route.

Today the company, run by West's son, has six small cruise ships. It has a legitimate claim to knowing Alaska from the insider's point of view, and the small vessels allow guests to get up close and personal to whales and other aquatic life, and the occasional bear on shore.

The ships are all less than 100 tons, which allows them unrestricted access to Glacier Bay; larger vessels must vie for a limited number of permits. As American-flagged vessels, they can sail from Seattle to Alaska without making a stop in Canada.

Other journeys include Tracy Arm for an upclose visit with South Sawyer Glacier, LeConte Bay, and narrow inlets off Glacier Bay. The line claims it has the only ships that regularly sail through Wrangell Narrows, rarely visited El Capitan, and Sea Otter Sound.

The company's longer tours—14 to 19 days—begin in Fairbanks or Anchorage and include rail, bus, and boat tours in central Alaska, and then include a flight to Juneau for a five-day cruise in the southeast portion of the state.

Alaska itineraries generally run from about April through October, after which time the ships migrate south to California and down to Mexico for explorations of Baja California.

California trips include San Francisco to the Napa-Carneros-Sonoma wine region and a visit to Old Sacramento.

In recent winters, the company has based the Spirit of Endeavour in Cabo San Lucas to explore the Sea of Cortés in Mexico, home to many species of wildlife, including visits to remote desert beaches. Available shore excursions include a visit to Copper Canyon with a trip on the South Orient Express; the railroad, which took almost 100 years to build, travels from sea level to almost 8,000 feet, across 36 bridges and through 86 tunnels, including a 360-degree spiral through a mile-long tunnel.

The Alaska Sightseeing/Cruise West Experience

Four vessels include bow landing platforms, permitting the ships to offload passengers in many locations without having to use tenders. (This harkens back to the sternwheeler riverboats of the American heartland.)

Passengers are generally permitted to visit the bridge while the ships are underway, which allows guests to chat with the captain and consult charts and radar screens.

The dining room emphasizes the cuisine of the Pacific Northwest. Orders for dinner entrees are often taken the night before the meal; special requests can often be met.

These are decidedly casual cruises, with an open seating for meals and little in the way of entertainment—except for the spectacular passing scenery. And aside from your cabin, there are not many quiet hideaways away from the other guests. When the ship overnights in a port, the concierge will make dinner reservations and provide transportation to shore points.

Spirit of '98

Econoguide rating:	★★★
Ship size:	**Small**
Category:	**Adventure**
Price range:	**Opulent $$$$**
Registry:	United States
Year built:	1984 (As *Pilgrim Belle* of American Cruise Line; later the *Colonial Explorer* of Exploration Cruise Line; and *Victorian Empress* of St. Lawrence Cruises. Refurbished 1995.)
Itinerary:	Spring, in Columbia and Snake rivers; summer, Alaska's Inside Passage; fall, California Wine Country
Information:	(800) 888-9378
Website:	www.cruisewest.com
Passenger capacity:	96 (double occupancy)
Crew:	26
Passenger-to-Crew Ratio:	3.7:1
Tonnage:	96
Length:	192 feet
Beam:	40 feet
Draft:	9.3 feet
Cruising speed:	13 knots
Guest decks:	4
Total cabins:	49
Outside:	48
Inside:	0
Suites:	1
Wheelchair cabins:	1
Cuisine:	Dining rooms has single, open seating
Style:	Casual
Price notes:	Two single cabins available, 125 percent to 175 percent supplement
Tipping suggestions:	$10 pp/pd

A modern-day recreation of a Victorian-era riverboat, with nice attention to detail. The *Spirit of '98* was built to resemble old-time coastal cruising vessels; her Gay Nineties interior includes carved cabinetry, etched glass and plush upholstery, In the summer of 1997, the ship helped lead a centennial celebration of the Klondike Gold Rush.

In the summer, the *Spirit of '98* travels the Inside Passage between Seattle and Juneau, moving to the California Wine Country in the fall.

Staterooms on this ship are among the largest in the Alaska Sightseeing/Cruise West fleet.

In the summer of 1999, the *Spirit of '98* suffered an unpleasant encounter with a rock about 16 miles into Tracy Arm in Alaska's Inside Passage. There were no reports of injuries or fuel spills, and all 93 passengers were transferred to another boat by inflatable rafts.

The ship was about 100 yards from shore in the passage when it struck a rock and began taking on water. Some of the ship's crew members remained aboard to operate pumps, and with the aid of the U.S. Coast Guard and another cruise ship, the *Regal Princess,* the flooding was controlled and the ship was rescued.

Spirit of Alaska

Econoguide rating:	★★★
Ship size:	**Small**
Category:	**Adventure**
Price range:	**Opulent $$$$**
Registry:	United States
Year built:	1980 (Built as *Pacific Northwest Explorer* of Exploration Cruise Lines)
Sister ship:	*Spirit of Columbia*
Itinerary:	Spring and fall, Columbia and Snake rivers; summer, Alaska's Inside Passage
Information:	(800) 888-9378
Website:	www.cruisewest.com
Passenger capacity:	78 (double occupancy)
Crew:	21
Passenger-to-Crew Ratio:	3.7:1
Tonnage:	97
Length:	143 feet
Beam:	28 feet
Draft:	7.5 feet
Cruising speed:	12 knots
Guest decks:	4
Total cabins:	39
Outside:	27
Inside:	12
Suites:	3
Wheelchair cabins:	0
Cuisine:	Single, open seating dining room
Style:	Casual
Tipping suggestions:	$10 pp/pd

The *Spirit of Alaska* cruises Prince William Sound in the summer and the Columbia and Snake rivers in the spring and fall. Guests are accommodated in staterooms that range from lower-deck, inside cabins that have two single beds to upper-deck cabins that have double beds or two single beds, as well as view windows. *Spirit of Alaska* is the twin sister to the *Spirit of Columbia.*

Spirit of Columbia

Econoguide rating:	★★★
Ship size:	**Small**
Category:	**Adventure**
Price range:	**Opulent $$$$**
Registry:	United States
Year built:	1979 (As *New Shoreham II.* Refurbished 1995)
Sister ship:	*Spirt of Alaska*
Itinerary:	Spring, British Columbia and islands of the Pacific Northwest; summer, Prince William Sound; fall, British Columbia

Information:	(800) 888-9378
Website:	www.cruisewest.com
Passenger capacity:	78 (double occupancy)
Crew:	21
Passenger-to-Crew Ratio:	3.7:1
Tonnage:	98
Length:	143 feet
Beam:	28 feet
Draft:	6.5 feet
Cruising speed:	9 knots
Guest decks:	3
Total cabins:	38
Outside:	27
Inside:	11
Suites:	4
Wheelchair cabins:	0
Cuisine:	Single, open seating dining room
Style:	Casual
Tipping suggestions:	$10 pp/pd

The *Spirit of Columbia* sails weekly in the summer between Ketchikan and Juneau. In the Spring and Fall, the Spirit of Columbia cruises Canada's Inside Passage round trip from Seattle.

The ship, sister to the *Spirit of Alaska,* carries 78 guests.

Spirit of Discovery

Econoguide rating:	★★★
Ship size:	**Small**
Category:	**Adventure**
Price range:	**Opulent $$$$**
Registry:	United States
Year built:	1976 (As *Independence* for American Cruise Line, later *Columbia.* Refurbished 1992)
Itinerary:	Spring and fall, Columbia and Snake rivers; summer, Alaska's Inside Passages
Information:	(800) 888-9378
Website:	www.cruisewest.com
Passenger capacity:	84 (double occupancy)
Crew:	21 American
Passenger-to-Crew Ratio:	4:1
Tonnage:	94
Length:	166 feet
Beam:	37 feet
Draft:	7.5 feet
Cruising speed:	13 knots
Guest decks:	3
Total cabins:	43
Outside:	43
Inside:	0
Suites:	0
Wheelchair cabins:	0
Cuisine:	Single, open seating dining room
Style:	Casual
Price notes:	Two single cabins available at 125 percent to 175 percent premium
Tipping suggestions:	$10 pp/pd

The *Spirit of Discovery* sails within Alaska between Ketchikan and Juneau in the summer, and in the fall cruises the Columbia and Snake rivers.

Spirit of Endeavor

Econoguide rating:	★★★★
Ship size:	**Small**
Category:	**Adventure**
Price range:	**Opulent $$$$**
Registry:	United States
Year built:	1983 (Built as *Newport Clipper* for Clipper Cruise Line, later *Sea Spirit*. Refurbished 1996, 1999)
Itinerary:	Winter, Baja Mexico; April to September, Alaska's Inside Passage; September to November, California Wine Country from San Francisco
Information:	(800) 888-9378
Website:	www.cruisewest.com
Passenger capacity:	102 (double occupancy)
Crew:	28
Passenger-to-Crew Ratio:	3.6:1
Tonnage:	95
Length:	217 feet
Beam:	37 feet
Draft:	8.5 feet
Cruising speed:	12 knots
Guest decks:	4
Total cabins:	51
Outside:	51
Inside:	0
Suites:	0
Wheelchair cabins:	0
Cuisine:	Single, open seating dining room
Style:	Casual
Price notes:	125 percent to 175 percent single supplement
Tipping suggestions:	$10 pp/pd

The *Spirit of Endeavour* is the flagship of the fleet; and it offers the line's largest public areas. The ship cruises the Inside Passage between Seattle and Juneau in the summer, moving to California Wine Country in the fall, and on to Baja Mexico's Sea of Cortés in the winter.

Spirit of Glacier Bay

Econoguide rating:	★★★
Ship size:	**Small**
Category:	**Adventure**
Price range:	**Premium $$$**
Registry:	United States
Year built:	1971 (As *New Shoreham I* for American Canadian Caribbean Line. Refurbished 1996)
Itinerary:	Summer, Alaska's Prince William Sound; spring and fall, Columbia and Snake rivers
Information:	(800) 888-9378
Website:	www.cruisewest.com
Passenger capacity:	54 (double occupancy)
Crew:	16
Passenger-to-Crew Ratio:	3.4:1

Tonnage:	97
Length:	125 feet
Beam:	28 feet
Draft:	6.5 feet
Cruising speed:	10 knots
Guest decks:	4
Total cabins:	27
Outside:	14
Inside:	13
Suites:	0
Wheelchair cabins:	0
Cuisine:	Single, open seating dining room
Style:	Casual
Price notes:	Single cabins at 125 percent to 175 percent premium
Tipping suggestions:	$10 pp/pd

The smaller *Spirit of Glacier Bay* operates on Prince William Sound cruises, making use of her 125-foot length and shallow draft to explore the nooks and crannies of those beautiful waters.

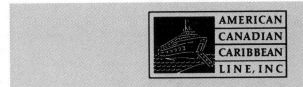

American Canadian Caribbean Line
461 Water St.
Warren, RI 02885
Information: (800) 556-7450
www.accl-smallships.com

American Canadian Caribbean Line Fleet

Grande Caribe. (1997) 100 passengers. 761 tons

Grande Mariner. (1998) 100 passengers. 781 tons

Niagara Prince. (1994) 84 passengers. 687 tons

A multinational name for a small but ambitious American-flagged cruise line. The line's three vessels sail a grand tour of the Americas, including the Mississippi, Great Lakes, Erie Canal, Newfoundland and Labrador, as well as the Caribbean and Central America to ports including the Virgin Islands, Antigua, Nassau, Trinidad and Tobago, Panama, Venezuela, Belize,Guatemala, and Hondura. Another interesting itinerary travels from Rhode Island to Buffalo, through New York City, Albany, and across the Erie Canal.

The twin flagships of the line are the *Grande Mariner* and the *Grande Caribe,* each having a capacity of 100 passengers. The third ship is the slightly smaller *Niagara Prince,* which carries 84 passengers.

ACCL was founded in 1966 by ship builder Luther Blount; all of the vessels are constructed at Blount Industries in Warren, Rhode Island. The company is one of the last working shipyards in New England building mid-sized metal boats, producing more than 300 ships since it began in 1949. In early 2000, Blount was still at the helm of the company, now in his 80s.

One of the goals of ACCL is to explore smaller waterways and ports. The vessels are custom-designed for that purpose, with shallow drafts and other features such as bow ramps for easy unloading of passengers directly to shore and an innovative retractable pilot house that permits the ships to sail under low bridges on waterways such as the Erie Canal. According to the company, Blount "seeks out unusual places and then builds the ships to take us there."

Cabins and public areas are simple and functional. There's no room service, no frills, no glitz, and a bring-your-own-bottle bar policy. The company's emphasis is much more on the destinations sailed by its ships than the ships themselves. Other nice features include glass-bottom launches on most trips.

Grande Caribe

Econoguide rating:	★★★
Ship size:	**Small**
Category:	**Adventure**
Price range:	**Premium $$$**
Registry:	United States
Year built:	1997
Itinerary:	Winter, in Panama; spring, in Intracoastal Waterway from Florida to Rhode Island; summer, in Atlantic Canada, and fall, Hudson River and Erie Canal
Information:	(800) 556-7450, (401) 247-0955
Website:	www.accl-smallships.com
Passenger capacity:	100 (double occupancy)
Crew:	17
Passenger-to-Crew Ratio:	6:1
Tonnage:	761 tons
Length:	183 feet
Beam:	40 feet
Draft:	6.6 feet
Cruising speed:	10 knots
Guest decks:	3
Total cabins:	50
Outside:	50
Inside:	0
Suites:	0
Wheelchair cabins:	Stair lifts
Cuisine:	One dining room on main deck accommodates all passengers for single-seating dining. Bring your own bottle.
Style:	Always casual
Price notes:	Single occupancy premium 175 percent in certain cabin classifications. Certain cabins on each vessel accommodate a third passenger at a 15 percent discount for each occupant.
Tipping suggestions:	Gratuities are left to discretion of guests

A comfortable soft adventure ship with some special features that are well-suited to small harbors and landings. The ship's small draft enables access to shallow rivers, canals and waterways; a retractable pilot house allows ships to maneuver under low bridges and locks. A bow ramp allows the ship to make its own landings on beaches and river banks.

ACCL brings along experts on wildlife, marine biology, flora and fauna and local indigenous cultures.

Like the other vessels in the ACCL fleet, this is a no-frills operation. You will not find room service, casinos, swimming pools, and formal dinners. The Vista View Lounge has a bring-your-own-bottle policy.

Grande Mariner

Econoguide rating:	★★★
Ship size:	**Small**
Category:	**Adventure**
Price range:	**Premium $$$**
Registry:	United States
Year built:	1998
Itinerary:	Winter, in Eastern Caribbean; spring and fall, in Intracoastal Waterway from Florida to Philadelphia and Rhode Island; summer, Erie Canal, New England, and Atlantic Canada
Information:	(800) 556-7450, (401) 247-0955
Website:	www.accl-smallships.com
Passenger capacity:	100 (double occupancy)
Crew:	17
Passenger-to-Crew Ratio:	6:1
Tonnage:	781 tons
Length:	183 feet
Beam:	40 feet
Draft:	6.6 feet
Cruising speed:	10 knots
Guest decks:	3
Total cabins:	50
Outside:	50
Inside:	0
Suites:	0
Wheelchair cabins:	Stair lifts
Cuisine:	One dining room on main deck accommodates all passengers for single-seating dining. Bring your own bottle.
Style:	Always casual
Price notes:	Single occupancy premium 175 percent in certain cabin classifications. Certain cabins on each vessel accommodate a third passenger at a 15 percent discount for each occupant
Tipping suggestions:	Gratuities are left to the discretion of guests.

The *Grande Mariner*'s philosophy and set of offerings are similar to those of the *Grande Caribe.*

Niagara Prince

Econoguide rating:	★★★
Ship size:	**Small**
Category:	**Adventure**
Price range:	**Premium $$$**
Registry:	United States
Year built:	1994
Information:	(800) 556-7450, (401) 247-0955
Website:	www.accl-smallships.com
Passenger capacity:	84 (double occupancy)
Crew:	17

Itinerary:	Winter, Belize and Guatemala; spring, Intracoastal Waterway from New Orleans to Texas; summer, Chicago and Great Lakes, Quebec City; fall, in Erie Canal
Passenger-to-Crew Ratio:	5:1
Tonnage:	687 tons
Length:	175 feet
Beam:	40 feet
Draft:	6.3 feet
Cruising speed:	10 knots
Guest decks:	3 decks
Total cabins:	42
Outside:	42
Inside:	0
Suites:	0
Wheelchair cabins:	Stair lifts
Cuisine:	One dining room on main deck accommodates all passengers for single-seating dining. Bring your own bottle.
Style:	Always casual
Price notes:	Single occupancy premium 175 percent. Certain cabins accommodate a third passenger at a 15 percent discount for each occupant.
Tipping suggestions:	Gratuities are left to discretion of guests

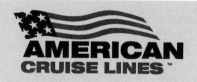

American Cruise Lines
One Marine Park
Haddam, CT 06438
Information: (860) 345-3311
www.americancruiselines.com

American Cruise Lines Fleet

American Eagle. (2000.) 49 passengers. 1,200 tons.

American Eagle began her coastal cruiser career in April of 2000, journeying up and down the Eastern Seaboard. Some trips explore from Connecticut to New York, and then up the Hudson to Albany. Other itineraries visit Block Island, Nantucket, Martha's Vineyard, New Bedford, and Newport. In her first season, she will head south in October to Chesapeake Bay and Williamsburg, South Carolina and then spend January through April operating from Fort Myers on Florida inland waterway cruises; returning to the northeast in June.

American Eagle

Econoguide rating:	★★★	
Ship size:	**Small**	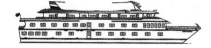
Category:	**Adventure**	
Price range:	**Premium $$$**	
Registry:	United States	
Year built:	2000	

Itinerary:	New England, Hudson River, East Coast
Information:	(860) 345-3311
Website:	www.americancruiselines.com
Passenger capacity:	49 (double occupancy)
Crew:	22 American
Passenger-to-Crew Ratio:	2.2:1
Tonnage:	1,200
Length:	162 feet
Beam:	39 feet
Draft:	7 feet
Cruising speed:	11 knots
Guest decks:	3 passenger decks and 1 sun deck
Total cabins:	31
Outside:	31
Inside:	0
Suites:	1
Wheelchair cabins:	0
Cuisine:	American cuisine.
Style:	Casual
Tipping suggestions:	$14.25 pp/pd

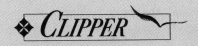

Clipper Cruise Line
7711 Bonhomme Ave.
St. Louis, MO 63105
Information: (800) 325-0010, (314) 727-2929
www.clippercruise.com

Clipper Cruise Line Fleet

Clipper Odyssey. (1989.) 120 passengers. 5,050 tons. Sails in Southeast Asia, Australia, New Zealand, and North Pacific.

Clipper Adventurer. (1975, rebuilt 1998) 122 passengers, 4,364 tons

Nantucket Clipper. (1984) 102 passengers, 1,471 tons

Yorktown Clipper. (1988) 138 passengers, 2,354 tons

The Clipper ships emphasize expeditions to unusual destinations; there are no casinos, Las Vegas-type shows, or glitzy gift shops aboard. And the accommodations and public rooms are comfortable but hardly posh.

The small ships travel to places as diverse as the hidden fjords of Alaska, Caribbean coves, the Intracoastal Waterway of the U.S. South, the coast of New England, the Guadalquiver River of Spain, and the icescapes of Antarctica.

The line's two U.S.-flagged ships, the *Nantucket Clipper* and the *Yorktown Clipper,* were designed with shallow draft and easy maneuverability for coastal trips along the mainland United States, Alaska, Canada, Mexico, the Caribbean, and Central and South America.

The *Clipper Adventurer* was built in 1975 as the Russian research vessel *Alla Tarasova;* and it has a hardened hull that allows her to navigate in rugged natural environments including ice fields. It was completely converted in 1998 for use as a small oceangoing cruiseship, with a remake of all of the cabins and public rooms; stabilizers were added later in the year. She includes a fleet of 10 Zodiac landing craft.

In late 1999, the company added a fourth ship. The *Clipper Odyssey* (originally the *Oceanic Odyssey*) is a small luxury vessel that has sailed in and around Bali, Singapore, and Australia for an Indonesian company since it was built in 1989. The 340-foot-long, 5,200-ton vessel can accommodate 120 passengers.

Plans call for cruises around Australia's Great Barrier Reef and New Zealand in early 2000, then heading off to China, Japan, and the islands of the North Pacific, including Russia's Kamchatka Peninsula for the summer. In the fall of 2000, she will return to Southeast Asia and Australia.

The *Clipper Adventurer's* cruise itineraries in 2000 include Antartica and the Falkland Islands; South America; the Mediterranean; the Kiel Canal and the Baltic; England, Scotland, Denmark, Iceland, and Greenland; across the Northwest Passage to Ottawa; Canada; Arctic and Maritime Canada; down the coast of North America, and back to South America for the fall of 2000.

The *Nantucket Clipper* and *Yorktown Clipper* were built specifically for the line, with shallow draft and quick maneuverability to provide access to secluded areas beyond the reach of the larger ships and mainstream tourism.

In 2000, the *Yorktown Clipper* was due to sail in Costa Rica and the Panama Canal; up the west coast to British Columbia and into Alaska's Inside Passage; through the Pacific Northwest, and in the inland waterways of Northern California before making her way back to the Caribbean for the winter.

The *Nantucket Clipper's* itineraries for 2000 include Colonial America with stops along the coasts of the Carolinas and Virginia; springtime in Chesapeake Bay; up the coast to New England and Nova Scotia; through Maritime Canada and the Thousand Islands; through French Canada and across the Great Lakes to Chicago; fall in New England; a trip up New York's Hudson River, turning around and continuing to Alexandria, Virginia, and passage along the Intracoastal Waterway enroute to the Caribbean for the winter.

The Clipper Experience

All of Clipper's voyages feature guest speakers, including naturalists, historians, and other experts. On cruises through the South, a Civil War historian gives lectures. On Alaskan cruises, guests are accompanied by a park ranger and naturalist.

Clipper Cruise Line was founded in 1982 in St. Louis. In 1996, Clipper was purchased by INTRAV, a deluxe-tour operator that was a sister company. In 1999, Clipper and INTRAV were in turn purchased by a Swiss company, Kuoni Travel Holding Ltd.

Clipper Adventurer

Econoguide rating:	★★★★
Ship size:	**Small**
Category:	**Adventure**
Price range:	**Premium $$$**
Registry:	Bahamas
Year built:	(Built as Russian research vessel *Alla Tarasova*. Rebuilt 1997–98)
Itinerary:	May to July, western Europe; July and August, Greenland and the Arctic; September to November, Mexico and the Americas; November to December, Europe; January Antarctica.
Information:	(800) 325-0010
Website:	www.clippercruise.com
Passenger capacity:	122 (double occupancy)
Crew:	72 International crew
Passenger-to-Crew Ratio:	1.7:1
Tonnage:	4,364 tons
Passenger Space Ratio:	35.8
Length:	338 feet
Beam:	53.2 feet
Draft:	15.3 feet
Cruising speed:	14 knots
Guest decks:	4
Total cabins:	61
Outside:	61
Inside:	0
Suites:	3
Cuisine:	American and Continental cuisine
Style:	Casual and comfortable. No formal clothing or evening wear required
Price notes:	Single occupancy premium approximately 150 percent
Tipping suggestions:	$9 pp/pd

A relatively new vessel, especially after its 1998 conversion from its former life as a Russian research ship, the *Clipper Adventurer* in some ways harks back to the style at the heyday of the steamship era in the 1930s and 1940s.

Public rooms are small and club-like, including the Clipper Club & Bar, and an intimate Library/Card Room. The ship includes a covered promenade, sheltered from the weather. The windowed dining room accommodates all passengers at a single seating. The Main Lounge and Bar will accommodate a full passenger load.

I toured the ship soon after her arrival in America when she set anchor outside the harbor of Nantucket island. Most of her load of passengers clambered onto the ship's 10 Zodiacs for a choppy ride through October seas into town; others stayed onboard to listen to a lecture by a local artist.

An important part of the entertainment is educational—historians, naturalists and other experts are often on the cruises or come aboard in port. They replace variety shows and bingo. There's no gambling, no disco, and no television sets in the staterooms.

The cabins and public rooms were airy and well-appointed with Scandinavian furnishings. An attractive dining room offered windows on three sides. The bridge was open to visitors.

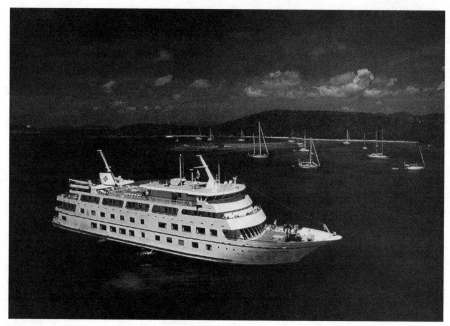

Clipper Cruise Line's Nantucket Clipper
Photo by Wolfgang Kaehler, courtesty Clipper Cruise Line

The *Clipper Adventurer's* cruise itineraries include expeditions to Antarctica, Greenland, Iceland, the Norwegian Arctic and Baffin Island, as well as visits to Portugal, Madeira, the Canary Islands, Morocco, Gibraltar, Spain, France, Belgium, Holland, Germany, Denmark, Poland, Lithuania, Latvia, Estonia, Russia, Finland, Sweden, England, Ireland, Scotland, Orkney Island, Shetland Islands, Norway, Newfoundland, Nova Scotia, the U.S. east coast, the Caribbean, the Orinoco and Amazon rivers, Brazil, Uruguay, and Argentina.

Nantucket Clipper

Econoguide rating:	★★★
Ship size:	**Small**
Category:	**Adventure**
Price range:	**Premium $$$**
Registry:	United States
Year built:	1984
Itinerary:	Spring and fall, Intracoastal waterway; June to August, Great Lakes and St. Lawrence River; winter, Caribbean; spring and fall, Eastern Seaboard
Information:	(800) 325-0010
Website:	www.clippercruise.com
Passenger capacity:	102 (double occupancy)
Crew:	32 American
Passenger-to-Crew Ratio:	3.2:1
Tonnage:	1,471
Length:	207 feet
Beam:	37 feet

Draft:	8 feet
Cruising speed:	8 knots
Guest decks:	4
Total cabins:	51
Outside:	51
Inside:	0
Suites:	0
Wheelchair cabins:	0
Cuisine:	American and Continental cuisine.
Style:	Casual and comfortable. No formal clothing or evening wear required.
Price notes:	Single occupancy premium 150 percent of category 2.
Tipping suggestions:	$9 pp/pd

It's a basic small ship for a cruise line that focuses more on ports of call and sights along the way than on interior flash.

An important part of the entertainment is educational; historians, naturalists and other experts often are on the cruises, replacing variety shows, disco dancing, bingo, and gambling. In some ports, local musicians or artisans come aboard.

The young chefs are recruited from the Culinary Institute of America in upstate New York, the cabin and restaurant staff are bright-faced young (mostly) Americans who serve with casual friendliness.

Yorktown Clipper

Econoguide rating:	★★★
Ship size:	**Small**
Category:	**Adventure**
Price range:	**Premium $$$**
Registry:	United States
Year built:	1988
Itinerary:	May to July and September to November, Alaska, British Columbia and West Coast; March to April and November, Central America and Mexico's Baja Peninsula
Information:	(800) 325-0010
Website:	www.clippercruise.com
Passenger capacity:	138 (double occupancy)
Crew:	40 American
Passenger-to-Crew Ratio:	3.4:1
Tonnage:	2,354
Length:	257 feet
Beam:	43 feet
Draft:	8 feet
Cruising speed:	10 knots
Guest decks:	4
Total cabins:	69
Outside:	69
Inside:	0
Suites:	0
Wheelchair cabins:	0
Cuisine:	American and Continental cuisine
Style:	Casual and comfortable. No formal clothing or evening wear required.
Price notes:	Single occupancy premium 150 percent
Tipping suggestions:	$9 pp/pd

A relaxed country club atmosphere on an unpretentious small ship. The excitement comes from the ports of call and waterways. Again, historians, naturalists and other experts often are on the cruises, and local musicians, artisans, and representatives come aboard in some ports.

Delta Queen Coastal Voyages

Delta Queen Coastal Voyages
Robin Street Wharf
1380 Port of New Orleans Place
New Orleans, LA 70130-1890
Information: (504) 586-0631

Delta Queen Coastal Voyages Fleet

Unnamed coastal packet. (Spring 2001) 226 passengers. 1,580 tons

Delta Queen Coastal Voyages plans to set sail in 2001 with the first of as many as five new small coastal ships, inspired by the classic coastal packet steamers such as those of the Fall River Line, a famous fleet of East Coast vessels that flourished between 1847 and 1937.

The diesel-powered vessels, about 1,580 tons in capacity, will be 300 feet in length, and have a beam of 50 feet, and a 12.5-foot draft. Plans call for 114 passenger staterooms, including two Outside Owner's Suites, 99 outside staterooms, and 13 inside staterooms.

Although they're designed to echo classic old ships and include New England Federal and nautical decor, these new packets will be thoroughly modern with satellite television, VCRs, ship-to-shore telephone service, and other amenities.

The Dining Room will feature fine art and elaborate architectural embellishments; the Main Deck room will seat 144 guests for each of two seatings. The Grand Saloon will feature a dance floor, crystal basket lighting, an ornate stamped metal ceiling, and a row of tall windows along both sides; the room will be used for lectures, cabaret shows, and other entertainment.

On the East Coast, passengers will be able to explore the yachting meccas of Nova Scotia and New Brunswick, the northeast harbors of Boston, Martha's Vineyard, and New York, and from Chesapeake Bay down to Baltimore, Annapolis, Washington, D.C., Norfolk, Charleston, Savannah, and Florida.

Later ships will cruise in the Pacific Northwest, along the navigable paths of the Lewis & Clark expeditions on the Columbia River, past spectacular gorges, and through the lush Willamette River valley, which marks the end of the Oregon trail.

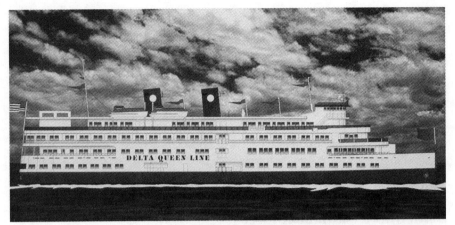

A model of the Delta Queen's planned coastal ship
Delta Queen Steamship Co.

In California, itineraries will include the Pacific Coast, Napa Valley wineries, Gold Country, Yosemite National Forest, Sacramento, and San Francisco.

The new cruise line is an offshoot of American Classic Voyages Co., which also operates the Delta Queen Steamboat Co., American Hawaii Cruises, and the United States Line.

Unnamed coastal packet (Preview, Spring 2001)

Econoguide rating:	**N/A**
Ship size:	**Small**
Category:	**Adventure**
Price range:	N/A
Registry:	United States
Year built:	2001
Itinerary:	Eastern Seaboard, Great Lakes, Caribbean, Mexico
Information:	(504) 586-0631
Website:	To be announced
Passenger capacity:	226 (double occupancy)
Crew:	To be announced
Passenger-to-Crew Ratio:	N/A
Tonnage:	1,580
Length:	300 feet
Beam:	50 feet
Draft:	12.5 feet
Cruising speed:	13 knots
Guest decks:	4
Total cabins:	114
Outside:	99
Inside:	40
Suites:	2
Wheelchair cabins:	2
Cuisine:	American regional cuisine
Style:	Casual by day, semi-formal night
Tipping suggestions:	To be announced

The Delta Queen Steamboat Co.

Delta Queen Steamboat Co.
Robin Street Wharf
1380 Port of New Orleans Place
New Orleans, LA 70130-1890
Information: (800) 543-7637
www.deltaqueen.com

Delta Queen Steamboat Fleet

Delta Queen. (1927) 174 passengers. 3,360 tons

American Queen. (1995) 436 passengers. 3,707 tons

Mississippi Queen. (1976, refurbished 1996) 414 passengers. 3,364 tons

Columbia Queen. (2000) 161 passengers. 1,599 tons

The Delta Queen Co. is the oldest U.S. flag cruise line, tracing its lineage back to 1890 when a young riverboat captain bought his first paddlewheeler.

The fleet founded by Capt. Gordon Greene and his wife Mary Becker Greene, also a licensed steamboat captain, eventually included 30 boats.

The flagship of today's fleet is the *Delta Queen,* a National Historic Landmark. She was launched in 1927, built with the finest woods available, including teak, oak, birch, and Oregon cedar; within she features Tiffany-styled stained glass windows and gleaming brass fixtures.

The larger *Mississippi Queen* was launched in 1976, and the even larger *American Queen* in 1995. In 2000, the fleet was joined by a new, small gem, the *Columbia Queen*, which will sail on the rivers of the Northwest.

These are real paddlewheelers—the main source of propulsion is that large, red contraption at the stern. (They are updated a bit with bow thrusters located below the waterline for maneuvering. They employ modern navigational devices as well.)

At the peak of the Steamboat era, from about 1811 to the turn of the century, there were more than 10,000 of these vessels on U.S. rivers.

Today, the Delta Queen Steamboat Company's boats explore the inner passage of America, on 10 major waterways. The main road, of course, is the Mississippi, which meanders some 2,350 miles from its mouth below New Orleans to St. Paul in Minnesota.

Ports on the lower Mississippi include New Orleans and Baton Rouge, Natchez and Vicksburg, Miss., and Memphis, Tenn. On the upper Mississippi, the steamboat ports include Cape Girardeau, St. Louis, and Hannibal, Mo.; Davenport and Dubuque, Iowa; and Red Wing and Minneapolis/St. Paul, Minn.

Other waterways plied by the Queens include the Ohio River as far as Pittsburgh; the Tennessee River to Chattanooga, Tenn. and Decatur, Ala.; the

Cumberland River to Nashville, Tenn.; the Arkansas River to Pine Bluff, Little Rock, and Fort Smith; the Kanawha River to Charleston, W. Va.; the Red River to Natchitoches and Shreveport, La., and the Intracoastal Waterway to destinations such as Port of Iberia, La., and Port Arthur and Galveston, Texas.

Onboard an old style steamboat, the master of ceremonies is the "Interlocutor;" and on the ships in the Delta Queen fleet, he oversees a cast of musicians and singers that pays tribute to American music from Stephen Foster to Dixieland Jazz to Bluegrass to Broadway.

For many, the meal service onboard the steamboats is worth the trip, even though it would not qualify as haute cuisine. The boats feature regional American specialties such as Bayou Stuffed Catfish, Cincinnati Five-Way Chili, Minnesota Wild Rice Soup, fried green tomatoes, and other down-home cooking.

The line also has an interesting mix of theme cruises, from Big Band to '50s Rock to Elvis and Mark Twain (not together). Several voyages are "tramping" itineraries; on these, the boat will stop at the whim of the captain.

The annual Great Steamboat Race of 2000, between the Delta Queen and Mississippi Queen, a most casual event, is scheduled to begin on June 24 in New Orleans and finish in St. Louis on July 5.

In 2000, the two larger ships, *Mississippi Queen* and *American Queen*, add musical revues: "Hooray for Hollywood," a collection of songs from the Silver Screen, and "Once More with Feeling," a journey through the past century of American popular song. Other continuing revues include "Dancing on Air," a simulated radio broadcast from the golden days of radio of the 1930s, featuring actual period music and actual radio commercials of the era.

Delta Queen

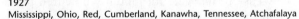

Econoguide rating:	★★★★
Ship size:	**Small**
Category:	**Adventure**
Price range:	**Premium $$$**
Registry:	United States
Year built:	1927
Itinerary:	Mississippi, Ohio, Red, Cumberland, Kanawha, Tennessee, Atchafalaya rivers, intracoastal waterways in Louisiana and Texas
Information:	(800) 543-7637
Website:	www.deltaqueen.com
Passenger capacity:	174 (double occupancy)
Crew:	75 American
Passenger-to-Crew Ratio:	2.32:1
Tonnage:	3,360
Passenger Space Ratio:	19.3
Length:	285 feet
Beam:	60 feet
Draft:	9 feet
Cruising speed:	10 miles per hour
Guest decks:	4
Total cabins:	87
Outside:	87
Inside:	0
Suites:	4
Wheelchair cabins:	0
Cuisine:	American regional cuisine

Style:	Casual by day, semi-formal at night
Price notes:	Single occupancy premium 150 percent to 175 percent
Tipping suggestions:	$10 pp/pd

Here's a chance to sail aboard a floating National Historic Landmark. The *Delta Queen* was launched in Stockton, Calif. in 1928 at a then-impressive cost of $1 million.

She boasts a fully welded steel hull; her superstructure and paddlewheel are made of various woods, reinforced with steel. The plates for the steel hulls were fabricated in Scotland and then shipped to California for assembly.

The ship operated as a coastal steamboat between San Francisco and Sacramento from 1927 through 1940. During World War II, painted Navy gray, the Delta Queen was operated as a U.S. Navy ferry in San Francisco bay.

After the war, the *Delta Queen* was auctioned off for $46,250 (a fraction of its original cost) by the government and purchased by Tom Greene, president of the Cincinnati-based Greene Line Steamers.

The next problem: getting the ship from California to the inland rivers. A huge watertight crate was constructed to protect the *Delta Queen* from the ocean, and she set off on a 5,000-mile-voyage from San Francisco—under tow, through the Panama Canal, north into the Gulf of Mexico, and finally up the Mississippi River to New Orleans—arriving May 21, 1947. There she was uncrated before setting off to Pittsburgh under steam for a major facelift.

The interior was restored and reconfigured for new staterooms and dining rooms. The *Delta Queen*'s steam calliope was recovered from the sunken show boat Water Queen, and installed on the paddlewheeler in 1947.

The *Delta Queen*'s twin, the *Delta King,* is a floating hotel in Sacramento.

The 44-ton paddlewheel is driven by a pair of steam engines with a combined 2,000 horsepower that is capable of producing a top speed of nearly 10 miles per hour. The ship's wooden superstructure was almost her undoing in the late 1960s, but the steamboat was granted by Congress an exemption from Federal safety legislation. The boat also does not have elevators and is not especially easy to navigate for mobility-impaired passengers; the *Mississippi Queen* and *American Queen* are more accommodating in this regard.

Most cruises include a historian, "riverlorian," or naturalist. Theme cruises in recent years included Mardi Gras, Spring Pilgrimage, Kentucky Derby, Cajun Culture, Mark Twain, Dickens on the Strand, and Old-Fashioned Holidays. There are no childrens' programs on the steamboats.

American Queen

Econoguide rating:	★★★★	
Ship size:	**Small**	
Category:	**Adventure**	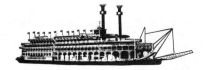
Price range:	**Premium $$$**	
Registry:	United States	
Year built:	1995	
Itinerary:	Mississippi and Ohio rivers	

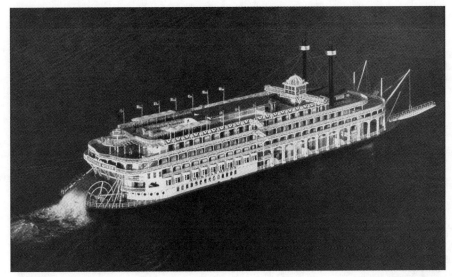

American Queen
Delta Queen Steamboat Co.

Information:	(800) 543-7637
Website:	www.deltaqueen.com
Passenger capacity:	436 (double occupancy)
Crew:	180 American
Passenger-to-Crew Ratio:	2.4:1
Tonnage:	3,707
Length:	418 feet
Beam:	89.4 feet
Draft:	8.6 feet
Cruising speed:	11 miles per hour, average 7 miles per hour
Guest decks:	6
Total cabins:	222
Outside:	168
Inside:	54
Suites:	24
Wheelchair cabins:	9
Cuisine:	American regional cuisine
Style:	Casual by day, semi-formal evenings
Price notes:	Single occupancy premium 150 percent to 175 percent
Tipping suggestions:	$10 pp/pd

The largest steamboat ever built, constructed in 1995 as a recreation of the opulent nineteenth century floating palaces. She stands 97 feet tall when her twin-fluted stacks are fully extended; the stacks and the pilot house can be lowered to 55 feet to pass beneath low bridges.

The ship is furnished largely with antique furniture, vintage artwork, photographs and books. Her J. M. White Dining Room has filigree woodwork, stunning chandeliers, and a full view of the riverside. The two-story Grand Saloon has private box seats in the mezzanine, in the style of an 1890s opera house. Other public rooms include the delicate Ladies' Parlor, the leather-upholstered Gentlemen's Card Room, and the Engine Room Bar. The ship's library has more than 600 volumes, including many classic, turn-of-the-century books.

The ship still uses steam to propel its 30-foot-wide 45-ton paddlewheel; the builders refurbished a pair of 1930s-era steam engines that originally drove the U.S. Army Corps of Engineers dredge *Kennedy.*

Nearly every cruise has a theme; recent cruises included Dixie Fest, Gardens of the River, the Civil War, 1950s Rockin' on the River, Fall Foliage, and Old-Fashioned Thanksgiving, and Southern Christmas holidays.

Historians, "riverlorians," and naturalists present talks about the history, culture and lore of the river. There are no childrens' programs.

Mississippi Queen

Econoguide rating:	★★★★
Ship size:	**Small**
Category:	**Adventure**
Price range:	**Premium $$$**
Registry:	United States
Year built:	1976 (Refurbished 1996)
Itinerary:	Mississippi, Ohio, Cumberland rivers
Information:	(800) 543-7637
Website:	www.deltaqueen.com
Passenger capacity:	416 (double occupancy)
Crew:	156 American
Passenger-to-Crew Ratio:	2.6:1
Tonnage:	3,364
Length:	382 feet
Beam:	68 feet
Draft:	9 feet
Cruising speed:	11 miles per hour
Guest decks:	7
Total cabins:	208
Outside:	135
Inside:	73
Suites:	26
Wheelchair cabins:	1
Cuisine:	American regional cuisine
Style:	Casual by day, semi-formal night
Tipping suggestions:	$8.50 pp/pd

The *Mississippi Queen* is a modern recreation of a classic steamboat, built in 1976 and refurbished in 1996 in Victorian style.

The boat was built at the former Howard Shipyard in Jeffersonville, Ill. where, beginning in 1834, more than 4,800 steamboats were built, including the famous J. M. White in 1878.

Half of the 208 staterooms offer a private veranda. All of the cabins are named after river towns, old riverboats, and historic Civil War sites. The *Mississippi Queen*'s calliope, with 44 whistles, is the world's largest.

The two-story Paddlewheel Lounge, decorated as an 1890s saloon, offers ragtime, Dixieland, and banjo music. In the Forward Cabin Lounge is a grand silver water cooler of the style of the Reed & Barton cooler that adorned the famed J. M. White steamboat. At midship, the Grand Staircase is topped with a trompe l'oeil ceiling of cherubs frolicking among the clouds.

Historians, "riverlorians", and naturalists accompany most cruises. In 1999, theme cruises include Big Band; Mardi Gras, Spring Pilgrimage, Kentucky Derby, Korean War Years, the Great Steamboat Race, and Old-Fashioned Thanksgiving and Southern Christmas holidays. There are no childrens' programs on the steamboats.

Columbia Queen

Econoguide rating:	★★★★
Ship size:	**Small**
Category:	**Adventure**
Price range:	**Premium $$$**
Registry:	United States
Year built:	2000
Itinerary:	Columbia, Snake, and Willamette rivers from Portland, Oregon
Information:	(800) 543-7637
Website:	www.deltaqueen.com
Passenger capacity:	161 (double occupancy)
Crew:	80 American
Passenger-to-Crew Ratio:	2:1
Tonnage:	1,599
Length:	218 feet
Beam:	60 feet
Draft:	12 feet
Cruising speed:	10 to 12 knots
Guest decks:	4
Total cabins:	81
Outside:	56
Inside:	25
Suites:	0
Wheelchair cabins:	1 cabin. Vessel is wheelchair accessible
Cuisine:	American regional cuisine
Style:	Casual by day, semi-formal evenings
Price notes:	Single occupancy premium 150 percent to 175 percent
Tipping suggestions:	$8.50 pp/pd

The newest riverboat in the fleet will begin service from its home port of Portland, Oregon in April of 2000. Seven-night cruises travel the Columbia River west to its mouth at Astoria, and then back upriver to Hood River, through the dramatic Columbia River Gorge, The Dalles, and through the Cascade Mountains to Pasco, Washington and as far east as Lewiston, Idaho before heading back to Portland.

The thoroughly modern version of an old riverboat includes 17 rooms with French balconies. The elegant two-tier Astoria Room is dining room, show room, and theater for the guests. Another attractive room is the Back Porch, aft on the Observation deck. On nice days, the French doors and windows are open to the fresh Pacific Northwest air.

Vacations are sold as eight-night trips including an overnight in Portland before departure.

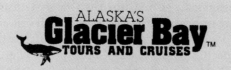

Glacier Bay Tours and Cruises
226 Second Ave.
Seattle, WA 98119
Information: (800) 451-5952, (206) 623-7110
www.glacierbaytours.com

The Glacier Bay Fleet

Executive Explorer. (1986) 49 passengers. 98 tons

Wilderness Adventurer. (1983) 74 passengers. 98 tons

Wilderness Discoverer. (1993) 86 passengers. 95 tons

Wilderness Explorer. (1969) 36 passengers. 98 tons

A small fleet of intimate "soft adventure" ships, now owned by an Alaskan company; Glacier Bay makes the most of its shallow-draft vessels to explore some of the more remote inlets of our most isolated state. The ships visit Alaska's Inside Passage, Glacier Bay National Park, Tracy Arm Fjord, and Admiralty Island National Monument.

All voyages include the option for sea kayaking and onshore hiking.

Executive Explorer

Econoguide rating:	★★★
Ship size:	**Small**
Category:	**Adventure**
Price range:	**Opulent $$$$**
Registry:	United States
Year built:	1986
Itinerary:	May to September from Ketchikan or Juneau to Alaska's Inside Passage, Glacier Bay National Park, and Tracy Arm Fjord
Information:	(800) 451-5952
Website:	www.glacierbaytours.com
Passenger capacity:	49 passengers (double occupancy)
Crew:	18 American
Passenger-to-Crew Ratio:	2.7:1
Tonnage:	98
Length:	98.5 feet
Beam:	36.75 feet
Draft:	8 feet
Cruising speed:	18 knots
Guest decks:	4
Total cabins:	25
Outside:	25
Inside:	0
Suites:	0
Wheelchair cabins:	0

Cuisine:	Alaskan cuisine
Style:	Casual
Price notes:	Single occupancy premium 175 percent of cabin category chosen. Triple and Quad rates upon request
Tipping suggestions:	$10 pp/pd

A twin-hulled catamaran that looks as if a cruise line ship had been shortened by a deli slicer, the *Executive Explorer* makes the most of its shape, offering large windows from cabins and dining rooms and views from the top-level open deck. The catamaran design allows the ship to cruise faster than many other smaller ships.

A typical itinerary includes the Tracy Arm Fjord and a close-up encounter with the Sawyer Glaciers, a cruise of Lynn Canal to Haines and the Gold Rush town of Skagway, a visit to Glacier Bay, a stop in the former Russian capital of Sitka, and a stop at the tiny Tlingit native village of Kake.

Wilderness Adventurer

Econoguide rating:	★★★
Ship size:	**Small**
Category:	**Adventure**
Price range:	**Premium $$$**
Registry:	United States
Year built:	1983 (As *Caribbean Prince* of American Canadian Caribbean Line)
Itinerary:	From Juneau through Alaska's Inside Passage; Glacier Bay, Chichagof and Baranof Islands; Tracy Arm Fjord; Mexico's Sea of Cortés from January to March
Information:	(800) 451-5952
Website:	www.glacierbaytours.com
Passenger capacity:	72 passengers (double occupancy)
Crew:	19 American
Passenger-to-Crew Ratio:	3.8:1
Tonnage:	89
Length:	156.6 feet
Beam:	38 feet
Draft:	6.5 feet
Cruising speed:	10 knots
Guest decks:	4. Kayak launch platform
Total cabins:	34
Outside:	All outside; B cabins have no windows
Inside:	0
Suites:	0
Cuisine:	Alaskan cuisine
Style:	Casual
Price notes:	Single supplement 175 percent of cabin category chosen. Triple rates on request.
Tipping suggestions:	$10 pp/pd

The *Wilderness Adventurer* carries a fleet of stable, two-person sea kayaks for up-close exploration of Southeast Alaska's spectacular shoreline. The ship also has a bow ramp for easy access to the shore.

The ship had a minor mishap in June of 1999 in Glacier Bay National Park and Reserve, going aground and spilling more than 200 gallons of fuel.

Wilderness Discoverer

Econoguide rating:	★★★
Ship size:	**Small**
Category:	**Adventure**
Price range:	**Premium $$$**
Registry:	United States
Year built:	1993 (As *Mayan Prince* for American Canadian Caribbean Line)
Itinerary:	Alaska's Inside Passage and Glacier Bay
Information:	(800) 451-5952
Website:	www.glacierbaytours.com
Passenger capacity:	88 passengers (double occupancy)
Crew:	19. American
Passenger-to-Crew Ratio:	4.6:1
Tonnage:	95
Length:	169 feet
Beam:	38 feet
Cruising speed:	12 knots
Guest decks:	4
Total cabins:	42
Outside:	All are outside, but category B staterooms have no windows
Inside:	0
Suites:	0
Cuisine:	Alaskan specialties
Style:	Casual
Price notes:	Single supplement 175 percent. Triple rate on request.
Tipping suggestions:	$10 pp/pd

Wilderness Explorer

Econoguide rating:	★★★
Ship size:	**Small**
Category:	**Adventure**
Price range:	**Premium $$$**
Registry:	United States
Year built:	1969
Itinerary:	Alaska's Inside Passage, Glacier Bay, Tracy Arm Fjord
Information:	(800) 451-5952
Website:	www.glacierbaytours.com
Passenger capacity:	34 (double occupancy)
Crew:	13 American
Passenger-to-Crew Ratio:	2.6:1
Tonnage:	98
Length:	112 feet
Beam:	22 feet
Cruising speed:	9 knots
Guest decks:	3. Kayak launch platform
Total cabins:	17
Outside:	All outside
Inside:	0
Suites:	0
Cuisine:	Alaskan cuisine
Style:	Casual
Price notes:	Single supplement 175 percent
Tipping suggestions:	$10 pp/pd

Luxury lies beyond the windows, not in the small but comfortable cabins and public rooms. *Wilderness Explorer* ran aground in an inlet 70 miles west of Juneau in July of 1999; there were no injuries and the ship was repaired.

S V E N · O L O F   L I N D B L A D ' S
SPECIAL👁EXPEDITIONS

Lindblad Special Expeditions
720 Fifth Ave.
New York, NY 10019
Information: (800) 397-3348
www.expeditions.com

Lindblad Special Expeditions Fleet

Sea Bird. (1981) 70 passengers. 100 tons.

Sea Lion. (1982) 70 passengers 100 tons.

The Lindblad family has been taking travelers to extraordinary destinations since 1979, visiting Alaska, the Pacific Northwest, Baja California, Central and South America, the Galapagos Islands, Western Europe, Egypt, the Baltics, Antarctica, the Mediterranean, Australia, and New Zealand.

The company traces its roots to Lars-Eric Lindblad, who began a travel agency in 1958 specializing in visits to far-flung places such as Antarctica, the Galapagos, China, Mongolia, Tibet, and Africa. Today, the company is run by his son, Sven-Olof.

The company's fleet of ocean-going vessels carry between 30 and 110 passengers; the ships are equipped with Zodiac landing craft and some also carry sea kayaks. These are tours for active travelers—swimmers, kayakers, snorkelers, hikers, and observers of all sorts. The onboard entertainment consists of naturalists and scientists who explain the views all around.

The company's 70-passenger *Sea Bird* and *Sea Lion,* which visit Alaska, the Columbia and Snake Rivers of the Pacific Northwest, Baja California, and southern Florida, are covered in this book. Lindblad also owns the 80-passenger expedition ship *Polaris,* which sails in Central and South America, and the 110-passenger *Caledonian Star,* which sails in the Mediterranean, the Caribbean, South America, and Antarctica.

On these small ships, the accommodations and public areas can best be described as casual and intimate. There are open sun decks for observation, a dining room, and a lounge. Don't look for a casino, hydrotherapy pool, or a virtual reality/multimedia entertainment center; the excitement is outside.

Sea Bird

Econoguide rating:	★★★
Ship size:	**Small**
Category:	**Adventure**
Price range:	**Premium $$$**
Registry:	United States
Year built:	1981

Itinerary:	Alaska, Pacific Northwest, Baja California
Information:	(800) 397-3348
Website:	www.expeditions.com
Passenger capacity:	70 (double occupancy)
Crew:	21 American
Passenger-to-Crew Ratio:	2.5:1
Tonnage:	100
Length:	152 feet
Beam:	31 feet
Draft:	8 feet
Cruising speed:	12 knots
Guest decks:	4
Total cabins:	37
Outside:	37
Inside:	0
Suites:	0
Wheelchair cabins:	Main deck, category 3 cabins. No elevators onboard.
Cuisine:	Continental
Style:	Informal
Price notes:	Single occupancy premium about 150 percent
Tipping suggestions:	$9 pp/pd

This is a comfortable transport to some of the most remote places on earth. Guests venture out in Zodiac landing craft to view whales and explore onshore happenings. Most voyages carry naturalists and other lecturers.

Sea Lion

Econoguide rating:	★★★
Ship size:	**Small**
Category:	**Adventure**
Price range:	**Premium $$$**
Registry:	United States
Year built:	1982
Itinerary:	Alaska, Pacific Northwest, Baja California
Information:	(800) 397-3348
Website:	www.expeditions.com
Passenger capacity:	70 (double occupancy)
Crew:	21 American
Passenger-to-Crew Ratio:	3.3:1
Tonnage:	100
Length:	152 feet
Beam:	31 feet
Draft:	8 feet
Cruising speed:	12 knots
Guest decks:	4
Total cabins:	37
Outside:	37
Inside:	0
Suites:	0
Wheelchair cabins:	Main deck, category 3 cabins. No elevators onboard.
Cuisine:	Continental
Style:	Informal
Price notes:	Single occupancy premium about 150 percent
Tipping suggestions:	$9 pp/pd

Chapter 16
Sailing Vessels

Sea Cloud Cruises
Star Clippers
Windjammer Barefoot Cruises
Windstar Cruises

Sea Cloud Cruises
32-40 North Dean St.
Englewood Cliffs, NJ 07631
Information: (888) 732-2568, (201) 227-9404
www.seacloud.com

Sea Cloud Cruises Fleet

Sea Cloud. (1931) 69 passengers, 2,532 tons

Sea Cloud II. (2000) 96 passengers, 3,000 tons

The four-masted barque *Sea Cloud* was built in 1931 for cereal food heiress Marjorie Merriweather Post by her husband, Wall Street broker Edward F. Hutton. Post, famous for her parties and social events, turned the ship into a gathering place for royalty, heads of state, and society hobnobbers.

After a half century of various adventures, including a stint as a weather observation and submarine spotting ship during World War II and as a notorious party boat for a Panamanian dictator and his son, *Sea Cloud* was restored to her former glory within and without.

More than a football field long, the ship is a place of marble and teak and gold-plated fixtures; several of the original owners' cabins include fireplaces. Dining includes fine wine and beer at lunch, often served beneath a canopy on deck, and dinner in the elegant dining parlor.

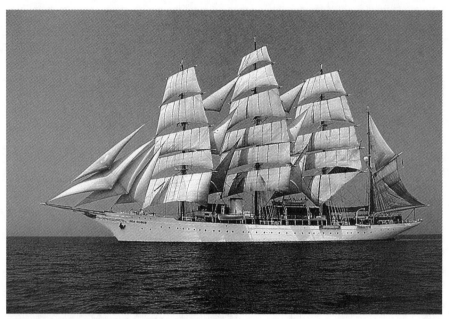

The classic Sea Cloud *under full sail*
Sea Cloud Cruises

The ship was rescued from oblivion by a group of German businessmen who bankrolled her restoration. Modern updates include air conditioning, some additional cabins, and the latest radar, satellite, and communications gear. But lucky guests are very much at sea in a classic with the feel of the Thirties and before.

In 2000, the fleet will double with the addition of *Sea Cloud II*, a new ship built in the style of her famous cousin. The new ship is slightly larger and includes some more modern features and amenities. She will follow a similar schedule, sailing in the Caribbean in the winter and the Mediterranean in the summer.

Sea Cloud

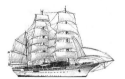

Econoguide rating:	★★★★
Ship size:	**Tall Ship**
Category:	**Adventure**
Price range:	**Moderate $$**
Registry:	Malta
Year built:	1931 (As S.V. *Hussar.*) Refurbished 1979, 1993
Itinerary:	Caribbean from Antigua, Mediterranean
Information:	(888) 732-2568
Web site:	www.seacloud.com
Passenger capacity:	69
Crew:	60
Passenger-to-Crew Ratio:	1.15:1
Tonnage:	2,532
Length:	360 feet

Beam:	50 feet
Draft:	17 feet
Cruising speed:	12 knots under power
Guest decks:	3
Total cabins:	34
Outside:	34
Inside:	0
Suites:	0
Wheelchair accessibility:	0
Cuisine:	Nouvelle cuisine; wines included.
Style:	Informal
Tipping suggestions:	$10–$12 pp/pd

If you're very lucky, you'll find yourself in cabin No. 1, Marjorie Post's own cabin, a seagoing palace complete with a fireplace and bathroom of Carrara marble, mahogany furniture, Louis Philippe chairs, and an antique French bed. But even the lesser cabins are rather grand, outfitted in marble and fine furniture. The restaurant, created from the ship's original saloon, is like a fine private club. Passengers receive rotating invitations to sit at the captain's table.

Sea Cloud II

Econoguide rating:	★★★★	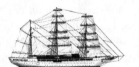
Ship size:	**Tall Ship**	
Category:	**Adventure**	
Price range:	**Moderate $$**	
Registry:	Malta	
Year built:	2000	
Itinerary:	Caribbean, Mediterranean	
Information:	(888) 732-2568	
Web site:	www.seacloud.com	
Passenger capacity:	96	
Crew:	60	
Passenger-to-Crew Ratio:	1.6:1	
Tonnage:	3,000	
Length:	384	
Beam:	53 feet	
Draft:	18 feet	
Cruising speed:	14 knots under power	
Guest decks:	4	
Total cabins:	48	
Outside:	48	
Inside:	0	
Suites:	0	
Wheelchair accessibility:	0	
Cuisine:	Nouvelle cuisine, wines included	
Style:	Informal	
Tipping suggestions:	$10–$12 pp/pd	

The irreplaceable *Sea Cloud* gained a new cousin, the *Sea Cloud II* in mid-2000. The new ship offers 48 cabins under a set of rigging that includes 24 sails on masts reaching 174 feet into the sky. Public rooms include an elegant restaurant, lounge, fitness room, and sauna. She also offers a watersports platform.

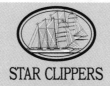

STAR CLIPPERS

Star Clippers
4101 Salzedo St.
Coral Gables, FL 33146
Information: (800) 442-0551
www.star-clippers.com

Star Clippers Fleet

Royal Clipper. (2000) 228 passengers. 5000 tons.

Star Clipper. (1992) 170 passengers. 2,298 tons.

Star Flyer. (1991) 170 passengers. 2,298 tons.

The Star Clipper fleet are modern re-creations of the classic clipper sailing ships that were the wonders of the seventeenth century. The clippers were called the "greyhounds" of the sea at their heyday; the largest of the ships was the *Great Republic*, built in 1853, at 308 feet. Many of the ships sailed from Great Britain or the United States to Asia; the end of the clipper age arrived with the opening of the Suez Canal in 1869, which made the steamboat more cost-effective.

Swedish businessman Mikael Krafft brought the Clipper ship back from extinction in 1991 when construction began in Belgium on what would be the largest clipper ship in history, the 360-foot-long *Star Flyer*, later joined by an identical twin, *Star Clipper*. In 2000, the even larger and more opulent 439-foot *Royal Clipper* joined the fleet. Her 226-foot-high mainmast is taller than almost any cruise liner on the seas.

Plans call for the *Royal Clipper* to be based in Barbados for the winter and will the Atlantic to the Mediterranean in April, returning in October. The *Star Clipper* resides full-time in the Caribbean, sailing to the Leeward, Windward, and Grenadine islands. The *Royal Clipper* is based in the Mediterranean for the summer, moving to the Far East and the Andaman Sea for the winter.

Although the ships are quite modern in their appointments, these are not computerized cruise ships with a sail on top for old-time's sake. The crew—and the passengers—are pressed into service to handle 40,000 square feet of sails on four masts on the *Star Clipper* and *Star Flyer*, and

Open space on small ships. Most of the sailing vessels in this chapter do not have a passenger space ratio listed; smaller ships are configured differently from sprawling cruise ships, doing without open atriums and making multiple use of dining rooms and theaters.

56,000 square feet on five masts on the *Royal Clipper*. Under a strong wind astern, the ships have reached speeds of as much as 17 knots, about the same as a modern cruise ship.

Rooms are attractive and tidy, most with small portholes; a few of the upper deck cabins have doors that open directly onto the Main Deck. The best views are found up on the large Sun Decks of the ships, outfitted with deck chairs and lounging spaces alongside several pools. The captain meets with guests every morning to discuss the day's schedule and tell stories of sailing lore and technique.

And one of the real treats of these ships is to pose for pictures for passengers along the rails of modern megaships in the harbor; the Star Clippers are among the prettiest sights they're likely to find at sea.

Royal Clipper

Econoguide rating:	★★★★
Ship size:	**Tall Ship**
Category:	**Adventure**
Price range:	**Moderate $**
Registry:	Luxembourg
Year built:	2000
Itinerary:	Caribbean, Mediterranean
Information:	(800) 442-0551
Web site:	www.star-clippers.com
Passenger capacity:	228
Crew:	105
Passenger-to-Crew Ratio:	2.2:1
Tonnage:	5,000
Length:	439 feet
Beam:	54 feet
Draft:	18.5 feet
Cruising speed:	Approximately 11 knots under sail
Guest decks:	5
Total cabins:	98
Outside:	42
Inside:	6
Suites:	2
Wheelchair accessibility:	0
Cuisine:	International and regional
Style:	Informal
Price notes:	Single occupancy premium 150 percent
Tipping suggestions:	$8 pp/pd

This is not your basic little sailboat. In fact, it's the world's largest sailing ship. Her dimensions follow those of the famed clipper ship *Preussen*, which dominated the world's sail cargo routes from 1902 to 1908.

Cabins are trimmed in mahogany and brass, with marble bathrooms, and color televisions. The three-level dining room is a step back into the Edwardian age. The ceiling above the Piano Bar is the glass bottom of the largest of three swimming pools. The lounge also offers submarine portholes, illuminated after dusk by underwater floodlights.

Each of the five masts includes a passenger lookout platform part of the way up; there's a settee in place, and stewards will deliver refreshments to the perch on call.

A small fleet of boats is available to passengers from the water sports platform that is lowered into the sea from the stern.

Star Clipper

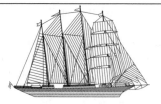

Econoguide rating:	★★★★
Ship size:	**Tall Ship**
Category:	**Adventure**
Price range:	**Moderate $**
Registry:	Luxembourg
Year built:	1992
Itinerary:	Caribbean, Mediterranean
Information:	(800) 442-0551
Web site:	www.star-clippers.com
Passenger capacity:	170
Crew:	72
Passenger-to-Crew Ratio:	2.4:1
Tonnage:	2,298
Length:	360 feet
Beam:	50 feet
Draft:	18.5 feet
Cruising speed:	11 knots under sail
Guest decks:	4
Total cabins:	85
Outside:	81
Inside:	4
Suites:	0
Wheelchair accessibility:	0
Cuisine:	International and regional
Style:	Informal
Price notes:	Single occupancy premium 150 percent
Tipping suggestions:	$8 pp/pd

Star Flyer

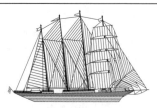

Econoguide rating:	★★★★
Ship size:	**Tall Ship**
Category:	**Adventure**
Price range:	**Moderate $**
Registry:	Luxembourg
Year built:	1991
Itinerary:	Caribbean, Mediterranean
Information:	(800) 442-0551
Web site:	www.star-clippers.com
Passenger capacity:	170
Crew:	72
Passenger-to-Crew Ratio:	2.4:1
Tonnage:	2,298
Length:	360 feet
Beam:	50 feet
Draft:	18.5 feet

Cruising speed:	11 knots under sail
Guest decks:	4
Total cabins:	85
Outside:	81
Inside:	4
Suites:	0
Wheelchair accessibility:	0
Cuisine:	International and regional
Style:	Informal
Price notes:	Single occupancy premium 150 percent
Tipping suggestions:	$8 pp/pd

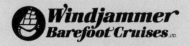

**Windjammer Barefoot Cruises
P.O. Box 190-200
Miami, FL 33119-0120
Information: (800) 327-2601
www.windjammer.com**

Windjammer Barefoot Cruises Fleet

Flying Cloud. (1935) 66 passengers. 400 tons.

Legacy. (1959) 122 passengers. 1,740 tons.

Mandalay. (1923) 72 passengers. 420 tons.

Polynesia. (1938) 126 passengers. 430 tons.

Yankee Clipper. (1927) 64 passengers. 327 tons.

Amazing Grace. (1955) 94 passengers. 1,585 tons

Windjammer is the largest operator of tall ships in the world, with six ships in its fleet that have passenger capacities of 64 to 126, sailing year-round in the Caribbean.

According to company lore, Mike Burke woke up in Miami in 1947 with a headache and a 19-foot sloop, purchased sometime during the night with $600 in Navy pay. The boat, christened *Hangover*, became the basis for the Windjammer empire.

Each of the ships has an interesting story of its own, the oldest dating back more than 75 years. The vessels have been refurbished and accommodations brought up to modern standards.

Windjammer suffered a major loss in 1998 with the destruction of the *Fantome* during Hurricane Mitch off Central America; the ship's passengers had been safely deposited in port, but the crew of 31 perished when the ship

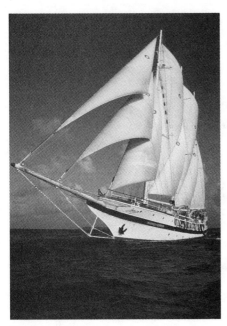

Yankee Clipper
Windjammer Barefoot Cruises

headed out to sea to attempt to out-run the storm to safety.

The fleet includes some true classics:

Mandalay, considered one of the most luxurious yachts in the world when she was built in 1923 as a three-masted Barquentine for financier E. F. Hutton and his wife Marjorie Merri-weather Post.

Flying Cloud, built in 1935 as a cadet training ship for the French Navy, and later serving as a decoy and spy ship for the Allied Forces, participating in the sinking of two Japanese sub-marines during World War II.

Legacy, the flagship of the fleet, built in 1959 as a meteorological research and exploration ship for the French government.

Polynesia, a four-masted schooner built in Holland in 1938 for the Por-tuguese Grand Banks cod fishing fleet.

Yankee Clipper, one of the only armor-plated private yachts in the world, was built in 1927 for German arms maker Alfred Krupp. She was confiscated by the United States after World War II, was later acquired by the Vanderbilt family and raced off California.

Amazing Grace, the sixth ship in the fleet, is a former Scottish service ship built in 1955 that provided supplies to North Sea lighthouses. The motorized vessel today supplies the six sailing vessels in the Windjammer fleet, carry-ing passengers on a full itinerary of Caribbean stops.

The Windjammer Experience

None of the ships could qualify as luxury liners, and cabins and public rooms are small and simple. The atmosphere is decidedly relaxed, sometimes verg-ing on non-stop partying. Some cruises have lifestyle themes such as nudism, singles, swingers, and gays. Be sure to inquire whether any such gathering is planned on the cruise you might select.

The loss of the *Fantome* has cut back on the company's itineraries. The handsome ship, built in 1927 as a destroyer for the Italian Navy and later reconstructed as a private floating palace for the Duke of Westminster, had sailed in and around Belize in the summer and fall and out of Antigua for much of the remainder of the year.

Windjammer has been experiencing increasing bookings in recent years and before the accident had announced plans to add three ships in the next decade and as many as five during the next 15 years.

One interesting offering is a "stowaway" onboard the ship the night before departure. For a reasonable fee, guests can spend the night onboard the ship and partake of dinner, rum swizzles, a steel drum band party, and breakfast.

Flying Cloud

Econoguide rating:	★★★
Ship size:	**Tall Ship**
Category:	**Adventure**
Price range:	**Budget $**
Registry:	Equatorial Guinea
Year built:	1935 (Joined Windjammer fleet in 1968. Refurbished 1968)
Itinerary:	Caribbean
Information:	(800) 327-2601
Web site:	www.windjammer.com
Passenger capacity:	66 (double occupancy)
Crew:	28
Passenger-to-Crew Ratio:	2.4:1
Tonnage:	400
Length:	208 feet
Beam:	32 feet
Draft:	16 feet
Cruising speed:	6 knots
Guest decks:	3
Total cabins:	33
Outside:	33
Inside:	0
Suites:	0
Wheelchair accessibility:	0
Cuisine:	Island/Continental. Most dinners served family-style; some buffets.
Style:	Informal
Price notes:	Stowaway aboard ship night before sailing for $55 pp including meals.
Tipping suggestions:	$7 pp/pd

Built in 1935 as a cadet training ship for the French Navy, the three-masted barquentine *Oiseau des Isles* (Bird of the Islands) sailed the French Polynesian islands during World War II as a decoy and spy ship for the Allied Forces. Premier Charles DeGaulle decorated her for her assistance in sinking two Japanese submarines.

Used as a cargo vessel by a Mexican company after the war, she joined the Windjammer fleet in 1968 and was renamed *Flying Cloud*. Refurbishments included installation of teak decks, an elevated charthouse, and new riggings that resemble legendary pirate ships. Also added was a honeymoon deluxe suite that has a private entrance.

The *Flying Cloud* sails weekly from Tortola on Drake's Passage and Treasure Isles itineraries.

Legacy

Econoguide rating:	★★★
Ship size:	**Tall Ship**
Category:	**Adventure**
Price range:	**Moderate $$**
Registry:	Equatorial Guinea

Year built:	1959 (Acquired by Windjammer in 1989. Refurbished 1989)
Itinerary:	Puerto Rico to Virgin Passage and Blackbeard's Backyard
Information:	(800) 327-2601
Web site:	www.windjammer.com
Passenger capacity:	122 (double occupancy)
Crew:	43
Passenger-to-Crew Ratio:	2.8:1
Tonnage:	1,740
Length:	294 feet
Beam:	40 feet
Draft:	23 feet
Cruising speed:	12 knots
Guest decks:	4
Total cabins:	61
Outside:	61
Inside:	0
Suites:	0
Wheelchair accessibility:	0
Cuisine:	Island/Continental, served family-style
Style:	Informal
Price notes:	Single occupancy 175 percent premium. Reduced rates for children younger than 12 years of age sharing cabin. Stowaway aboard ship night before sailing for $55 pp including meals.
Tipping suggestions:	$7 pp/pd

The youngest antique in the Windjammer fleet, the four-masted barquentine was built in 1959 as the *France II* as a meteorological research and exploration vessel for the French government. She was acquired in 1989 by Windjammer and converted into a traditional Tall Ship.

Legacy sails from Fajardo, Puerto Rico, to the serene Virgin Passage and exotic Blackbeard's Backyard.

Mandalay

Econoguide rating:	★★★
Ship size:	**Tall Ship**
Category:	**Adventure**
Price range:	**Budget $**
Registry:	Equatorial Guinea
Year built:	1923 (*Hussar, Vema.* Joined fleet in 1982. Refurbished 1982)
Itinerary:	Grenada or Antigua to Windward and Leeward Islands
Information:	(800) 327-2601
Web site:	www.windjammer.com
Passenger capacity:	72 (double occupancy)
Crew:	28
Passenger-to-Crew Ratio:	2.6:1
Tonnage:	420
Length:	236 feet
Beam:	33 feet
Draft:	15 feet
Cruising speed:	10 knots
Guest decks:	3
Total cabins:	36
Outside:	30
Inside:	0
Suites:	6
Wheelchair accessibility:	0

Cuisine:	Island/Continental family-style dinners
Style:	Informal
Price notes:	Single occupancy 175 percent premium. Reduced rates for children under 12 years of age sharing cabin. Stowaway aboard ship night before sailing for $55 pp including meals.
Tipping suggestions:	$7 pp/pd

Built in 1923 as *Hussar*, a three-masted Barquentine for financier E. F. Hutton and his wife, Marjorie Merriweather Post; the wealthy couple traded up to a new vessel now sailing for Sea Cloud Cruises as *Sea Cloud*.

In the 1930s, the vessel was sold to shipping magnate George Vettlesen and renamed *Vema*. Beginning in 1953, she took on a new role as a floating laboratory for Columbia University's Lamont-Doherty Geological Observatory, sailing more than 1 million miles studying the ocean floor and gathering important research in confirmation of the continental drift theory.

The ship joined the Windjammer fleet in 1982, and was renamed *Mandalay* and renovated throughout. All cabins are outside and have a porthole or window; two deck cabins have private verandas.

The *Mandalay* sails a varied schedule from Grenada and Antigua, with six- and 13-day voyages in the Windward and Leeward islands.

Polynesia

Econoguide rating:	★★★
Ship size:	**Tall Ship**
Category:	**Adventure**
Price range:	**Budget $**
Registry:	Equatorial Guinea
Year built:	1938 (*Argus*. Acquired by Windjammer in 1975. Refurbished 1975)
Itinerary:	Leeward and Windward Islands from St. Maarten
Information:	(800) 327-2601
Web site:	www.windjammer.com
Passenger capacity:	126 (double occupancy)
Crew:	45
Passenger-to-Crew Ratio:	2.8:1
Tonnage:	430
Length:	248 feet
Beam:	36 feet
Draft:	18 feet
Cruising speed:	8 knots
Guest decks:	4
Total cabins:	57
Outside:	55
Inside:	0
Suites:	2
Wheelchair accessibility:	0
Cuisine:	Island/Continental. Dinners usually family-style, occasionally buffet.
Style:	Informal
Price notes:	Single occupancy 175 percent premium. Reduced rates for children under 12 years of age sharing cabin. Stowaway aboard ship night before sailing for $55 pp including meals.
Tipping suggestions:	$7 pp/pd

Built in Holland in 1938, this four-masted schooner, originally named

Argus, was at one time the swiftest and most profitable of the Portuguese cod fishing fleet on the Grand Banks. The ship was purchased and brought out of retirement in 1975; renamed *Polynesia,* renovations included installation of a teak deck, exotic wood paneling, and a dining salon with each table depicting one of the islands on Polynesia's itinerary.

Polynesia sails from St. Maarten to the Leeward Islands and Westward Islands of the French West Indies. It is one of Windjammer's most popular vessels, hosting special singles' cruises and theme cruises.

Yankee Clipper

Econoguide rating:	★★★
Ship size:	**Tall Ship**
Category:	**Adventure**
Price range:	**Budget $**
Registry:	Equatorial Guinea
Year built:	1927 (As *Cressida,* then *Pioneer;* acquired by Windjammer in 1965. Refurbished 1965)
Itinerary:	Grenadine Passage and Spice Islands from Grenada
Information:	(800) 327-2601
Web site:	www.windjammer.com
Passenger capacity:	64 (double occupancy)
Crew:	24
Passenger-to-Crew Ratio:	2.7:1
Tonnage:	327
Length:	197 feet
Beam:	30 feet
Draft:	17 feet
Cruising speed:	14 knots
Guest decks:	3
Total cabins:	32
Outside:	32
Inside:	0
Suites:	0
Wheelchair accessibility:	0
Cuisine:	Island/continental, usually family-style
Style:	Informal
Price notes:	Single occupancy 175 percent premium. Reduced rates for children under 12 years of age sharing cabin. Stowaway aboard ship night before sailing for $55 pp including meals.
Tipping suggestions:	$7 pp/pd

This is an updated antique, one of the fastest tall ships at sea, often sailing at 14 knots.

One of the only armor-plated private yachts in the world, the *Cressida* was built in Kiel, Germany in 1927 by German industrialist and manufacturer Alfred Krupp. After World War II the U.S. Coast Guard confiscated the schooner as a war prize.

Acquired by the Vanderbilts and renamed *Pioneer,* she was raced off Newport Beach, California, where she was considered one of the fastest Tall Ships on the West Coast.

Pioneer was purchased by Windjammer's Mike Burke in 1965, and following extensive renovations renamed her *Yankee Clipper.* In 1984, she was completely restored to her former majesty with refurbishments totaling $4 million. The work included a new set of three masts, a new engine room with custom-designed navigation and communication and weather-monitoring devices.

Amazing Grace

Econoguide rating:	★★★
Ship size:	**Medium**
Category:	**Adventure**
Price range:	**Budget $**
Registry:	Equatorial Guinea
Year built:	1955 (As the *Pharos,* a British Navy motor vessel)
Itinerary:	13-day island-hopping tour from Grand Bahama or Trinidad to provision sailing ships in Bahamas and Caribbean
Information:	(800) 327-2601
Web site:	www.windjammer.com
Passenger capacity:	94 (double occupancy)
Crew:	40
Passenger-to-Crew Ratio:	2.3:1
Tonnage:	1,585
Length:	257 feet
Beam:	40 feet
Draft:	17 feet
Cruising speed:	14 knots
Guest decks:	5
Total cabins:	48
Outside:	46
Inside:	1
Suites:	1
Wheelchair accessibility:	0
Cuisine:	Island/Continental. Dinners family-style, occasionally buffet
Style:	Very informal
Price notes:	Single occupancy 175 percent premium
Tipping suggestions:	$7 pp/pd

The motorized service vessel for the Windjammer fleet, *Amazing Grace* permits passengers to hitch a ride on her circuit through the Caribbean and the Bahamas.

Built in 1955 as the Scottish lighthouse service ship *Pharos,* she hosted Queen Elizabeth and other members of the Royal Family. Acquired by Windjammer in 1985, *Amazing Grace* delivers provisions to the six tall ships in the fleet on 13-day tours.

Restored to her original British charm, the ship features a smoking lounge, antique fireplaces, and a piano room.

Only the top-priced cabins have private bathrooms; other cabins share facilities on the same level. The Owner's Suite, named Burke's Berth, has a large sitting room separated from the stateroom by a set of aquariums. The bath, which includes a hot tub, is built with marble and teak.

Amazing Grace sails from Trinidad to Grand Bahama, reversing course every two weeks.

WINDSTAR°CRUISES
A HOLLAND AMERICA LINE COMPANY

Windstar Cruises
300 Elliott Ave. West
Seattle, WA 98119
Information: (800) 258-7245, (206) 281-3535
www.windstarcruises.com

Windstar Cruises Fleet

Wind Song. (1987) 148 passengers. 5,350 tons

Wind Spirit. (1988) 148 passengers. 5,350 tons

Wind Star. (1986) 148 passengers. 5,350 tons

Wind Surf. (1990) 312 passengers. 14,745 tons

In November of 1986, the first commercial sailing vessel built in 60 years left the dock in Le Havre, France. Although the *Wind Star* had the appearance of a classic sailing schooner, the ship—and the three others in the Windstar fleet, are decidedly modern-day creations. Computers controls the rigging; the huge booms are motor-controlled with high-tech sensors to trim the angle of the sail. Some 21,000 square feet of white sail unfurls at the push of a button. The angle of heel is kept at a maximum of six degrees by a computerized stabilizing system that pumps thousands of gallons of water from side to side with changes in the wind.

Today the *Wind Star* is joined by sister ships *Wind Song*, and *Wind Spirit*, and the larger *Wind Surf*. The latter ship, a five-masted sail cruise ship, was originally the *Club Med I*; it was rebuilt for Windstar and made her maiden voyage as the *Wind Surf* in mid-1998.

The ships have auxiliary engines that are used when wind conditions are not favorable and for maneuvering in some harbors. Windstar says, though, that almost half the time at sea is spent under sail.

The Windstar Experience

These are not the ships that Charles Dickens or Herman Melville wrote about. Cabin amenities include a color television and video player, CD player, refrigerator, and direct-dial telephones. Cuisine onboard the ships is directed by Joachim Splichal, chef and owner of Patina Restaurant in Los Angeles, with regional specialties and fine wines. Splichal created 180 signature dishes for Windstar vessels, ranging from rich Continental fare to Sail Light Menus.

When possible, Windstar shops the local markets for fresh native foods, including cheeses, mangoes, spices, and local fish. Ambience is casual, with no assigned seating and no dress codes for dining.

The ships offer complimentary watersport activities, including water skiing, sailboarding, kayaking, and snorkeling. Scuba diving is available for an additional charge.

The company's ships sail in the Caribbean in the winter and spring, including Panama Canal passages. The *Wind Song, Wind Spirit,* and *Wind Surf* move to the Mediterranean for summer cruises from Athens, Rome, Lisbon, Barcelona, and Nice, while the *Wind Star* remains in Barbados.

The Windstar cruises include a wide range of shore excursions from the ordinary to the extraordinary, including an exploration of Costa Rica's rain forests where guests will "zip-line" on a pulley and cable from tree to tree way above the forest floor. Other on-shore activities include sea kayaking, cultural odysseys, and river float expeditions.

Windstar was purchased by Holland America in 1988; Holland America was in turn purchased by Carnival Corporation in 1989.

Look for A.S.A.P. early booking discounts reduced prices by as much as 40 percent off brochure prices. In 2000, the company introduced a new program that offered deep discounts on airfare to Europe, reducing the cost of travel in peak season for Windstar cruises. And new itineraries were added in the Andalusia and Provence regions of Portugal, Spain, and France, and new itineraries in the Pacific for 2001.

Wind Song

Econoguide rating:	★★★★
Ship size:	**Tall Ship**
Category:	**Adventure**
Price range:	**Opulent $$$$**
Registry:	Bahamas
Year built:	1987 (Refurbished 1996, 1999)
Sister ships:	*Wind Spirit* and *Wind Star*
Itinerary:	Trans-Atlantic (between Lisbon & Caribbean), Caribbean Lesser Antilles, Costa Rica, Panama Canal, Greek Islands
Information:	(800) 258-7245
Web site:	www.windstarcruises.com
Passenger capacity:	148 (double occupancy)
Crew:	88
Passenger-to-Crew Ratio:	1.7:1
Tonnage:	5,350
Passenger Space Ratio:	36.1
Length:	360 feet (waterline); 440 including bowsprit
Beam:	52.1 feet
Draft:	14 feet
Cruising speed:	8.5 knots to 14 knots, depending on wind. 8.5 knots to 10 knots with engines only
Guest decks:	4, plus flying bridge
Total cabins:	73
Outside:	74
Inside:	0
Suites:	1 Owner's Suite
Wheelchair accessibility:	0
Cuisine:	Includes Sail Light menus and vegetarian
Style:	Casually elegant
Price notes:	Single occupancy premium is 175 percent to 200 percent
Tipping suggestions:	Tipping not required

Wind Spirit

Econoguide rating:	★★★★
Ship size:	**Tall Ship**
Category:	**Adventure**
Price range:	**Opulent $$$$**
Registry:	Bahamas
Year built:	1988 (Refurbished 1999)
Sister ships:	*Wind Song* and *Wind Star*
Itinerary:	Virgin Islands, Lesser Antilles, Trans-Atlantic between Lisbon and Caribbean
Information:	(800) 258-7245
Web site:	www.windstarcruises.com
Passenger capacity:	148 (double occupancy)
Crew:	88
Passenger-to-Crew Ratio:	1.7:1
Tonnage:	5,350
Passenger Space Ratio:	36.1
Length:	360 feet (waterline); 440 including bowsprit
Beam:	52.1 feet
Draft:	14 feet
Cruising speed:	Up to 14 knots, depending on wind. 8.5 knots to 10 knots with engines
Guest decks:	4, plus flying bridge
Total cabins:	74
Outside:	73
Inside:	0
Suites:	1
Wheelchair accessibility:	0
Cuisine:	Includes Sail Light menus and vegetarian
Style:	Casually elegant
Price notes:	Single occupancy premium 175 percent to 200 percent
Tipping suggestions:	Tipping not required.

Wind Star

Econoguide rating:	★★★★
Ship size:	**Tall Ship**
Category:	**Adventure**
Price range:	**Opulent $$$$**
Registry:	Bahamas
Year built:	1986 (Refurbished 1999)
Sister ships:	*Wind Song* and *Wind Spirit*
Itinerary:	Fall and winter in Mexican Riviera, Belize, and Honduras; Summer and spring trans-Atlantic between Lisbon and Caribbean
Information:	(800) 258-7245
Web site:	www.windstarcruises.com
Passenger capacity:	148 (double occupancy)
Crew:	88
Passenger-to-Crew Ratio:	1.7:1
Tonnage:	5,350
Passenger Space Ratio:	36.1
Length:	360 feet (waterline); 440 including bowsprit
Beam:	52.1 feet
Draft:	14 feet
Cruising speed:	8.5 knots to 14 knots, depending on wind. 8.5 knots to 10 knots with engines only. Stabilized with 2 sets of Denny Brown stabilizers and a 142,653-gallon/540 CBM sea water hydraulic ballast system to limit heel when sails are up.
Guest decks:	4, plus flying bridge
Total cabins:	74

Outside:	73
Inside:	0
Suites:	1
Wheelchair cabins:	0
Cuisine:	Includes Sail Light menus and vegetarian
Style:	Casually elegant
Price notes:	Single occupancy premium 175 percent to 200 percent
Tipping suggestions:	Tipping not required

A trio of football-field-sized sailboats, with four 200-foot-tall masts and six self-furling, computer-operated Dacron sails.

Modern amenities include a restaurant that accommodates all passengers at one sitting, a discotheque, CD and video libraries, water sports platform, salt-water pool, hot tub, casino, and fitness center.

Children—especially infants and toddlers—are not encouraged aboard the cruises.

Wind Surf

Econoguide rating:	★★★★
Ship size:	**Tall Ship**
Category:	**Adventure**
Price range:	**Opulent $$$$**
Registry:	Bahamas
Year built:	1990 (As *Club Med I*. Refurbished 1999)
Itinerary:	Spring and fall, Western Mediterranean and trans-Atlantic; spring and summer, French and Italian Riviera; winter, in Caribbean Lesser Antilles
Information:	(206) 258-7245
Web site:	www.windstarcruises.com
Passenger capacity:	312 (double occupancy)
Crew:	163 International
Passenger-to-Crew Ratio:	1.9:1
Tonnage:	14,745
Passenger Space Ratio:	47.3
Length:	535 feet, 617 feet, including bowsprit
Beam:	66 feet
Draft:	16.5 feet
Cruising speed:	10 knots to 15 knots, depending on wind. 12 knots under power
Guest decks:	7
Total cabins:	156
Outside:	125
Inside:	0
Suites:	31
Wheelchair accessibility:	0
Cuisine:	Sail Light menus and vegetarian
Style:	Casually elegant
Price notes:	Single occupancy premium 175 percent to 200 percent
Tipping suggestions:	Tipping not required

This is not a simple sailboat. The seven-deck *Wind Surf* was born as the *Club Med I,* a thoroughly modern sailing and party vessel.

The ship includes two restaurants, The Restaurant and the smaller Veranda Bistro, which can accommodate all passengers at one seating with no assigned tables.

Windstar refurbished the *Club Med* to reduce the number of cabins, adding a deck of 400-square-foot suites.

Seven triangular, self-furling computer-operated Dacron sails offer 26,881 square feet of surface area. Depending on destination and wind conditions, the ship is typically under sail about half the time, relying on its engines at other times.

The ship includes an open-air sports platform that has snorkeling gear, sailboards, water skis, kayaks, and sailboats.

Children—especially infants and toddlers—are not encouraged aboard the cruises. Windstar ships have no elevators, and, therefore, are not suitable for people in wheelchairs.

Chapter 17
A History of Cruising

Today's cruise industry can trace its lineage back to the nineteenth century, when passenger ships were a means of transportation—primarily from Europe to the United States, and from Europe to and from its far-flung colonies in Asia and Africa.

But the arrival of commercial jet airplanes in the late 1950s marked the beginning of the end for the trans-Atlantic and trans-Pacific liners. Many of the big ships went to the breakers to be cut up for salvage.

But not that long afterwards, a new concept took hold—the cruise ship. Here the ship itself took center stage, as a floating resort hotel.

The Atlantic Ferry

By the middle of the nineteenth century, the traffic from Europe to America (and to a lesser extent the other direction) was so steady the route across the North Atlantic became known as the "Atlantic Ferry."

The race was literally on, as shipbuilders pushed for larger and faster ships. The queens of the line also became more and more opulent within, at least for the relatively few wealthy first-class passengers; at the same time, builders crammed more and more low-fare travelers into "steerage" areas, which were often more like bunkhouses than staterooms. (Steerage, though, was the source of much of the shipping lines' profits because of the sheer number of passengers crammed into that section.)

The first commercial steamship to cross the Atlantic was the *Savannah*, an American coastal packet ship designed as a sailing vessel in 1818 but refitted with an engine during construction. The ship made its first crossing in 1819, a 28-day voyage from Savannah to Ireland and Liverpool; the ship was never a commercial success.

The real beginnings of the Atlantic Ferry can be traced to Isambard Kingdom Brunel, chief engineer of the Great Western Railway in Great Britain. The rail line between Bristol and London was nearly finished in the 1830s, and Brunel decided to extend his company's reach across the pond. The ship he designed, the *Great Western*, left England for New York on April 8, 1838.

The Early Cunard Liners

In 1840, the Cunard Line began mail service across the Atlantic with a quartet of paddlewheel steamers that had auxiliary sails—the *Britannia, Acadia, Columbia*, and *Caledonia*. In 1858, Brunel's company launched the *Great Eastern*, an iron-hulled vessel that approached in size many of today's cruise ships, with a length of 692 feet.

For the next two decades, British and American interests competed for supremacy as merchant marine powers. During the U.S. Civil War, however, much of the American fleet was destroyed and Britain regained its leading role—a position it held for the rest of the nineteenth century.

German shipping lines held size and speed records near the end of the century, with vessels such as the 1,749-passenger *Kaiser Wilhelm der Grosse*. By 1898, the North German Lloyd line was carrying 28 percent of the passengers from Europe to New York.

The speed of the liners was limited because of the piston design of the steam engines. But by the 1890s, new technology using steam turbine engines began to be used, and these systems were more powerful and reliable.

The British, lead by the Cunard Line, sought to recapture preeminence with a set of superliners of the day. Cunard's *Lusitania* and the *Mauretania,* were launched in 1906. The *Mauretania* captured the Blue Riband for the fastest crossing in 1907, holding onto the honor until 1929. The *Lusitania* was sunk by a German submarine in 1915, an action that helped lead to the United States entry into World War II years later.

The *Titanic* and the Great War

About this same time, the White Star Line, direct competitor to Cunard, also commissioned a pair of superliners. The 45,324-ton *Olympic,* launched in 1911, was for a short period of time the largest ship ever built. That title was taken over by White Star's slightly larger *Titanic* in 1912. The *Titanic,* of course, came to an unhappy end on her maiden voyage in 1912.

After the end of World War I, Germany was removed from competition, with the three surviving German liners confiscated as war reparations.

In the postwar boom of the early 1920s, tourism grew markedly. Leaders include the French Line's *Ile de France* and the return of the German lines. The Great Depression slowed most but not all new construction, though.

In 1930, the French Line planned and launched the gigantic *Normandie,* considered one of the most beautiful ships ever built. She was also the first large ship to be built in accordance with the 1929 Convention for Safety of Life at Sea rules. The *Normandie*, which included 1,975 berths, used turboelectric engines which reached a speed of 32.1 knots during trials in 1935. The ship caught fire and sank at a New York dock in 1942 while being refitted as a troopship.

Cunard struck back with the *Queen Mary,* a 975-foot-long classic, which was launched in 1934. A sister ship, the 83,673-ton *Queen Elizabeth,* was launched in 1938, but served first as a troopship during World War II—along with most other civilian liners. After the war, it was completed as a luxury liner.

The Last Hurrah of the Liners

The last great American liner was the *United States,* launched in 1952; the ship had a top speed of 35.6 knots and captured the coveted Blue Riband from the *Queen Mary.*

But not soon afterward, the arrival of commercial air traffic across the Atlantic spelled the beginning of the end of the great liners. The propeller-driven DC-7 made the crossing at approximately 300 miles per hour, with a range of nearly 3,000 miles. By 1957, there were more passengers crossing the Atlantic by air than by sea.

About 1958, commercial jet planes began regular service, and regular transatlantic traffic by liner was entering its final days.

The True Tale of the *Titanic*

The *Titanic* was big, all right . . . although in today's terms she would merely be one of many large ships and not quite a Colossus.

The *Titanic* was the new flagship of the White Star Line. Work began in 1909, with the launch of the uncompleted hull two years later.

Titanic was 883 feet long, 92 feet wide, and 104 feet tall from keel to bridge. She was, at the time, the largest movable object ever made, standing taller than most buildings of the time.

The ship's construction featured a double hull of inch-thick steel plates. Below the waterline, the ship was divided into 16 supposedly watertight compartments that could be sealed off by massive doors by the closing of a switch on the bridge.

The *Titanic* also included an early Marconi radio system, allowing communication with other ships similarly equipped, as well as occasional connection with land-based stations.

Within, the *Titanic's* accommodations were among the most luxurious afloat, at least for those passengers booked into First Class. She was among the first ships with electric lighting in every room, as well as an indoor swimming pool, a squash court, and a gymnasium that had a mechanical horse and camel for exercise.

In an example of how everything old is someday considered a new idea, the *Titanic* offered two alternative restaurants in addition to the formal first-class dining saloon.

Down below, hundreds of immigrants were packed into steerage-class accommodations, which were nevertheless described as being of better quality than full-rate cabins on some other ships of the time.

The ship's designers had specified 32 lifeboats, which was probably not adequate for the ship's total capacity of 3,500 passengers and crew. White Star made the situation even worse by reducing the number of lifeboats to 20 for appearance sake. As the *Titanic* left on her maiden voyage, then, her lifeboats had a capacity of just 1,178 persons.

Titanic departed Southampton, England on April 10, 1912, stopping across the Channel in Cherbourg, France to pick up some additional passengers and calling the next day in Queenstown, Ireland for one more group. She headed out into the Atlantic on April 11, reaching her top speed of 22 knots; the *Titanic* was among the fastest ships of her time, but not expected to be the record holder.

The weather on the crossing was good. The winter of 1912 had been unusually moderate, making for good conditions at sea but also contributing to an unusually large amount of icebergs and floes breaking off the Arctic pack. In fact, *Titanic* may have received half a dozen or more warnings of ice in the North Atlantic. The captain, perhaps under pressure by executives of the ship line, continued to travel under full steam through the night of April 14.

At 11:40 P.M. that night, lookouts spotted a large iceberg ahead of the ship. The First Officer ordered the ship hard to port and the engines put into reverse, but the big ship was moving too fast and was too slow to turn; she struck a glancing blow against the side of the berg.

Five of the ship's watertight compartments were ruptured, and water spilled over the top of the other compartment doors and the *Titanic* was doomed.

Investigations claimed that the liner *Californian* was less than 20 miles away from the disaster and could have been on the scene in less than an hour, but its radio shack was not staffed during the night. Cunard's *Carpathia* finally arrived more than an hour after the ship went down, picking up most of the survivors in lifeboats.

In 1985, the wreck of the *Titanic* was located, split into two large pieces at a depth of about 13,000 feet. Surprisingly, no sign of the expected lengthwise gash in the side of the ship was found; scientists now believe the glancing blow against the iceberg popped open seams in the riveted hull plates of the ship and made a series of smaller gashes.

Glossary of Nautical Terms

OK, let's get one thing straight: It's a ship, not a boat. A boat is something you row across the pond, or sail across the river. A ship is a big vessel that has lots of cabins, many levels, a bingo parlor, a health club, and a rotating disco at the top of its massive funnel. You get the idea: Boat is little, ship is big.

If you really want to sound like a swabbie (the opposite of a landlubber), here is a guide to some nautical terms for the cruise vacationer.

Abeam. To the side of the ship, at a right angle to the keel that runs the length of the vessel.

Aft. At the stern (rear) of the ship, or rearward from your present location.

Amidships. At or near the middle of the ship.

Astern. Behind the stern of the ship.

Beam. The width of the ship at its broadest point, usually amidships.

Bearing. The compass direction of the ship in motion, or the direction toward a specified point.

Below. Any area beneath the main deck of the ship.

Berth. A dock or pier for the ship, or a bed for a passenger or crewman.

Bilge. The lowest interior space of the ship.

Boat station. The assigned assembly place for passengers and crew in a lifeboat drill or a true emergency.

Bow. The front of the ship.

Bridge. The principal navigation and control station.

Bulkhead. A vertical wall used to divide sections of the ship into waterproof and fire-resistant compartments.

Bunkers. Fuel storage areas.

Colors. The national flag or emblem flown by a particular vessel.

Companionway. An interior stairway.

Course. The bearing of the ship as underway, expressed in degrees.

Davit. The rope and pulley or motor system used to lower and raise lifeboats.

Draft. The distance from the ship's waterline to the lowest part of the keel; a ship cannot safely enter waters shallower than its draft.

Fantail. An overhang at the stern of the ship.

Fathom. A measurement of water depth equal to six feet.

Galley. The ship's kitchen.

Gangway. A walkway extended to connect the ship to shore.

Gross registered tonnes (GRT). A measurement of the total permanently enclosed spaces of the ship, excluding certain essential areas including the bridge

321

and galleys. 1 GRT=100 cubic feet of enclosed space. GRT was developed as a means of taxing vessels based on their cargo-carrying capacity.

Helm. The steering mechanism.

Hull. The body of the ship.

Knot. One nautical mile. This is based on a measure of one-sixtieth of a degree of the earth's circumference, which works out to 6,080.2 feet, or about 800 feet longer than a land-based mile. The term knot as a measure of speed refers to distance per hour; 20 knots means 20 knots per hour. Only a landlubber says "per hour." To convert knots to miles per hour, add about 15 percent. For example, 20 knots is equal to just over 23 miles per hour.

Leeward. The side of the ship or a body of land that is sheltered from the wind. The opposite is Windward.

Nautical Mile. A measurement of distance equal to one-sixtieth of a degree of the circumference of the earth, or about 6,080.2 feet.

Pilot. A specially trained guide to local waters sometimes taken aboard when a ship enters an unfamiliar or tricky harbor or area.

Pitch. The rise and fall of the ship's bow when it is underway.

Plimsoll Mark. A set of marks on the side of a vessel that show at least three depths—the maximum safe draft—the lowest the ship can safely sit in the water. One line is for summer when seas are generally calm in most parts of the world, another for winter when seas are usually rougher, and a third is a fresh water line to account for the fact that fresh water is significantly less buoyant than saltwater. The mark was named for nineteenth-century social reformer Samuel Plimsoll, who was concerned about ship disasters blamed on overloading by greedy owners.

Port. The left side of the ship when facing forward.

Quay. A berth or dock.

Rudder. A moveable extension of the ship that extends into the water and is used to steer the vessel.

Screw. A ship's propeller.

Stabilizer. An adjustable fin-like structure that extends from the side of a ship to minimize roll.

Starboard. The right side of the ship when facing forward.

Stern. The rearmost part of the ship.

Tender. A small boat used to transport passengers or crew to shore when the ship is anchored away from a dock.

Veranda. A private balcony for a passenger cabin, a feature of some of the most modern and luxurious vessels and generally located on the upper decks.

Wake. The track of disturbed water left behind a ship in motion.

Windward. The side of the ship or a body of land that is exposed to the wind.

And while I'm on the subject, here are a few terms from nautical sources that have become part of our common language.

The cat is out of the bag. The cat o'nine tails was used to whip sailors as punishment; when it was removed from its cloth bag, everyone knew what came next.

Jury rig. To put something together in a makeshift way. The term comes from "jury mast," a temporary mast constructed from any available spar.

Minding your Ps and Qs. The careful and neat sailor took care that his pigtail, or queue, which was kept in shape with a mousse of tar, did not soil his pea jacket.

Three sheets to the wind. On a small sailing vessel, three sheets (ropes) controlled the sails; if the sheets were loose the sails were out of control. Today, we apply the term to a sailor, or a landlubber, who is out of control with the assistance of drink.

The whole nine yards. A square-rigger sailing vessel had three masts with three yards (or sails) on each; if the captain was sailing hard, he was giving the vessel the whole nine yards.

Special Offers to Econoguide Readers

Look to your left, look to your right. One of you three people on vacation is paying the regular price for a cruise stateroom, airfare, hotels, meals, and shopping. One is paying premium price for a less-than-first rate package. And one pays a deeply discounted special rate.

Which one would you rather be?

In this book you've learned about strategies to obtain the lowest prices on cruise vacations, the best times to take a trip, and ideas on how to negotiate just about every element of travel.

And now, we're happy to present a special section of discount coupons for Econoguide readers.

All of the offers represent real savings. Be sure to read the coupons carefully, though, because of exclusions during holiday periods and other fine print. You'll find discounts from travel agencies as well as a selection of attractions in major cruise port cities.

The author and publisher of this book do not endorse any of the businesses whose coupons appear here, and the presence of a coupon in this section does not in any way affect the author's opinions expressed in this book.

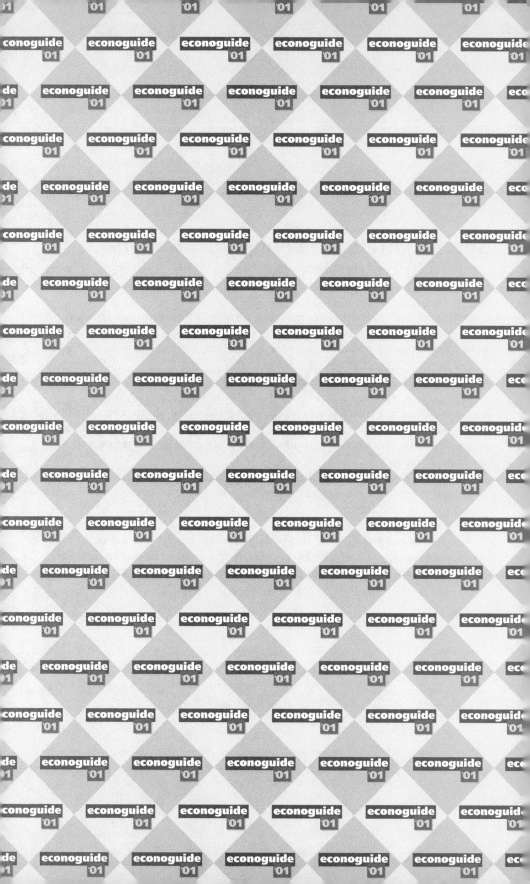

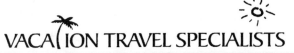

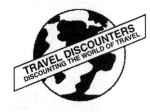

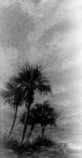

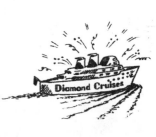

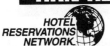

HRN REBATE COUPON

Coupon Rules:

1. Must return this coupon to receive rebate.
2. Coupon expires 12/31/01.
3. Rebate mailed after check-out.
4. Coupons non-combinable.
5. Not retroactive.
6. After check-out, send this coupon with self-addressed stamped envelope to: **HRN 8140 Walnut Hill Lane, Suite 203, Dallas, TX 75231.**
7. Rebate check mailed within 2-3 weeks.
8. One rebate per customer.

UP TO $50

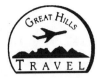
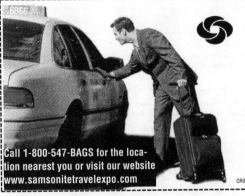
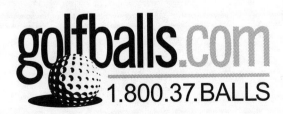

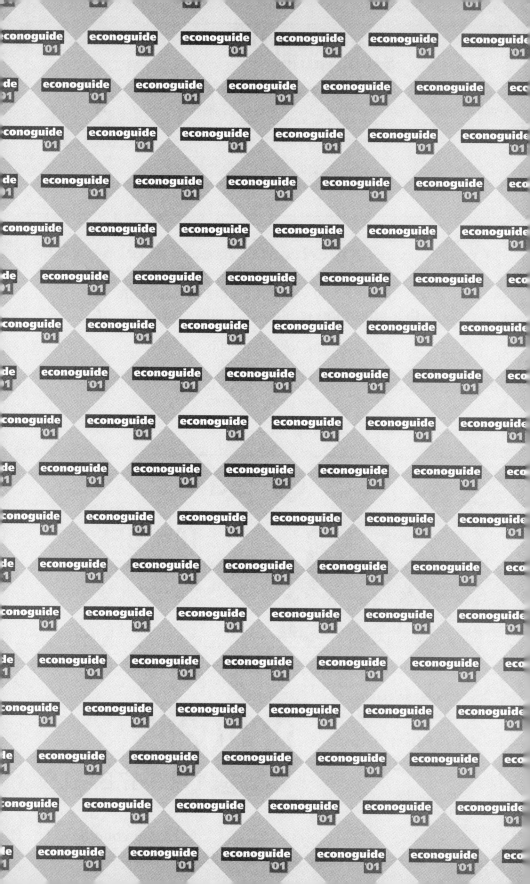

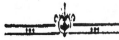
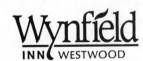

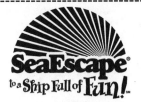
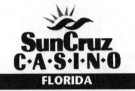
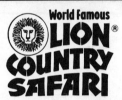
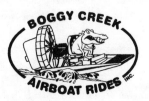

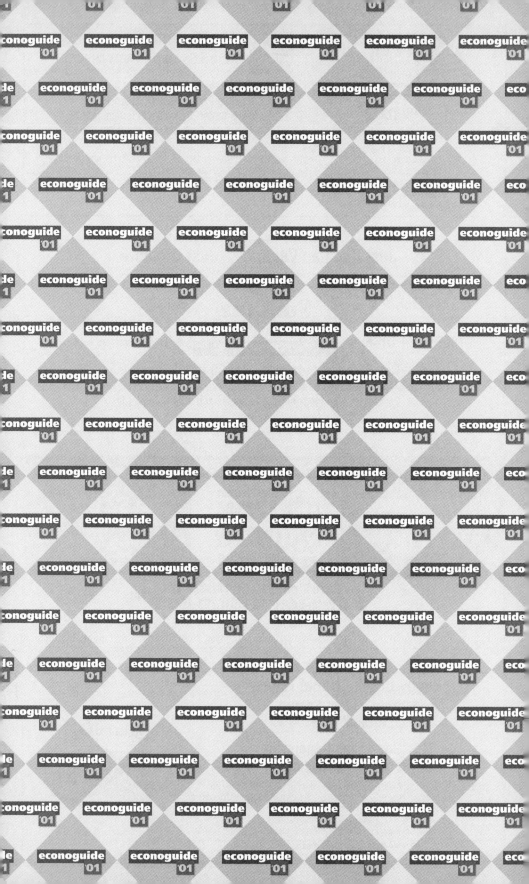

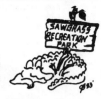

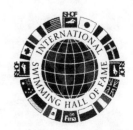

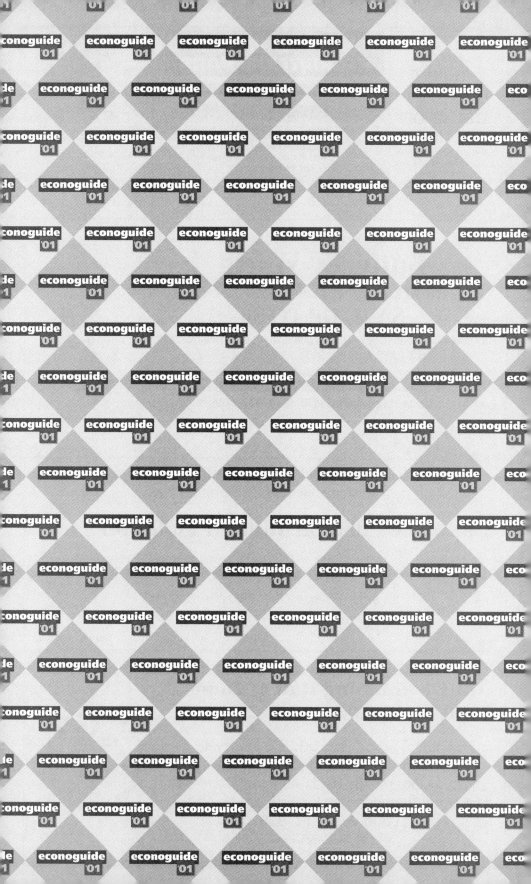

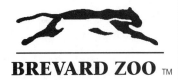
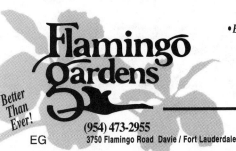
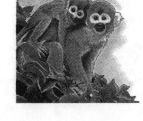

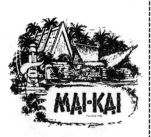
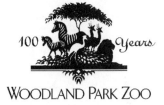
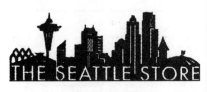
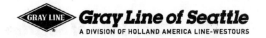

Econoguide Cruise Ratings and Index

Econoguide 2000–01: Best Cruise Lines

Carnival Cruise Lines
Celebrity Cruises
Costa Cruise Lines
Disney Cruise Line
Holland America Line
Norwegian Cruise Line
Princess Cruises
Royal Caribbean International

Econoguide 2000–01: Best Cruise Ships

★★★★★ *Carnival Destiny/Triumph/Victory*	Carnival Cruise Line
★★★★★ *Disney Magic/Disney Wonder*	Disney Cruise Line
★★★★★ *Grand Princess*	Princess Cruises
★★★★★ *Norwegian Sky*	Norwegian Cruise Line
★★★★★ *Voyager of the Seas/ Explorer of the Seas*	Royal Caribbean International

Econoguide 2000–01: Best Luxury Cruise Lines

Crystal Cruises
Radisson Seven Seas Cruises
Seabourn Cruise Line
Silversea Cruises

Econoguide 2000–01: Best Luxury Cruise Ships

★★★★★★ *Crystal Harmony/Symphony*	Crystal Cruises
★★★★★★ *Radisson Seven Seas Navigator/ Radisson Seven Seas Mariner*	Radisson Seven Seas Cruises
★★★★★★ *Seabourn Legend/Seabourn Pride*	Seabourn Cruise Line
★★★★★★ *Silver Cloud/Silver Wind/ Silver Shadow*	Silversea Cruises

Econoguide 2000–01: Best Adventure and Sailing Cruise Lines

Alaska Sightseeing/Cruise West
Clipper Cruise Line
Delta Queen Steamboat Company
Windstar Cruises

Econoguide 2000–01: Best Budget Cruise Line Values

Commodore Cruise Line
World Explorer Cruises

Index to Large Ships

Ship	Line	Econoguide Rating	Page
Big Red Boat I	Premier	★★	260
Big Red Boat II	Premier	★★	261
Big Red Boat III	Premier	★★	261
Big Red Boat IV	Premier	★★	262
Carnival Destiny	Carnival	★★★★★	136
Carnival Triumph	Carnival	★★★★★	137
Carnival Victory	Carnival	★★★★★	139
Caronia	Cunard	★★★★	171
Celebration	Carnival	★★★	147
Century	Celebrity	★★★★★	154
Columbus	Great Lakes	★★★★	255
CostaAtlantica	Costa	★★★★★	160
CostaRomantica	Costa	★★★★★	161
CostaVictoria	Costa	★★★★★	162
Crown Dynasty	Crown	★★★★	253
Crown Princess	Princess	★★★★	206
Crystal Harmony	Crystal	★★★★★★	165
Crystal Symphony	Crystal	★★★★★★	166
Dawn Princess	Princess	★★★★	204
Disney Magic	Disney	★★★★★	175
Disney Wonder	Disney	★★★★★	176
Dolphin IV	Cape Canaveral	★★	247
Ecstasy	Carnival	★★★★	141
Elation	Carnival	★★★★	142
Enchanted Capri	Commodore	★★★	252
Enchanted Isle	Commodore	★★★	250
Enchantment of the Seas	Royal Caribbean	★★★★	223
Explorer of the Seas	Royal Caribbean	★★★★★	220
Fantasy	Carnival	★★★★	140
Fascination	Carnival	★★★★	142
Galaxy	Celebrity	★★★★★	155
Grand Princess	Princess	★★★★★	202

Ship	Line	Econoguide Rating	Page
Grandeur of the Seas	Royal Caribbean	★★★★	224
Hanseatic	Radisson	★★★★★	211
Holiday	Carnival	★★★	146
Horizon	Celebrity	★★★★	156
Imagination	Carnival	★★★★	143
Independence	American Hawaii	★★★	245
Infinity	Celebrity	★★★★★	153
Inspiration	Carnival	★★★★	144
Jubilee	Carnival	★★★	148
Legend of the Seas	Royal Caribbean	★★★	227
Le Levant	Great Lakes	★★★★	255
Maasdam	Holland America	★★★★	183
Majesty of the Seas	Royal Caribbean	★★★	224
Melody	Mediterranean	★★	258
Mercury	Celebrity	★★★★★	155
Millennium	Celebrity	★★★★★	152
Monarch of the Seas	Royal Caribbean	★★★	225
Nieuw Amsterdam	Holland America	★★★	188
Noordam	Holland America	★★★	189
Nordic Empress	Royal Caribbean	★★★	229
Norway	NCL	★★★★	193
Norwegian Crown	NCL	★★★★	198
Norwegian Dream	NCL	★★★★	195
Norwegian Majesty	NCL	★★★★	197
Norwegian Sea	NCL	★★★	197
Norwegian Sky	NCL	★★★★★	194
Norwegian Wind	NCL	★★★★	196
Ocean Princess	Princess	★★★★	203
OceanBreeze	Imperial Majesty	★★	256
Paradise	Carnival	★★★★	145
Patriot	United States	★★★	267
Paul Gauguin	Radisson	★★★★★★	212
Queen Elizabeth 2	Cunard	★★★★	169
Radisson Diamond	Radisson	★★★★★★	213
Radisson Seven Seas Mariner	Radisson	★★★★★★	213
Radisson Seven Seas Navigator	Radisson	★★★★★★	214
Regal Empress	Regal	★★	265
Regal Princess	Princess	★★★★	207
Rhapsody of the Seas	Royal Caribbean	★★★★	221
Rotterdam	Holland America	★★★★★	187
Royal Princess	Princess	★★★	208
Ryndam	Holland America	★★★★	184
Seabourn Goddess I	Seabourn	★★★★★★	234

Index to Adventure Ships

Ship	Line	Econoguide Rating	Page
Sea Bird	Lindblad	★★★	297
Sea Lion	Lindblad	★★★	298
Spirit of '98	Alaska Sightseeing	★★★	273
Spirit of Alaska	Alaska Sightseeing	★★★	274
Spirit of Columbia	Alaska Sightseeing	★★★	274
Spirit of Discovery	Alaska Sightseeing	★★★	275
Spirit of Endeavor	Alaska Sightseeing	★★★★	276
Spirit of Glacier Bay	Alaska Sightseeing	★★★	276
Wilderness Adventurer	Glacier Bay	★★★	295
Wilderness Discoverer	Glacier Bay	★★★	296
Wilderness Explorer	Glacier Bay	★★★	296
Yorktown Clipper	Clipper	★★★	285

Index to Sailing Vessels

Ship	Line	Econoguide Rating	Page
Flying Cloud	Windjammer	★★★	307
Legacy	Windjammer	★★★	307
Mandalay	Windjammer	★★★	308
Polynesia	Windjammer	★★★	309
Royal Clipper	Star Clipper	★★★★	303
Sea Cloud	Sea Cloud	★★★★	300
Sea Cloud II	Sea Cloud	★★★★	301
Star Clipper	Star Clipper	★★★★	304
Star Flyer	Star Clipper	★★★★	304
Wind Song	Windstar	★★★★	313
Wind Spirit	Windstar	★★★★	314
Wind Star	Windstar	★★★★	314
Wind Surf	Windstar	★★★★	315
Yankee Clipper	Windjammer	★★★	310

Index to Cruise Lines

Quick-Find Index